D0188223

Maternity & Newborn Nursing

Shannon E. Perry, RN, PhD, FAAN
Professor Emerita, School of Nursing
San Francisco State University
San Francisco, California

Kitty Cashion, RN, BC, MSN
Clinical Nurse Specialist
University of Tennessee Health Science Center
Department of Obstetrics and Gynecology
Division of Maternal-Fetal Medicine
Memphis, Tennessee

Deitra Leonard Lowdermilk, RNC, PhD, FAAN
Clinical Professor Emerita, School of Nursing
University of North Carolina at Chapel Hill
Chapel Hill, North Carolina

Kathryn Rhodes Alden, EdD, MSN, RN, IBCLC
Clinical Associate Professor, School of Nursing
University of North Carolina at Chapel Hill
Chapel Hill, North Carolina

ELSEVIER
MOSBY

2ND EDITION

ELSEVIER
MOSBY

3251 Riverport Lane
St. Louis, MO 63043

CLINICAL COMPANION FOR MATERNITY & NEWBORN NURSING,
2nd Edition   ISBN: 978-0-323-07799-6
Copyright © 2012 by Mosby, Inc., an affiliate of Elsevier Inc.

Notice

Previous edition copyrighted 2007
Nursing Diagnoses–Definitions and Classifications 2009-2011 © 2009, 2007, 2005, 2003, 2001, 1998, 1996, 1994 NANDA International. Used by arrangement with Wiley – Blackwell Publishing, a company of John Wiley and Sons, Inc.

ISBN: 978-0-323-07799-6

Executive Editor: Robin Carter
Managing Editor: Laurie K. Gower
Publishing Services Manager: Jeff Patterson
Design Direction: Karen Pauls
Cover Illustration: Sally Wern Comport

Working together to grow
libraries in developing countries
www.elsevier.com | www.bookaid.org | www.sabre.org

ELSEVIER BOOK AID International Sabre Foundation

Printed in the United States of America

Last digit is the print number: 9   8   7   6   5   4   3   2

Preface

Purpose

This Clinical Companion was written for nursing students and practicing nurses. Its handy size makes it a portable reference book that can easily be carried to the clinical area where information that relates to hands-on practice is most useful. The authors explain essential background information and describe expected medical interventions, and nursing assessments and interventions. This Clinical Companion complements the tenth edition of *Maternity & Women's Health Care* by Lowdermilk, Perry, Cashion, and Alden as well as the eighth editon of Lowdermilk, Perry, and Cashion, *Maternity Nursing,* but it can be used alone by nurses who need a review or a quick reference.

Content and Organization

This companion book is divided into eight sections:

Section 1: *Pregnancy,* includes antepartum assessment, fetal assessment, maternal and fetal nutrition, and nursing care during pregnancy.

Section 2: *Selected Pregnancy Complications,* addresses therapeutic management and nursing considerations of the most commonly occurring pregnancy complications.

Section 3: *Intrapartum,* describes management of discomfort, fetal assessment, and nursing care during labor and birth.

Section 4: *Selected Childbirth Complications,* addresses therapeutic management and nursing considerations of the most commonly occurring complications of labor and birth.

Section 5: *Postpartum,* describes nursing care required during the normal postpartum period including care of the breastfeeding mother and infant and contraception.

Section 6: *Selected Postpartum Complications,* describes therapeutic management and nursing considerations of the most commonly occurring postpartum complications.

Section 7: *The Newborn,* describes assessment and care of the newborn and nutrition and formula feeding.

Section 8: *Selected Newborn Complications,* addresses problems of the newborn related to gestational age and acquired and congenital problems. Nursing considerations related to grieving the loss of a newborn are included.

Guides for some of the most common procedures in maternal-newborn nursing are included in each section. Tools for assessment are included where relevant, as are patient teaching boxes.

Appendices include laboratory values for pregnant and nonpregnant women, medication guides, and useful words and phrases in English-Spanish translations. A bibliography is included for reference.

Pregnancy

PRENATAL PERIOD

The prenatal period is a time of physical and psychologic preparation for birth and parenthood.

- Pregnancy lasts 9 calendar months. Health care providers use lunar months, not calendar months, to determine fetal age and to discuss the pregnancy.
- A lunar month lasts 28 days, or 4 weeks.
  - ❏ Normal (term) pregnancy lasts about 10 lunar months, 40 weeks, or 280 days.
- Health care providers refer to early, middle, and late pregnancy as trimesters.
  - ❏ The first trimester—weeks 1 through 13
  - ❏ The second trimester—weeks 14 through 26
  - ❏ The third trimester—weeks 27 through 40

Diagnosis of Pregnancy

- Women may suspect pregnancy when they miss a menstrual period. Many women come to the first prenatal visit after a positive home pregnancy test.
- Great variability is possible in the subjective and objective symptoms of pregnancy; therefore, the diagnosis of pregnancy may be uncertain for a time. Many indicators are clinically useful in the diagnosis of pregnancy, and they are classified as presumptive, probable, or positive (Box 1-1).

Estimating Date of Birth

- One formula used to calculate the estimated date of birth (EDB) is Nägele's rule.
  - ❏ Determine the first day of the last menstrual period (LMP), subtract 3 calendar months and add 7 days, *or*
  - ❏ Add 7 days to the LMP and count forward 9 calendar months.

BOX 1-1

Signs of Pregnancy

PRESUMPTIVE SIGNS*
- Breast changes
- Amenorrhea
- Nausea, vomiting
- Urinary frequency
- Fatigue
- Quickening

PROBABLE SIGNS (OBJECTIVE SIGNS DETECTED BY AN EXAMINER)
- Goodell sign—*softening of cervix*
- Chadwick sign—*Bluish discoloration of cervix, vagina, + labia*
- Hegar sign—*softening in the consistency of the uterus; cervix + uterus seem to be 2 seperate regions → pertains to uterine isthmus*
- Positive pregnancy test (serum/urine)
- Braxton Hicks contractions
- Ballottement → *Pushing against uterine wall w/ a finger inserted in vagina and feeling a return impact of the displaced fetus*

POSITIVE SIGNS
- Visualization of fetus by real-time ultrasound examination
- Fetal heart tones detected by ultrasound examination
- Visualization of fetus by radiographic study
- Fetal heart tones detected by Doppler ultrasound stethoscope
- Fetal heart tones detected by fetal stethoscope
- Fetal movements palpated by examiner
- Fetal movements visible

*Presumptive signs of pregnancy can be caused by conditions other than gestation. Therefore, these signs alone are not reliable for diagnosis.

- Most women give birth during the period extending from 7 days before to 7 days after the EDB.

Gravidity and Parity

Box 1-2 defines terms related to gravidity and parity.

NURSING ALERT *Information related to obstetrics may be noted in a woman's records in a variety of ways because no one standardized system exists. Until such a system is in place, the nurse should understand the documentation system used by the health care facility.*

BOX 1-2

Definitions Related to Gravidity and Parity
- *Gravida:* a woman who is pregnant
- *Gravidity:* pregnancy
- *Late preterm:* a pregnancy that ends between 34 and 36 6/7 wk of gestation
- *Multigravida:* a woman who has had two or more pregnancies
- *Multipara:* a woman who has completed two or more pregnancies to 20 or more wk of gestation
- *Nulligravida:* a woman who has never been pregnant
- *Nullipara:* a woman who has not completed a pregnancy with a fetus or fetuses who have reached 20 wk of gestation
- *Parity:* the number of pregnancies in which the fetus or fetuses have reached 20 wk of gestation when they are born, not the number of fetuses (e.g., twins) born. Whether the fetus is born alive or is stillborn (fetus who shows no signs of life at birth) does not affect parity.
- *Postdate or postterm:* a pregnancy that goes beyond 42 wk of gestation
- *Preterm:* a pregnancy that has reached 20 wk of gestation but ends before completion of 37 wk of gestation
- *Primigravida:* a woman who is pregnant for the first time
- *Primipara:* a woman who has completed one pregnancy with a fetus or fetuses who have reached 20 wk of gestation
- *Term:* a pregnancy from the completion of wk 37 of gestation to the end of wk 42 of gestation
- *Viability:* capacity to live outside the uterus; there are no clear limits of gestational age or weight but it is rare for a fetus to survive before 22 to 24 wk of gestation and weighing less than 500 g

Sources: Cunningham, F., Leveno, K., Bloom, S., Hauth, J., Rouse, D., & Spong, C. (2010). *Williams obstetrics* (23rd ed.). New York: McGraw-Hill; Katz, V. (2007). Spontaneous and recurrent abortions. In V. Katz, G. Lentz, R. Lobo, & D. Gershenson (Eds.), *Comprehensive gynecology* (5th ed.). Philadelphia: Mosby.

- Gravidity and parity may be described with only two digits: The first digit represents the number of pregnancies the woman has had, including the present one, and parity is the number of pregnancies that have reached 20 or more weeks of gestation. For example, if the woman had twins at 36 weeks with her first pregnancy, parity would still be counted as one birth (gravida 1, para 1).
- Another system which is commonly used consists of five digits separated by hyphens to describe obstetric history: gravidity—number

of term births—number of preterm births—number of abortions (miscarriage or elective termination of pregnancy)—number of children currently living.

- ❏ The acronym GTPAL (gravidity, term, preterm, abortions, living children) may be helpful in remembering this system of notation.
- ❏ For example, if a woman pregnant only once gives birth at week 34 and the infant survives, the abbreviation that represents this information is "1-0-1-0-1." During her next pregnancy, the abbreviation is "2-0-1-0-1."

Adaptation to Pregnancy

Pregnancy affects all family members; each member must adapt to the pregnancy and interpret its meaning in light of his or her own needs. The following descriptions are based on the traditional North American model and may not apply to families who do not fit that model.

- Women of all ages use the months of pregnancy to adapt to the maternal role, a complex process of social and cognitive learning.
- Developmental tasks of the mother include accepting the pregnancy, identifying with the role of mother, reordering the relationships between herself and her mother and between herself and her partner, establishing a relationship with the unborn child, and preparing for the birth experience.
  - ❏ Mood swings, irritability, and ambivalence about the pregnancy are normal responses in early pregnancy whether the pregnancy was planned or not.
  - ❏ Although the woman's relationship with her mother is significant in considering her adaptation in pregnancy, the most important person to the pregnant woman is usually the father of her child.
- Emotional attachment begins during the prenatal period as women use fantasizing and daydreaming to prepare for motherhood. The mother-child relationship progresses through pregnancy.
- Many women actively prepare for birth by reading books, viewing films, attending parenting classes, and talking to other women.
- Toward the end of the third trimester, most women become impatient for labor to begin, whether the birth is anticipated with joy, dread, or both. They have a strong desire to see the end of pregnancy.

- The sexual relationship is affected by physical, emotional, and interactional factors, including myths about sex during pregnancy, sexual dysfunction, and physical changes in the woman.
- Developmental tasks experienced by the expectant father include acknowledgment of the biologic fact of pregnancy, adjustment to the reality of pregnancy, and acceptance of the pregnancy. In the last trimester the father becomes actively involved in both the pregnancy and his relationship with his child. He begins to think of himself as a father.
  - ❑ Some men experience pregnancy-like symptoms, such as nausea, weight gain, and other physical symptoms. This phenomenon is known as the couvade syndrome.
  - ❑ As the expected date of birth approaches, many men experience anticipation and anxiety. Major concerns are getting the woman to a health care facility in time for the birth and not appearing ignorant. The man also may have fears concerning safe passage of his child and partner and the possible death or complications of his partner and child.
- Parents may occasionally show or voice disappointment over the gender of the child. Negative responses are usually temporary.
- Siblings' responses to pregnancy vary with their age and dependency needs.
  - ❑ The 1-year-old infant seems largely unaware of the process.
  - ❑ Toddlers may exhibit more clinging behavior and revert to dependent behaviors in toilet training or eating.
  - ❑ By age 3 or 4 years, children like to be told the story of their own beginning and accept its being compared with the present pregnancy. They like to listen to the fetal heartbeat and feel the baby moving in utero.
  - ❑ School-age children take a more clinical interest in their mother's pregnancy. They may want to know in more detail, "How did the baby get in there?" and "How will it get out?"
  - ❑ Early and middle adolescents preoccupied with the establishment of their own sexual identity may have difficulty accepting the overwhelming evidence of the sexual activity of their parents.
  - ❑ Late adolescents do not appear to be unduly disturbed. They are busy making plans for their own lives.
- Box 1-3 lists suggestions for sibling preparation.

BOX 1-3

Tips for Sibling Preparation

PRENATAL

- Take your child on a prenatal visit. Let the child listen to the fetal heartbeat and feel the baby move.
- Involve the child in preparations for the baby, such as helping decorate the baby's room.
- Move the child to a bed (if still sleeping in a crib) at least 2 mo before the baby is due.
- Read books, show videos or DVDs, and take the child to sibling preparation classes, including a hospital tour.
- Answer your child's questions about the coming birth, what babies are like, and any other questions.
- Take your child to the homes of friends who have babies so that the child has realistic expectations of what babies are like.

DURING THE HOSPITAL STAY

- Have someone bring the child to the hospital to visit you and the baby (unless you plan to have the child attend the birth).
- Do not force interactions between the child and the baby. The child will often be more interested in seeing you and being reassured of your love.
- Help the child explore the infant by showing how and where to touch the baby.
- Give the child a gift (from you or from you, the father, and the baby).

GOING HOME

- Leave the child at home with a relative or babysitter.
- Have someone else carry the baby from the car so that you can hug the child first.

ADJUSTMENT AFTER THE BABY IS HOME

- Arrange for a special time with the child alone with each parent.
- Do not exclude the child during infant feeding times. The child can sit with you and the baby and feed a doll or drink juice or milk or sit quietly with a game.
- Prepare small gifts for the child so that when the baby gets gifts the sibling will not feel left out. The child can also help open the baby gifts.
- Praise the child for acting age appropriately (so that being a baby does not seem better than being older).

- Most grandparents are delighted at the prospect of a new baby in the family. The grandparents' presence and support can strengthen family systems by widening the circle of support and nurturance.
  - ❏ Grandparents may need information about changes in maternity care and childbirth practices that have occurred since they had their children.

CARE MANAGEMENT

The purpose of prenatal care is to identify existing risk factors and other deviations from normal so that pregnancy outcomes can be enhanced. Major emphasis is placed on preventive aspects of care.

Prenatal Visit Schedule

- In traditional prenatal care the initial visit usually occurs in the first trimester, with monthly visits through week 28 of pregnancy. Thereafter, visits are scheduled every 2 weeks until week 36 and then every week until birth. Research supports a model of fewer prenatal visits, and in some practices there is a growing tendency to have fewer visits with women who are at low risk for complications.
- CenteringPregnancy, a care model that is gaining in popularity, is group prenatal care in which authority is shifted from the provider to the woman and other women who have similar due dates. Most care takes place in the group setting after the first visit. At each meeting the first 30 minutes is spent in completing assessments (by the woman and by the health care provider), and the rest of the time is spent in group discussion of specific issues such as discomforts of pregnancy and preparation for labor and birth. Families and partners are encouraged to participate.
- In CenteringPregnancy, the first visit is scheduled within the first trimester (12 weeks). Thereafter, women are seen every 4 weeks from week 16 to week 28 and every 2 weeks during weeks 29 through 40.

Initial Visit

- The initial evaluation includes a comprehensive health history emphasizing the current pregnancy, previous pregnancies, the family, a psychosocial profile, a physical assessment, diagnostic testing, and an overall risk assessment.

❑ *Current pregnancy.* The presumptive signs of pregnancy may be of great concern to the woman. A review of her symptoms and how she is coping with them helps establish a database to develop a plan of care. Some early teaching may be provided at this time.

❑ *Childbearing and female reproductive system history.* The woman's age at menarche, menstrual history, and contraceptive history; the nature of any infertility or gynecologic conditions; sexually transmitted infections (STIs); sexual history; and details of all her pregnancies, including the present pregnancy, and their outcomes. Date of the last Papanicolaou (Pap) test and the result. Date of her LMP to establish the EDB.

❑ *Medical history.* Physical conditions or surgical procedures that can affect the pregnancy or that can be affected by the pregnancy. Description of the nature of previous surgical procedures, especially reproductive ones. Presence of any handicapping conditions.

❑ *Nutritional history.* A dietary assessment to identify special dietary practices, food allergies, eating behaviors, the practice of pica, and other factors related to her nutritional status.

craving and chewing substances w/ no nutrition value (ice, clay, soil, paper)

❑ *History of drug and herbal preparations use.* Past and present use of legal (over-the-counter [OTC] and prescription medications; herbal preparations; caffeine; alcohol; nicotine) and illegal (e.g., marijuana, cocaine, heroin) drugs. Informed consent must be obtained before testing for drug use.

❑ *Family history.* Information about familial or genetic disorders or conditions that could affect the present health status of the woman or her fetus.

❑ *Social, experiential, and occupational history.* Situational factors, such as the family's ethnic and cultural background and socioeconomic status. Woman's past and present work settings.

❑ *History or risk of physical abuse.* The likelihood of abuse by the partner increases during pregnancy; sexual assault by the partner is common. Assess for reports of physical blows directed to the head, breasts, abdomen, and genitalia.

❑ *Review of systems.* Identify and describe preexisting or concurrent problems in any of the body systems; assess her mental status. For each sign or symptom described, obtain the following data: body location, quality, quantity, chronology, aggravating or alleviating factors, and associated manifestations (onset, character, course).

- ❑ *Physical examination.* Record vital signs and height and weight. Each examiner develops a routine for proceeding with the physical examination; most choose the head-to-toe progression.
- ■ One vaginal examination during pregnancy is recommended; others are done if medically indicated.
  - ❑ *Laboratory tests.* Tests are listed in Table 1-1.

TABLE 1-1

Laboratory Tests in the Prenatal Period

Laboratory Test	Purpose
Hemoglobin, hematocrit, WBC, differential	Detects anemia; detects infection
Hemoglobin electrophoresis	Identifies women with hemoglobinopathies (e.g., sickle cell anemia, thalassemia)
Blood type, Rh, and irregular antibody	Identifies those fetuses at risk for developing erythroblastosis fetalis or hyperbilirubinemia in neonatal period
Rubella titer	Determines immunity to rubella
Tuberculin skin testing; chest film after 20 wk of gestation in women with reactive tuberculin tests	Screens for exposure to tuberculosis
Urinalysis, including microscopic examination of urinary sediment; pH, specific gravity, color, glucose, albumin, protein, RBCs, WBCs, casts, acetone; hCG	Identifies women with glycosuria, renal disease, hypertensive disease of pregnancy; infection; occult hematuria
Urine culture	Identifies women with asymptomatic bacteriuria
Renal function tests: BUN, creatinine, electrolytes, creatinine clearance, total protein excretion	Evaluates level of possible renal compromise in women with a history of diabetes, hypertension, or renal disease
Pap test	Screens for cervical intraepithelial neoplasia; if a liquid-based test is used, may also screen for HPV

(handwritten: → hemolytic anemia)

Continued

TABLE 1-1	

Laboratory Tests in the Prenatal Period—cont'd

Laboratory Test	Purpose
Cervical culture for *Neisseria gonorrhoeae, Chlamydia*	Screens for asymptomatic infection in high risk women
Rectovaginal culture	Screens for GBS infection; done at 35-37 wk
RPR, VDRL, or FTA-ABS	Identifies women with untreated syphilis
HIV antibody,* hepatitis B surface antigen, toxoplasmosis	Screens for specific infections
MSAFP/Quad Screen	Screens for NTDs, Down syndrome; performed at 15-20 wks (16-18 wks is ideal)
1-hr glucose tolerance	Screens for gestational diabetes; done at initial visit for women with risk factors; done at 24-28 wk for at risk pregnant women who tested negative at the initial screening; women who are low risk by history and clinical risk factors are usually not screened
3-hr glucose tolerance	Diagnoses gestational diabetes in women with elevated glucose level after 1-hr screen; must have two elevated readings for diagnosis
Cardiac evaluation: ECG, chest x-ray film, and echocardiogram	Evaluates cardiac function in women with a history of hypertension or cardiac disease

*Universal opt-out screening is recommended for HIV.

BUN, Blood urea nitrogen; *ECG,* electrocardiogram; *FTA-ABS,* fluorescent treponemal antibody absorption test; *GBS,* group B streptococci; *hCG,* human chorionic gonadotropin; *HIV,* human immunodeficiency virus; *HPV,* human papillomavirus; *MSAFP,* maternal serum alpha-fetoprotein; *NTD,* neural tube defects; *RBC,* red blood cell; *RPR,* rapid plasma reagin; *VDRL,* Venereal Disease Research Laboratory; *WBC,* white blood cell.

Follow-up Visits

- The pattern of interviewing the woman first and then assessing physical changes and performing laboratory tests is maintained.
- At each visit the woman is asked to summarize relevant events that have occurred since the previous visit. She is asked about

her general emotional and physiologic well-being, complaints, problems, and questions she may have. Personal and family needs are identified and explored. The woman's physical systems are reviewed. Any suspicious signs or symptoms are assessed in depth.

- At each visit, physical parameters are measured.
  - ❏ Take the blood pressure using the same arm at every visit, with the woman sitting, using a cuff of appropriate size.
  - ❏ Weight: Note the appropriateness of the gestational weight gain in relation to her body mass index (BMI).
  - ❏ Note the location and degree of edema.
  - ❏ Examination of the abdomen: The woman lies on her back with her arms by her side and head supported by a pillow. The bladder should be empty. Abdominal inspection is followed by measurement of the height of the fundus.

NURSING ALERT   *Be alert for supine hypotension. When a woman is lying on her back, the weight of the abdominal contents may compress the vena cava and aorta, causing a decrease in blood pressure and a feeling of faintness. If this occurs, turn the woman onto her side until her symptoms are gone and her vital signs stabilize.*

- Monitor for a range of signs and symptoms that indicate potential complications in addition to hypertension. (See the Signs of Potential Complications box.)
- Assess fetal heart tones (FHTs) at each visit usually beginning toward the end of the first trimester when they can be heard with an ultrasound fetoscope or an ultrasound stethoscope.
- The fundal height, measurement of the height of the uterus above the symphysis pubis, is used as one indicator of fetal growth. The measurement also provides a gross estimate of the duration of pregnancy. From approximately 18 to 32 weeks of gestation with an empty bladder at the time of measurement, the height of the fundus in centimeters is approximately the same as the number of weeks of gestation (±2).
  - ❏ A stable or decreased fundal height may indicate intrauterine growth restriction (IUGR).
  - ❏ An excessive increase could indicate a multifetal gestation (more than one fetus) or hydramnios.

Signs of Potential Complications

SIGNS AND SYMPTOMS	POSSIBLE CAUSES
FIRST TRIMESTER	
Severe vomiting	Hyperemesis gravidarum
Chills, fever	Infection
Burning on urination	Infection
Diarrhea	Infection
Abdominal cramping, vaginal bleeding	Miscarriage, ectopic pregnancy
SECOND AND THIRD TRIMESTERS	
Persistent, severe vomiting	Hyperemesis gravidarum, hypertension, preeclampsia
Sudden discharge of fluid from vagina before 37 wk	Preterm premature rupture of membranes (preterm PROM)
Vaginal bleeding, severe abdominal pain	Miscarriage, placenta previa, placental abruption
Chills, fever, burning on urination, diarrhea	Infection
Severe backache or flank pain	Kidney infection or stones, preterm labor
Change in fetal movements: absence of fetal movements after quickening, any unusual change in pattern or amount	Fetal jeopardy or intrauterine fetal death
Uterine contractions, pressure, cramping before 37 wk	Preterm labor
Visual disturbances: blurring, double vision, or spots	Hypertensive conditions, preeclampsia
Swelling of face or fingers and over sacrum	Hypertensive conditions, preeclampsia
Headaches: severe, frequent, or continuous	Hypertensive conditions, preeclampsia
Muscular irritability or convulsions	Hypertensive conditions, preeclampsia
Epigastric or abdominal pain (perceived as heartburn or severe stomachache)	Hypertensive conditions, preeclampsia, placental abruption
Glycosuria, positive glucose tolerance test	Gestational diabetes mellitus

- Fetal gestational age is determined from the menstrual history, contraceptive history, pregnancy test result, and the following findings obtained during the clinical evaluation:
  - First uterine evaluation: date, size
  - Fetal heart (FH) first heard: date, method (Doppler stethoscope, fetoscope)
  - Date of quickening
  - Current fundal height, estimated fetal weight (EFW)
  - Current week of gestation by history of LMP and/or ultrasound examination
  - Ultrasound examination: date, week of gestation, biparietal diameter (BPD)
  - Reliability of dates
- Quickening ("feeling of life"), the mother's first perception of fetal movement, usually occurs between weeks 16 and 20 of gestation. Multiparas often perceive fetal movement sooner than primigravidas, as early as 14 weeks.
- Ultrasound examination in early pregnancy may be used to establish the duration of pregnancy if the woman cannot give a precise date for her LMP or if the size of the uterus does not conform to the EDB as calculated by Nägele's rule. Ultrasound also provides information about the well-being of the fetus. The use of ultrasound has become routine in the United States.
- Regular fetal movement is a reliable indicator of fetal health. The mother is instructed to note the extent and timing of fetal movements and to report immediately if the pattern changes or if movement ceases.

Laboratory Tests

See Table 1-1 for diagnostic tests used to assess the health status of both the pregnant woman and the fetus.

Interventions

Education About Maternal and Fetal Changes

Expectant parents are typically curious about the growth and development of the fetus and the subsequent changes that occur in the mother's body. Mothers are sometimes more tolerant of the discomforts related to the continuing pregnancy if they understand the underlying causes. Educational literature that describes fetal and maternal changes can be used to explain changes as they occur. Educational material may include electronic and written materials appropriate to the pregnant woman's or couple's literacy level and experience and the agency's resources. To be most effective, it is important that these materials reflect the pregnant woman's or couple's ethnicity, culture, and literacy level.

Teaching for Self-Management

The expectant mother needs information about many subjects. Several topics that may cause concerns are discussed in the following sections.

- *Nutrition.* Teaching may include discussion about foods high in iron, those that contain folic acid, and the importance of taking prenatal vitamins, limiting caffeine intake, and avoiding drinking alcohol.
  - ❑ Refer women to a registered dietitian if a need for in-depth counseling is identified.
- *Personal hygiene.* During pregnancy the sebaceous (sweat) glands are highly active because of hormonal influences, and women often perspire freely.
  - ❑ Baths and warm showers can be therapeutic because they relax tense, tired muscles; help counter insomnia; and make the pregnant woman feel fresh.
  - ❑ Tub bathing is permitted even in late pregnancy because little water enters the vagina unless under pressure. However, late in pregnancy, when the woman's center of gravity lowers, she is at risk for falling.
  - ❑ Tub bathing is contraindicated after rupture of the membranes.
- *Preventing urinary tract infections.* Instruct women to inform their health care provider if blood or pain occurs with urination. Instruct in the following preventive measures:
  - ❑ Use good handwashing techniques before and after urinating; wipe the perineum from front to back. Use soft, absorbent toilet tissue, preferably white and unscented; harsh, scented, or printed toilet paper may cause irritation.
  - ❑ Avoid using bubble bath or other bath oils because these may irritate the urethra.
  - ❑ Wear cotton crotch underpants and pantyhose and avoid wearing tight-fitting slacks or jeans for long periods; anything that allows a buildup of heat and moisture in the genital area may foster the growth of bacteria.
  - ❑ Advise the woman to drink at least 2 L (eight glasses) of liquid, preferably water, each day to maintain an adequate fluid intake that ensures frequent urination.
  - ❑ Pregnant women should not limit fluids in an effort to reduce the frequency of urination.

- ❑ Inform women that if the urine looks dark (concentrated), they must increase their fluid intake.
- ❑ Consuming yogurt and acidophilus milk may help prevent urinary tract and vaginal infections.
- ❑ Review healthy urination practices with the woman.
  - Do not ignore the urge to urinate, because holding urine lengthens the time bacteria are in the bladder and allows them to multiply.
  - Always urinate before going to bed at night.
  - Because bacteria can be introduced during intercourse, urinate before and after intercourse, and then drink a large glass of water to promote additional urination.
- ■ *Preparing for breastfeeding.* A woman's decision about the method of infant feeding often is made before pregnancy. The pregnant woman is encouraged to breastfeed. Support for the woman and her partner should be provided, whichever method of feeding is selected.
  - ❑ Women with inverted nipples need special consideration if they are planning to breastfeed. The pinch test is done to determine whether the nipple is everted or inverted.
    - To perform the pinch test, have the woman place her thumb and forefinger on her areola and gently press inward. The nipple will either stand erect or invert. Most nipples will stand erect.
    - Breast shells, small plastic devices that fit over the nipples, may be recommended for women who have flat or inverted nipples. Breast shells should be worn for 1 to 2 hours daily during the last trimester of pregnancy, for gradually increasing periods of time.
  - ❑ Teach the woman to cleanse the nipples with warm water to keep the ducts from being blocked with dried colostrum. Soap, ointments, alcohol, and tinctures should not be applied because they remove protective oils that keep the nipples supple and prevent cracking of the nipples during early lactation.
- ■ *Dental care.* Dental care during pregnancy is especially important because nausea during pregnancy may lead to poor oral hygiene, allowing dental caries to develop. A fluoride toothpaste should be used daily. Dental surgery is not contraindicated during pregnancy. If dental treatment is necessary, the woman will be most comfortable having it done during the second trimester because the uterus is outside the pelvis but not so large as to cause discomfort while she sits in a dental chair.

■ *Physical activity.* See the Teaching for Self-Management box: Exercise Tips for Pregnant Women.

Teaching for Self-Management

Exercise Tips for Pregnant Women

■ *Consult your health care provider* when you know or suspect you are pregnant. Discuss your health and pregnancy history, your current exercise regimen, and the exercises you would like to continue throughout pregnancy.

■ *Seek help* in determining an exercise routine that is well within your limit of tolerance, especially if you have not been exercising regularly.

■ *Consider decreasing weight-bearing exercises* (jogging, running) and concentrating on non–weight-bearing activities such as swimming, cycling, or stretching. If you are a runner, starting in your seventh month, it is advisable to walk instead.

■ *Avoid risky activities* such as surfing, mountain climbing, skydiving, and racquetball because such activities, which require precise balance and coordination, may be dangerous. Avoid activities that require holding your breath and bearing down (Valsalva maneuver). Jerky, bouncy motions also should be avoided.

■ *Exercise regularly* every day if possible, as long as you are healthy, to improve muscle tone and increase or maintain your stamina. Exercising sporadically may put undue strain on your muscles.

■ *Thirty minutes* of moderate physical exercise is recommended. This activity can be broken up into shorter segments with rest in between. For example, exercise for 10 to 15 min, rest for 2 to 3 min, then exercise for another 10 to 15 min.

■ *Decrease your exercise level* as your pregnancy progresses. The normal alterations of advancing pregnancy, such as decreased cardiac reserve and increased respiratory effort, may produce physiologic stress if you exercise strenuously for a long time.

■ *Take your pulse* every 10 to 15 min while you are exercising. If it is more than 140 beats/min, slow down until it returns to a maximum of 90 beats/min. You should be able to converse easily while exercising. If you cannot, you need to slow down.

■ *Avoid becoming overheated* for extended periods. It is best not to exercise for more than 35 min, especially in hot, humid weather. As your body temperature rises, the heat is transmitted to your fetus. Prolonged or repeated elevation of fetal temperature may result in birth defects, especially during the first 3 mo. Your temperature should not exceed 38° C.

Exercise Tips for Pregnant Women—cont'd

■ *Avoid the use of hot tubs and saunas.*

■ *Warm-up and stretching exercises* prepare your joints for more strenuous exercise and lessen the likelihood of strain or injury to your joints. After the fourth month of gestation you should not perform exercises flat on your back.

■ *A cool-down period* of mild activity involving your legs after an exercise period will help bring your respiration, heart, and metabolic rates back to normal and prevent the pooling of blood in the exercised muscles.

■ *Rest for 10 min after exercising,* lying on your side. As the uterus grows, it puts pressure on the vena cava, a major vein in your abdomen, which carries blood to your heart. Lying on your side removes the pressure and promotes return circulation from your extremities and muscles to your heart, thereby increasing blood flow to your placenta and fetus. You should rise gradually from the floor to prevent dizziness or fainting (orthostatic hypotension).

■ *Drink two or three 8-oz glasses of water* after you exercise to replace the body fluids lost through perspiration. While exercising, drink water whenever you feel thirsty.

■ *Increase your caloric intake* to replace the calories burned during exercise and provide the extra energy needs of pregnancy. (Pregnancy alone requires an additional 340-452 kcal/day.) Choose high-protein foods such as fish, milk, cheese, eggs, and meat.

■ *Take your time.* This is not the time to be competitive or train for activities requiring speed or long endurance.

■ *Wear a supportive bra.* Your increased breast weight may cause changes in posture and put pressure on the ulnar nerve.

■ *Wear supportive shoes.* As your uterus grows, your center of gravity shifts and you compensate for this by arching your back. These natural changes may make you feel off balance and more likely to fall.

■ *Stop exercising immediately* if you experience shortness of breath, dizziness, numbness, tingling, pain of any kind, more than four uterine contractions per hour, decreased fetal activity, or vaginal bleeding, and consult your health care provider.

Sources: American College of Obstetricians and Gynecologists (ACOG). (2002). Exercise during pregnancy and the postpartum period. ACOG Committee Opinion No. 267. *Obstetrics & Gynecology, 77*(1), 79-81; Kramer, M., & McDonald, S. (2006). Aerobic exercise for women during pregnancy. *The Cochrane Database of Systematic Reviews, 2006,* 2, CD000180; Morris, S., & Johnson, N. (2005). Exercise in pregnancy: A critical appraisal of the literature. *Journal of Reproductive Medicine, 50*(3), 181-188.

■ *Posture and body mechanics.* Skeletal and musculature changes and hormonal changes (relaxin) in pregnancy may predispose the woman to backache and possible injury. See the Teaching for Self-Management box: Posture and Body Mechanics for strategies to prevent or relieve backache.

■ *Rest and relaxation.* The pregnant woman is encouraged to plan regular rest periods, particularly as pregnancy advances.

Text continued on p. 28

Teaching for Self-Management

Posture and Body Mechanics

TO PREVENT OR RELIEVE BACKACHE
■ Do pelvic tilt:
  ❑ Pelvic tilt (rock) on hands and knees and while sitting in straight-back chair
  ❑ Pelvic tilt (rock) in standing position against a wall or lying on floor
  ❑ Perform abdominal muscle contractions during pelvic tilt while standing, lying, or sitting to help strengthen the rectus abdominis muscle.
■ Use good body mechanics.
■ Use leg muscles to reach objects on or near the floor. Bend at the knees, not from the back. Knees are bent to lower body to squatting position. Feet are kept 12 to 18 inches apart to provide a solid base to maintain balance.
■ Lift with the legs. To lift heavy object (e.g., young child), one foot is placed slightly in front of the other and kept flat as woman lowers herself onto one knee. She lifts the weight, holding it close to her body and never higher than the chest. To stand up or sit down, she places one leg slightly behind the other as she raises or lowers herself.

TO RESTRICT THE LUMBAR CURVE
■ For prolonged standing (e.g., ironing, employment), place one foot on low footstool or box; change positions often.
■ Move car seat forward so that knees are bent and higher than hips. If needed, use a small pillow to support the lower back area.
■ Sit in chairs low enough to allow both feet to be placed on the floor, preferably with knees higher than hips.

TO PREVENT ROUND LIGAMENT PAIN AND STRAIN ON ABDOMINAL MUSCLES
■ Implement suggestions given in Table 1-2.

TABLE 1-2

Discomforts Related to Pregnancy

Discomfort	Physiology	Teaching for Self-Management
FIRST TRIMESTER		
Breast changes, new sensations: pain, tingling, tenderness	Hypertrophy of mammary glandular tissue and increased vascularization, pigmentation, and size and prominence of nipples and areolae caused by hormonal stimulation	Wear supportive maternity bras with pads to absorb discharge, may be worn at night; wash with warm water and keep dry; breast tenderness may interfere with sexual expression or foreplay but is temporary
Urgency and frequency of urination	Vascular engorgement and altered bladder function caused by hormones; bladder capacity reduced by enlarging uterus and fetal presenting part	Empty bladder regularly; perform Kegel exercises; limit fluid intake before bedtime; wear perineal pad; report pain or burning sensation to primary health care provider
Languor and malaise; fatigue (early pregnancy, most commonly)	Unexplained; may be caused by increasing levels of estrogen, progesterone, and hCG or by elevated BBT, psychologic response to pregnancy and its required physical and psychologic adaptations	Rest as needed; eat well-balanced diet to prevent anemia

Continued

TABLE 1-2

Discomforts Related to Pregnancy—cont'd

Discomfort	Physiology	Teaching for Self-Management
FIRST TRIMESTER—cont'd		
Nausea and vomiting, morning sickness—occurs in 50%-75% of pregnant women; starts between first and second missed periods and lasts until about fourth missed period; may occur any time during day; fathers also may have symptoms	Cause unknown; may result from hormonal changes, possibly hCG; may be partly emotional, reflecting pride in, ambivalence about, or rejection of pregnant state	Avoid empty or overloaded stomach; maintain good posture—give stomach ample room; stop smoking; eat dry carbohydrate on awakening; remain in bed until feeling subsides, or alternate dry carbohydrate every other hour with fluids such as hot herbal decaffeinated tea, milk, or clear coffee until feeling subsides; eat five to six small meals per day; avoid fried, odorous, spicy, greasy, or gas-forming foods; consult primary health care provider if intractable vomiting occurs
Ptyalism (excessive salivation) may occur starting 2 to 3 wk after first missed period	Possibly caused by elevated estrogen levels; may be related to reluctance to swallow because of nausea	Use astringent mouthwash, chew gum, eat hard candy as comfort measures
Gingivitis and epulis (hyperemia, hypertrophy, bleeding, tenderness of the gums); condition will disappear spontaneously 1 to 2 mo after birth	Increased vascularity and proliferation of connective tissue from estrogen stimulation	Eat well-balanced diet with adequate protein and fresh fruits and vegetables; brush teeth gently and observe good dental hygiene; avoid infection; see dentist

Nasal stuffiness; epistaxis (nosebleed)	Hyperemia of mucous membranes related to high estrogen levels	Use humidifier; avoid trauma; normal saline nose drops or spray may be used
Leukorrhea: often noted throughout pregnancy	Hormonally stimulated cervix becomes hypertrophic and hyperactive, producing abundant amount of mucus	Not preventable; do not douche; wear perineal pads; perform hygienic practices such as wiping front to back; report to primary health care provider if accompanied by pruritus, foul odor, or change in character or color
Psychosocial dynamics, mood swings, mixed feelings	Hormonal and metabolic adaptations; feelings about female role, sexuality, timing of pregnancy, and resultant changes in life and lifestyle	Participate in pregnancy support group; communicate concerns to partner, family, and health care provider; request referral for supportive services if needed (financial assistance)
SECOND TRIMESTER		
Pigmentation deepens; acne, oily skin	Melanocyte-stimulating hormone (from anterior pituitary)	Not preventable; usually resolves during puerperium → period of about 6 weeks PP
Spider nevi (angiomas) appear over neck, thorax, face, and arms during second or third trimester	Focal networks of dilated arterioles (end arteries) from increased concentration of estrogens	Not preventable; they fade slowly during late puerperium; rarely disappear completely

Continued

TABLE 1-2

Discomforts Related to Pregnancy—cont'd

Discomfort	Physiology	Teaching for Self-Management
SECOND TRIMESTER—cont'd		
Pruritus (noninflammatory)	Unknown cause; various types: nonpapular; closely aggregated pruritic papules Increased excretory function of skin and stretching of skin possible factors	Keep fingernails short and clean; contact primary health care provider for diagnosis of cause Not preventable; use comfort measures for symptoms such as Keri baths; distraction; tepid baths with sodium bicarbonate or oatmeal added to water; lotions and oils; change of soaps or reduction in use of soap; loose clothing; see health care provider if mild sedation is needed
Palpitations	Unknown; should not be accompanied by persistent cardiac irregularity	Not preventable; contact primary health care provider if accompanied by symptoms of cardiac decompensation
Supine hypotension (vena cava syndrome) and bradycardia	Induced by pressure of gravid uterus on ascending vena cava when woman is supine; reduces uteroplacental and renal perfusion	Side-lying position or semi-sitting posture, with knees slightly flexed (see Nursing Alert, p. 11)

Faintness and, rarely, syncope (orthostatic hypotension) may persist throughout pregnancy	Vasomotor lability or postural hypotension from hormones; in late pregnancy may be caused by venous stasis in lower extremities	Moderate exercise, deep breathing, vigorous leg movement; avoid sudden changes in position and warm crowded areas; move slowly and deliberately; keep environment cool; avoid hypoglycemia by eating five or six small meals per day; wear elastic hose; sit as necessary; if symptoms are serious, contact primary health care provider
Food cravings	Cause unknown; craving influenced by culture or geographic area	Not preventable; satisfy craving unless it interferes with well-balanced diet; report unusual cravings to primary health care provider
Heartburn (pyrosis or acid indigestion): burning sensation, occasionally with burping and regurgitation of a little sour-tasting fluid	Progesterone slows GI tract motility and digestion, reverses peristalsis, relaxes cardiac sphincter, and delays emptying time of stomach; stomach displaced upward and compressed by enlarging uterus	Limit or avoid gas-producing or fatty foods and large meals; maintain good posture; sip milk for temporary relief; drink hot herbal tea; primary health care provider may prescribe antacid between meals; contact primary health care provider for persistent symptoms
Constipation	GI tract motility slowed because of progesterone, resulting in increased resorption of water and drying of stool; intestines compressed by enlarging uterus; predisposition to constipation because of oral iron supplementation	Drink 8 to 10 glasses of water per day; include roughage in diet; engage in moderate exercise; maintain regular schedule for bowel movements; use relaxation techniques and deep breathing; do not take stool softener, laxatives, mineral oil, other drugs, or enemas without first consulting primary health care provider

Continued

TABLE 1-2

Discomforts Related to Pregnancy—cont'd

Discomfort	Physiology	Teaching for Self-Management
SECOND TRIMESTER—cont'd		
Flatulence with bloating and belching	Reduced GI motility because of hormones, allowing time for bacterial action that produces gas; swallowing air	Chew foods slowly and thoroughly; avoid gas-producing foods, fatty foods, large meals; exercise; maintain regular bowel habits
Varicose veins (varicosities): may be associated with aching legs and tenderness; may be present in legs and vulva; hemorrhoids are varicosities in perianal area	Hereditary predisposition; relaxation of smooth muscle walls of veins because of hormones causing tortuous dilated veins in legs and pelvic vasocongestion; condition aggravated by enlarging uterus, gravity, and bearing down for bowel movements; thrombi from leg varices rare but may occur in hemorrhoids	Avoid obesity, lengthy standing or sitting, constrictive clothing, and constipation and bearing down with bowel movements; moderate exercise; rest with legs and hips elevated; wear support stockings; thrombosed hemorrhoid may be evacuated; relieve swelling and pain with warm sitz baths, local application of astringent compresses
Leukorrhea: often noted throughout pregnancy	Hormonally stimulated cervix becomes hypertrophic and hyperactive, producing abundant amount of mucus	Not preventable; do not douche; maintain good hygiene; wear perineal pads; report to primary health care provider if accompanied by pruritus, foul odor, or change in character or color
Headaches (through wk 26)	Emotional tension (more common than vascular migraine headache); eye strain (refractory errors); vascular engorgement and sinus congestion resulting from hormone stimulation	Conscious relaxation; contact primary health care provider for constant "splitting" headache to assess for preeclampsia

Carpal tunnel syndrome (involves thumb, second, and third fingers, lateral side of little finger)	Compression of median nerve resulting from changes in surrounding tissues; pain, numbness, tingling, burning; loss of skilled movements (typing); dropping of objects	Not preventable; elevate affected arms; splinting of affected hand may help; regressive after pregnancy; surgery is curative
Periodic numbness, tingling of fingers (acrodysesthesia) occurs in 5% of pregnant women	Brachial plexus traction syndrome resulting from drooping of shoulders during pregnancy (occurs especially at night and early morning)	Maintain good posture; wear supportive maternity bra; condition will disappear if lifting and carrying baby does not aggravate it
Round ligament pain (tenderness)	Stretching of ligament caused by enlarging uterus	Not preventable; rest, maintain good body mechanics to avoid overstretching ligament; relieve cramping by squatting or bringing knees to chest; sometimes heat helps
Joint pain, backache, and pelvic pressure; hypermobility of joints	Relaxation of symphyseal and sacroiliac joints because of hormones, resulting in unstable pelvis; exaggerated lumbar and cervicothoracic curves caused by change in center of gravity resulting from enlarging abdomen	Maintain good posture and body mechanics; avoid fatigue; wear low-heeled shoes; abdominal supports may be useful; conscious relaxation; sleep on firm mattress; apply local heat or ice; get back rubs; do pelvic tilt exercises; rest; condition will disappear 6 to 8 wk after birth

Continued

TABLE 1-2

Discomforts Related to Pregnancy—cont'd

Discomfort	Physiology	Teaching for Self-Management
THIRD TRIMESTER		
Shortness of breath and dyspnea occur in 60% of pregnant women	Expansion of diaphragm limited by enlarging uterus; diaphragm is elevated about 4 cm; some relief after lightening	Good posture; sleep with extra pillows; avoid overloading stomach; stop smoking; contact health care provider if symptoms worsen to rule out anemia, emphysema, and asthma
Insomnia (later weeks of pregnancy)	Fetal movements, muscle cramping, urinary frequency, shortness of breath, or other discomforts	Reassurance; conscious relaxation; back massage or effleurage; support of body parts with pillows; warm milk or warm shower before retiring
Psychosocial responses: mood swings, mixed feelings, increased anxiety	Hormonal and metabolic adaptations; feelings about impending labor, birth, and parenthood	Reassurance and support from significant other and health care providers; improved communication with partner, family, and others
Urinary frequency and urgency return	Vascular engorgement and altered bladder function caused by hormones; bladder capacity reduced by enlarging uterus and fetal presenting part	Empty bladder regularly, Kegel exercises; limit fluid intake before bedtime; reassurance; wear perineal pad; contact health care provider for pain or burning sensation
Perineal discomfort and pressure	Pressure from enlarging uterus, especially when standing or walking; multifetal gestation	Rest, conscious relaxation, and good posture; contact health care provider for assessment and treatment if pain is present

Braxton Hicks contractions	Intensification of uterine contractions in preparation for work of labor	Reassurance; rest; change of position; practice breathing techniques when contractions are bothersome; effleurage; differentiate from preterm labor
Leg cramps (gastrocnemius spasm), especially when reclining	Compression of nerves supplying lower extremities because of enlarging uterus; reduced level of diffusible serum calcium or elevation of serum phosphorus; aggravating factors: fatigue, poor peripheral circulation, pointing toes when stretching legs or when walking, drinking more than 1 L (1 qt) of milk per day	Check for Homans sign; if negative, use massage and heat over affected muscle; dorsiflex foot until spasm relaxes; stand on cold surface; oral supplementation with calcium carbonate or calcium lactate tablets; aluminum hydroxide gel, 30 ml, with each meal removes phosphorus by absorbing it (consult primary health care provider before taking these remedies)
Ankle edema (nonpitting) to lower extremities	Edema aggravated by prolonged standing, sitting, poor posture, lack of exercise, constrictive clothing, or hot weather	Ample fluid intake for natural diuretic effect; put on support stockings before arising; rest periodically with legs and hips elevated; exercise moderately; contact health care provider if generalized edema develops; diuretics are contraindicated

BBT, Basal body temperature; *GI*, gastrointestinal; *hCG*, human chorionic gonadotropin.

The side-lying position is recommended because it promotes uterine perfusion and fetoplacental oxygenation. Conscious relaxation is the process of releasing tension from the mind and body through deliberate effort and practice. The techniques for conscious relaxation are numerous and varied. Guidelines are given in Box 1-4.

- *Employment.* Employment usually has no adverse effects on pregnancy outcomes.
- *Safety.* Strategies to improve safety are described in the Teaching for Self-Management box: Safety During Pregnancy.
- *Clothing.* Comfortable, loose clothing and shoes are recommended. Avoid tight bras and belts, stretch pants, garters, tight-top knee socks, panty girdles, and other constrictive clothing because tight clothing over the perineum encourages vaginitis and miliaria (heat rash), and impaired circulation in the legs can cause varicosities. Platform shoes and high heels may cause the woman to lose her balance.
- *Travel.* Travel is not contraindicated for low risk pregnant women. However, women with high risk pregnancies are

---

BOX 1-4

Conscious Relaxation Tips

- **Preparation:** Loosen clothing, and assume a comfortable sitting or side-lying position with all parts of body well supported with pillows.
- **Beginning:** Allow yourself to feel warm and comfortable. Inhale and exhale slowly, and imagine peaceful relaxation coming over each part of the body, starting with the neck and working down to the toes. Often people who learn conscious relaxation speak of feeling relaxed even if some discomfort is present.
- **Maintenance:** Use imagery (fantasy or daydream) to maintain the state of relaxation. Using active imagery, imagine yourself moving or doing some activity and experiencing its sensations. Using passive imagery, imagine yourself watching a scene, such as a lovely sunset.
- **Awakening:** Return to the wakeful state gradually. Slowly begin to take in stimuli from the surrounding environment.
- **Further retention and development of the skill:** Practice regularly for some periods each day, for example, at the same hour for 10 to 15 min each day, to feel refreshed, revitalized, and invigorated.

Teaching for Self-Management

Safety During Pregnancy

- Changes in the body resulting from pregnancy include relaxation of joints, alteration to the center of gravity, faintness, and discomforts. Problems with coordination and balance are common. Therefore, the woman should follow these guidelines:
  - ❏ Use good body mechanics.
  - ❏ Use safety features on tools and vehicles (safety seat belts, shoulder harnesses, headrests, goggles, helmets) as specified.
  - ❏ Avoid activities requiring coordination, balance, and concentration.
  - ❏ Take rest periods; reschedule daily activities to meet rest and relaxation needs.
- Embryonic and fetal development is vulnerable to environmental teratogens. Many potentially dangerous chemicals are present in the home, yard, and workplace: cleaning agents, paints, sprays, herbicides, and pesticides. The soil and water supply may be unsafe. Therefore, the woman should follow these guidelines:
  - ❏ Read all labels for ingredients and proper use of the product.
  - ❏ Ensure adequate ventilation with clean air.
  - ❏ Dispose of wastes appropriately.
  - ❏ Wear gloves when handling chemicals.
  - ❏ Change job assignments or workplace as necessary.
  - ❏ Avoid travel to high altitude regions, which could jeopardize oxygen intake.

advised to avoid long-distance travel after fetal viability has been reached to avoid possible economic and psychologic consequences of giving birth to a preterm infant far from home.
- Women who contemplate foreign travel should be aware that many health insurance carriers do not cover a birth in a foreign setting or even hospitalization for preterm labor. In addition, vaccinations for foreign travel may be contraindicated during pregnancy.
  - ❏ Pregnant women who travel for long distances should schedule periods of activity and rest. While sitting, the woman can practice deep breathing, foot circling, and alternately contracting and relaxing different muscle groups. Women

riding in a car should wear automobile restraints and stop to walk every hour.

❏ Airline travel in large commercial jets usually poses little risk to the pregnant woman, but policies vary from airline to airline. The woman is advised to inquire about restrictions or recommendations from her carrier. Most health care providers allow air travel up to 36 weeks of gestation in women without medical or pregnancy complications. Metal detectors used at airport security checkpoints are not harmful to the fetus. Sitting in the cramped seat of an airliner for prolonged periods may increase the risk of superficial and deep vein thrombosis. Therefore, a pregnant woman is encouraged to take a walk around the aircraft during each hour of travel to minimize this risk.

■ *Medications and herbal preparations.* The possible teratogenicity of many medications, both prescription and OTC, is still unknown. This is especially true for new medications and combinations of drugs. The use of all drugs, including OTC medications, herbs, and vitamins, should be limited and a careful record kept of all therapeutic and nontherapeutic agents used. The woman should inform her health care provider of all the drugs she takes, including OTC medications, herbs, and vitamins.

■ *Immunizations.* Immunization with live or attenuated live viruses is contraindicated during pregnancy because of its potential teratogenicity. Live-virus vaccines include those for measles (rubeola and rubella), chickenpox, and mumps, as well as the Sabin (oral) poliomyelitis vaccine (no longer used in the United States). Vaccines that can be administered during pregnancy include tetanus, diphtheria, recombinant hepatitis B, and influenza because they are inactivated.

SAFETY ALERT *Pregnant women who become ill with seasonal respiratory influenza (flu) are more likely than other persons to develop serious complications, such as pneumonia. All women whose pregnancy will take place from November through March should be offered a flu vaccination.*

■ *Alcohol, cigarettes, caffeine, and drugs.* A safe level of alcohol consumption during pregnancy has not been established.

Complete abstinence is strongly advised. Cigarette smoking or continued exposure to secondhand smoke is associated with IUGR, an increased frequency of preterm labor, premature rupture of membranes (PROM), placental abruption, placenta previa, and fetal death. Most studies of human pregnancy have revealed no association between caffeine consumption and birth defects or low birth weight (LBW), although some have documented an increased risk for miscarriage or IUGR with caffeine intake greater than 200 mg/day. Because other effects are unknown, however, pregnant women are advised to limit their caffeine intake to no more than 200 mg/day. All drug use should be limited.

- *Recognizing potential complications.* One of the most important responsibilities of care providers is to alert the pregnant woman to signs and symptoms that indicate a potential complication of pregnancy (see the Signs of Potential Complications box on p. 12).
- *Sexual counseling.* Sexual counseling of expectant couples includes countering misinformation, providing reassurance of normality, and suggesting alternative behaviors. Because STIs may be transmitted to the woman and her fetus, condom use is recommended throughout pregnancy if the woman is at risk for acquiring an STI.

DISCOMFORTS RELATED TO PREGNANCY

Pregnant women have physical symptoms that would be considered abnormal in the nonpregnant state. Information about the physiology and prevention of and self-management for discomforts experienced during the three trimesters is given in Table 1-2.

ANTEPARTUM FETAL ASSESSMENT

The major expected outcome of all antepartum assessment is the detection of potential fetal compromise. Antepartum assessment is used primarily in women at risk for disrupted fetal oxygenation. In most cases, monitoring begins by 32 to 34 weeks of gestation and continues regularly until birth. Assessment tests should be selected based on their effectiveness, and the results must be interpreted in light of the complete clinical picture.

Biophysical Assessment

Daily Fetal Movement Count

Indication

Daily fetal movement count (DFMC, also called "kick counts") is frequently used to monitor the fetus in pregnancies complicated by conditions that may affect fetal oxygenation.

Procedure and Interpretation

- DFMC can be done at home, is noninvasive, is simple to understand, and usually does not interfere with a daily routine.
- Several different protocols may be used for counting.
  - ❑ Count fetal movement once each day for 60 minutes.
  - ❑ Count fetal movements two or three times daily for 60 minutes each time.
- The clinical value of the absolute number of fetal movements has not been established, *except* when fetal movements cease entirely for 12 hours. Fewer than three fetal movements within 1 hour usually warrants further evaluation.
- The presence of movements is generally a reassuring sign of fetal health.
- In assessing fetal movements, remember that they are usually not present during the fetal sleep cycle; also they may be temporarily reduced if the woman is taking depressant medications, drinking alcohol, or smoking a cigarette.
- Women should be taught the significance of the presence or absence of fetal movements, the procedure for counting that is to be used, how to record findings on a DFMC record, and when to notify their health care provider.

Ultrasonography

Indications

Diagnostic ultrasonography is an important, safe technique in antepartum fetal surveillance. It provides critical information to health care providers regarding fetal activity and gestational age, normal versus abnormal fetal growth curves, visual assistance with which invasive tests may be performed more safely, fetal and placental anatomy, and fetal well-being. Major indications for obstetric sonography appear by trimester in Table 1-3.

TABLE 1-3

Major Uses of Ultrasonography During Pregnancy

First Trimester	Second Trimester	Third Trimester
Confirm pregnancy	Establish or confirm dates	Confirm gestational age
Confirm viability	Confirm viability	Confirm viability
Determine gestational age	Detect polyhydramnios, oligohydramnios	Detect macrosomia
Rule out ectopic pregnancy	Detect congenital anomalies	Detect congenital anomalies
Detect multiple gestation	Detect intrauterine growth restriction (IUGR)	Detect IUGR
Determine the cause of vaginal bleeding	Assess placental placement	Determine fetal position
	Use for visualization during amniocentesis	Detect placenta previa or placental abruption
		Use for visualization during amniocentesis, external version
		Biophysical profile
		Amniotic fluid volume assessment
		Doppler flow studies
		Detect placental maturity

Procedure and Interpretation

- Ultrasound examination can be performed abdominally or transvaginally during pregnancy. Both methods produce a three-dimensional view from which a pictorial image is obtained. Newer machines produce a four-dimensional view.
- Abdominal ultrasonography is more useful after the first trimester when the pregnant uterus becomes an abdominal organ. For abdominal scans, the woman usually should have a full bladder to get a better image of the fetus. Transmission gel or paste is applied to the abdomen before a transducer is moved over the skin to enhance transmission and reception of the sound waves.

- Transvaginal ultrasonography, in which the probe is inserted into the vagina, is optimally used in the first trimester to detect ectopic pregnancies, monitor the developing embryo, help identify abnormalities, and help establish gestational age. A full bladder is not necessary. In some instances it may be used as an adjunct to abdominal scanning to evaluate preterm labor in second- and third-trimester pregnancies.
- Interpretation depends on why the scan was done.

Doppler Blood Flow Analysis
Indication

One of the major advances in perinatal medicine is the ability to study blood flow noninvasively in the fetus and placenta with ultrasound. Doppler blood flow analysis is a helpful tool in the management of pregnancies at risk because of hypertension, IUGR, diabetes mellitus, multiple fetuses, and preterm labor.

Procedure and Interpretation

- A pulsed Doppler device is positioned over the fetus, and umbilical and uterine artery blood flow is measured. A plot of velocity versus time and the shape of these waveforms can be analyzed to give information about blood flow and resistance in a given circulation.
- Velocity waveforms reported as systolic/diastolic (S/D) ratios can be first detected at 15 weeks of pregnancy. Because of the progressive decline in resistance in both the umbilical and uterine arteries, this ratio decreases as pregnancy advances.
- IUGR is seen more often in fetuses whose ratios remain elevated for their gestational age. Severely restricted uterine artery blood flow is indicated by absent or reversed flow during diastole. In postterm pregnancies, an elevated S/D ratio indicates a poorly perfused placenta. Abnormal results also are seen with certain chromosome abnormalities (trisomy 13 and trisomy 18) in the fetus and with lupus erythematosus in the mother. Exposure to nicotine from maternal smoking also has been reported to increase the S/D ratio.

Amniotic Fluid Volume Index

The amniotic fluid index (AFI) evaluates the quantity of amniotic fluid to determine adequate uteroplacental function. Decreased (oligohydramnios) or increased (hydramnios/polyhydramnios) amniotic fluid volume is frequently associated with fetal disorders. Oligohydramnios is associated with congenital anomalies (e.g., renal agenesis), growth restriction, and fetal distress during labor. Hydramnios/polyhydramnios is associated with neural tube defects, obstruction of the fetal gastrointestinal tract, multiple fetuses, and fetal hydrops.

Procedure and Interpretation

- The total amniotic fluid volume (AFV) can be evaluated by using ultrasound to measure the vertical depth (in centimeters) of the amniotic fluid in all four quadrants surrounding the maternal umbilicus. The measurements are totaled.
- A normal AFI is 10 cm or greater, with the upper range of normal around 25 cm. AFI values between 5 and 10 cm are considered to be low normal, whereas an AFI of less than 5 cm indicates oligohydramnios. With polyhydramnios the AFI is greater than 25 cm.

Biophysical Profile

The biophysical profile (BPP) is a noninvasive dynamic assessment of a fetus that is based on acute and chronic markers of fetal disease. Fetal heart rate (FHR) reactivity, fetal breathing movements (FBMs), fetal movement, and fetal tone reflect current central nervous system (CNS) status, whereas the AFV demonstrates the adequacy of placental function over a longer period.

Procedure and Interpretation

- An abdominal ultrasound scan is done to evaluate FBMs, fetal movements, fetal tone, and AFV; FHR and patterns are assessed by means of a nonstress test.
- BPP scoring and management is detailed in Tables 1-4 and 1-5.

Biochemical Assessment

Biochemical assessment involves biologic examination (e.g., as chromosomes in exfoliated cells) and chemical determinations (e.g., lecithin/sphingomyelin [L/S] ratio, bilirubin level, surfactant/albumin [S/A] ratio [TDx FLM assay]) (see Table 1-5). Procedures to obtain the needed specimens include amniocentesis, chorionic villus sampling, percutaneous umbilical blood sampling, and maternal blood sampling.

TABLE 1-4

Biophysical Profile Scoring

Biophysical Variable	Normal (Score = 2)	Abnormal (Score = 0)
Fetal breathing movements	At least one episode of >30 sec duration in 30 min observation	Absent or no episode of ≥30 sec duration in 30 min
Gross body movement	At least 3 discrete body/limb movements in 30 min (episodes of active continuous movement considered a single movement)	Up to two episodes of body/limb movements in 30 min
Fetal tone	At least one episode of active extension with return to flexion of fetal limb(s) or trunk, opening and closing of hand considered normal tone	Either slow extension with return to partial flexion or movement of limb in full extension or absent fetal movement
Reactive fetal heart rate	At least two episodes of acceleration of ≥15 beats/min and 15 sec duration associated with fetal movement in 30 min	Fewer than two accelerations or acceleration <15 beats/min in 30 min
Qualitative amniotic fluid volume	At least one pocket of amniotic fluid measuring 2 cm in two perpendicular planes	Either no amniotic fluid pockets or a pocket <2 cm in two perpendicular planes

Modified from Manning, F. (1992). Biophysical profile scoring. In S. Gabbe, J. Niebyl, & J. Simpson (Eds.), *Obstetrics: Normal and problem pregnancies* (5th ed.). Philadelphia: Churchill Livingstone.

Amniocentesis

Indications

- Amniocentesis is performed to obtain amniotic fluid, which contains fetal cells. Indications for the procedure include prenatal diagnosis of genetic disorders or congenital anomalies (neural tube defects in particular), assessment of pulmonary maturity, and diagnosis of fetal hemolytic disease.

TABLE 1-5

Biophysical Profile Management

Score	Interpretation	Management
10	Normal infant; low risk of chronic asphyxia	Repeat testing at weekly intervals; repeat twice weekly in diabetic women and women at 41 wk of gestation
8	Normal infant; low risk of chronic asphyxia	Repeat testing at weekly intervals; repeat testing twice weekly in diabetic women and women at 41 wk of gestation; oligohydramnios is an indication for delivery
6	Suspect chronic asphyxia	If 36 wk of gestation and conditions are favorable, deliver; if at >36 wk and L/S <2, repeat test in 4-6 hr; deliver if oligohydramnios is present
4	Suspect chronic asphyxia	If 36 weeks of gestation, deliver; if <32 wk of gestation, repeat score
0-2	Strongly suspect chronic asphyxia	Extend testing time to 120 min; if persistent score ≤4, deliver, regardless of gestational age

L/S, Lecithin/sphingomyelin.
Modified from Manning, F., Harman, C., Morrison, I., Menticoglou, S., Lange, I., & Johnson, J. (1990). Fetal assessment based on fetal biophysical profile scoring. *American Journal of Obstetrics and Gynecology, 162*(3), 703-709; Manning F. (1992). Biophysical profile scoring. In S. Gabbe, J. Niebyl, & J. Simpson (Eds.), *Obstetrics: Normal and problem pregnancies* (5th ed.). Philadelphia: Churchill Livingstone.

Procedure and Interpretation

- The examiner uses direct ultrasonographic visualization to insert a needle transabdominally into the uterus, withdraw amniotic fluid into a syringe, and perform various assessments. Amniocentesis is possible after week 14 of pregnancy, when the uterus becomes an abdominal organ and sufficient amniotic fluid is available for testing.
- Complications in the mother and fetus occur in less than 1% of the cases and include the following:
  - ❑ Maternal: hemorrhage, fetomaternal hemorrhage with possible maternal Rh isoimmunization, infection, labor, placental abruption, inadvertent damage to the intestines or bladder, and amniotic fluid embolism

❏ Fetal: death, hemorrhage, infection (amnionitis), direct injury from the needle, miscarriage or preterm birth and leakage of amniotic fluid

NURSING ALERT *Because of the possibility of fetomaternal hemorrhage, administering Rh_oD immunoglobulin to the woman who is Rh negative is standard practice after an amniocentesis.*

Table 1-6 lists possible findings and clinical significance of amniotic fluid analysis.

TABLE 1-6

Summary of Biochemical Monitoring Techniques

Test	Possible Findings	Clinical Significance
MATERNAL BLOOD		
Coombs' test	Titer of 1:8 and increasing	Significant Rh incompatibility
AFP	See below	
AMNIOTIC FLUID ANALYSIS		
Lung profile		Fetal lung maturity
L/S ratio	2 : 1	
Phosphatidylglycerol	Present	
S/A ratio (TDx FLM assay)	≥55 mg/g	
Creatinine	>2 mg/dl	Gestational age >36 wk
Bilirubin (ΔOD, 450/nm)	<0. 015	Gestational age >36 wk, normal pregnancy
	High levels	Fetal hemolytic disease in Rh isoimmunized pregnancies
Lipid cells	>10%	Gestational age >35 wk
AFP	High levels after 15 wks gestation	Open neural tube or other defect
Osmolality	Decline after 20 wks gestation	Advancing gestational age
Genetic disorders: Sex linked Chromosomal Metabolic	Dependent on cultured cells for karyotype and enzymatic activity	Counseling possibly required

AFP, Alpha-fetoprotein; *L/S,* lecithin-sphingomyelin; *S/A,* surfactant/albumin; *TDx FLM assay,* name of specific test used to determine S/A ratio.

Chorionic Villus Sampling

Indications

Chorionic villus sampling (CVS) is done for genetic studies. Because it offers diagnosis earlier in pregnancy and more rapid results, it is a popular technique for use in the first trimester, although some risks to the fetus exist. Indications for CVS are similar to those for amniocentesis, although CVS cannot be used for maternal serum marker screening because no fluid is obtained. CVS performed in the second trimester carries no greater risk of pregnancy loss than amniocentesis, and it is considered equal to amniocentesis in terms of diagnostic accuracy.

Procedure and Interpretation

- CVS is performed between 10 and 13 weeks of gestation and involves the removal of a small tissue specimen from the fetal portion of the placenta. Because chorionic villi originate in the zygote, this tissue reflects the genetic makeup of the fetus.
- CVS procedures can be accomplished either transcervically or transabdominally.
  - ❏ In transcervical sampling, the examiner uses continuous ultrasonographic guidance to introduce a sterile catheter into the cervix and aspirate a small portion of the chorionic villi with a syringe. The aspiration cannula and obturator must be placed at a suitable site, and rupture of the amniotic sac must be avoided.
  - ❏ If the abdominal approach is used, the examiner uses sterile conditions and ultrasound guidance to insert an 18-gauge spinal needle with stylet through the abdominal wall into the chorion frondosum. The stylet is then withdrawn, and the chorionic tissue is aspirated into a syringe.
- Complications occur rarely (in <1% of cases) but include vaginal spotting or bleeding immediately afterward, miscarriage, rupture of membranes, and chorioamnionitis.
- Controversy exists concerning fetal limb reduction defects associated with CVS. Any increased risk appears to exist before 10 weeks of gestation. For this reason CVS is usually not performed until after 9 menstrual weeks of gestation.
- Interpretation is based on what is being evaluated.

NURSING ALERT *Because of the possibility of fetomaternal hemorrhage, women who are Rh negative should receive Rh_0D immunoglobulin after CVS to prevent isoimmunization.*

Percutaneous Umbilical Blood Sampling
Indications

Percutaneous umbilical blood sampling (PUBS), or cordocentesis, is used for fetal blood sampling and transfusion via direct access to the fetal circulation. Indications for use of PUBS include prenatal diagnosis of inherited blood disorders, karyotyping of malformed fetuses, detection of fetal infection, and assessment and treatment of isoimmunization and thrombocytopenia in the fetus.

Procedure and Interpretation

- PUBS involves the insertion of a needle directly into a fetal umbilical vessel using ultrasound guidance.
- Generally a small amount of blood is removed and tested immediately by the Kleihauer-Betke procedure (Apt test) to ensure that it is fetal in origin.
- Complications that can occur include loss of the pregnancy, hematomas, bleeding from the puncture site in the umbilical cord, transient fetal bradycardia, and fetomaternal hemorrhage. Maternal complications are rare, but include hemorrhage and transplacental hemorrhage.
- Follow-up includes continuous FHR monitoring for 1 to 2 hours after the procedure.
- Interpretation is based on why PUBS was performed.

Maternal Assays

ALPHA-FETOPROTEIN
Indication

Maternal serum alpha-fetoprotein (MSAFP) levels have been used as a screening tool for neural tube defects (NTDs) in pregnancy. Through this technique, approximately 80% to 85% of all open NTDs and open abdominal wall defects can be detected early in pregnancy. Screening is recommended for all pregnant women.

Procedure and Interpretation

- MSAFP screening can be done with reasonable reliability anytime between 15 and 20 weeks of gestation (16 to 18 weeks is ideal).
- A blood sample is drawn and sent for analysis.

- Once the MSAFP is determined, it is compared with normal values for each week of gestation. Values also should be correlated with maternal age, weight, race, presence of a multifetal pregnancy, and whether the woman has insulin-dependent diabetes.
- Higher-than-normal levels are associated with NTDs.
- If findings are abnormal, follow-up procedures include genetic counseling for families with a history of NTD, repeated AFP, specialized ultrasound examination, and possibly amniocentesis.

MULTIPLE-MARKER SCREENS

Indications

These screening tests are done to diagnose chromosomal abnormalities in the fetus. Results are based on information obtained from the woman's history, maternal blood samples, and fetal ultrasound scans.

- First trimester screening for chromosomal abnormalities is done between 11 and 14 weeks of gestation. This screen includes measurement of two maternal biochemical markers, pregnancy-associated placental protein (PAPP-A) and human chorionic gonadotropin (hCG) or the free beta-human chorionic gonadotropin (β-hCG) subunit, and evaluation of fetal nuchal translucency (NT), an ultrasound measurement of fluid in the nape of the fetal neck, or a combination of both.
- The triple-screen is done between 16 and 18 weeks of gestation. It measures the levels of MSAFP, hCG, and unconjugated estriol in maternal blood.
- The quad-screen, also done between 16 and 18 weeks of gestation, adds an additional marker, a placental hormone called inhibin A, to the triple-screen to increase the accuracy of screening for Down syndrome (trisomy 21) in women less than 35 years of age.

Procedure and Interpretation

- A maternal blood sample is drawn and sent for analysis. An ultrasound is performed to measure the fetal NT.
- In the first trimester, hCG levels are higher than normal, whereas PAPP-A levels are lower than normal in the presence of a fetus with Down syndrome. About one third of all fetuses with an increased NT have a chromosome abnormality; half of these are trisomy 21.

- Triple- and quad-screen results
  - ❏ Low MSAFP and unconjugated estriol levels and high hCG levels are associated with trisomy 21.
  - ❏ Low values in all three markers are associated with trisomy 18.
  - ❏ Low inhibin A levels indicate the possibility of trisomy 21.
- The ability of multiple marker tests to detect chromosomal abnormalities depends on the accuracy of gestational age assessment. These tests are screening procedures only and are not diagnostic. A positive screening test result indicates an increased risk but is not diagnostic of trisomy 21 or another chromosomal abnormality. Women with positive results should be offered diagnostic testing by amniocentesis or fetal blood sampling for fetal karyotyping.

ANTEPARTAL ASSESSMENT USING ELECTRONIC FETAL MONITORING

Indications

First- and second-trimester antepartal assessment is directed primarily at the diagnosis of fetal anomalies. The goal of third-trimester testing is to determine whether the intrauterine environment continues to be supportive to the fetus. The testing is often used to determine the timing of childbirth for women at risk for uteroplacental insufficiency (UPI). Gradual loss of placental function results first in inadequate nutrient delivery to the fetus, leading to IUGR. Subsequently, respiratory function also is compromised, resulting in fetal hypoxia.

- The nonstress test (NST) and contraction stress test (CST), sometimes called the oxytocin challenge test (OCT), use the electronic fetal monitor for antepartal assessment in the late second and third trimesters.
- The NST is the most widely applied technique for antepartum evaluation of the fetus. It is an ideal screening test and is the primary method of antepartum assessment at most sites.
  - ❏ There are no contraindications for performing the NST, but results may not be conclusive if the gestational age is less than 26 weeks.
- The CST provides an earlier warning of fetal compromise than the NST and has fewer false-positive results. However, because it has several disadvantages, the test is infrequently used in current clinical practice.
  - ❏ In general, the CST cannot be performed on women who should not deliver vaginally at the time the test is performed.

❑ Absolute contraindications for the CST are preterm labor, placenta previa, vasa previa, cervical insufficiency, multiple gestation, and previous classic incision for cesarean birth.

❑ The CST is more time consuming and expensive than the NST. It is also an invasive procedure if oxytocin stimulation is required.

❑ Box 1-5 lists common indications for the NST and the CST.

Nonstress Test

Procedure and Interpretation

■ The woman is seated in a reclining chair (or in semi-Fowler position) with a slight lateral tilt to optimize uterine perfusion and avoid supine hypotension.

■ The FHR is recorded with a Doppler transducer, and a tocodynamometer is applied to detect uterine contractions or fetal movements.

■ The tracing is observed for signs of fetal activity and a concurrent acceleration of FHR.

■ The test is usually completed within 20 to 30 minutes, but it may take longer if the fetus must be awakened from a sleep state.

■ NST results are either reactive (Fig. 1-1) or nonreactive (Fig. 1-2). Box 1-6 describes interpretation of the NST.

BOX 1-5

Indications for Electronic Fetal Monitoring Assessment Using the Nonstress Test and the Contraction Stress Test

■ Maternal diabetes mellitus
■ Chronic hypertension
■ Hypertensive disorders in pregnancy
■ Intrauterine growth restriction
■ Sickle cell disease
■ Maternal cyanotic heart disease
■ Postmaturity
■ History of previous stillbirth
■ Decreased fetal movement
■ Isoimmunization
■ Hyperthyroidism
■ Collagen disease
■ Chronic renal disease

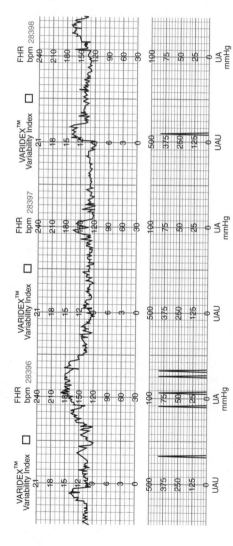

Fig. 1-1 Reactive nonstress test. (From Gabbe, S., Niebyl, J., & Simpson, J. [2007]. *Obstetrics: Normal and problem pregnancies* [5th ed.]. Philadelphia: Churchill Livingstone.)

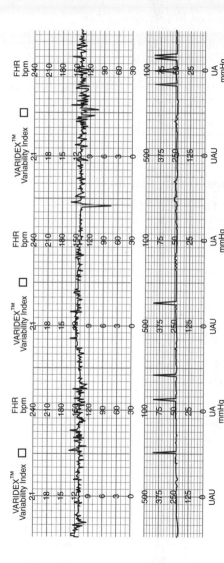

Fig. 1-2 Nonreactive nonstress test. (From Gabbe, S., Niebyl, J., & Simpson, J. [2007]. *Obstetrics: Normal and problem pregnancies* [5th ed.]. Philadelphia: Churchill Livingstone.).

BOX 1-6

Interpretation of the Nonstress Test

Reactive test: two accelerations in a 20-min period, each lasting at least 15 sec and peaking at least 15 beats/min above the baseline (before 32 wk of gestation, an acceleration is defined as an increase of at least 10 beats/min and lasting at least 10 sec)

Nonreactive test: a test that does not produce two or more qualifying accelerations in a 20-min period

Source: Tucker, S., Miller, L., & Miller, D. (2009). *Mosby's pocket guide to fetal monitoring: A multidisciplinary approach* (6th ed.). St. Louis: Mosby.

Vibroacoustic Stimulation

Vibroacoustic stimulation (also called fetal acoustic stimulation test) is another method of testing antepartum FHR response and is generally performed in conjunction with the NST. It uses a combination of sound and vibration to stimulate the fetus.

Procedure and Interpretation

- The test takes approximately 15 minutes to complete, with the fetus monitored for 5 to 10 minutes before stimulation to obtain a baseline FHR.
- If the fetal baseline pattern is nonreactive, the sound source (usually a laryngeal stimulator) is then activated for 3 seconds on the maternal abdomen over the fetal head. Monitoring continues for another 5 minutes, after which the monitor tracing is assessed.
- The desired result is a reactive NST. The test may be repeated at 1-minute intervals up to three times when there is no response. Further evaluation is needed with BPP or CST if the pattern is still nonreactive.

MATERNAL AND FETAL NUTRITION

Good nutrition before and after pregnancy and adequate weight gain during pregnancy are important preventive measures for problems such as LBW and prematurity. These problems can lead to higher neonatal and infant death rates as well as serious health impairments.

Nutrient Needs Before Conception

Women capable of becoming pregnant are advised to do the following:

- Take 0.4 mg of folic acid daily by eating fortified foods (ready-to-eat cereals and enriched grain products) or supplements in addition to a diet rich in folate (green leafy vegetables, whole grains, fruits) in order to prevent fetal NTDs. Women who have had a child with an NTD should take a 4-mg folic acid supplement daily.
- Achieve desirable body weight before conception in order to prevent maternal-fetal risks because of underweight or overweight status.

Nutrient Needs During Pregnancy

- Nutrient needs increase during the second and third trimesters as the uterine-placental-fetal unit develops, maternal breasts develop, and maternal blood volume and metabolic needs increase.
- Weight gain recommendations for pregnancy should be based on the woman's prepregnancy BMI (www.nhlbi.nih.gov/guidelines/obesity/bmi_tbl.pdf). Prepregnant BMI classifications and weight gain recommendations for women with single fetuses are as follows:
  - ❏ Underweight (BMI <18.5), 12.5 to 18 kg (28 to 40 lb)
  - ❏ Normal (BMI 18.5 to 24.9), 11.5 to 16 kg (25 to 35 lb)
  - ❏ Overweight (BMI 25 to 29.9), 7 to 11.5 kg (15 to 25 lb)
  - ❏ Obese (BMI >30), 5 to 9 kg (11 to 20 lb)
- During the first trimester of a singleton pregnancy, the average total weight gain is only 1 to 2 kg. The following weekly gains are recommended for the remainder of the pregnancy:
  - ❏ Underweight BMI, 0.5 kg (1.1 lb)
  - ❏ Normal weight BMI, 0.4 kg (0.88 lb)
  - ❏ Overweight BMI, 0.3 kg (0.66 lb)
  - ❏ Obese BMI, 0.2 kg (0.44 lb)
- The reasons for inadequate or excessive weight gain can include inadequate or excessive dietary intake, measurement or recording errors, and differences in the weight of clothing or the time of day. An exceptionally high gain is likely to result from the accumulation of fluids, and a gain of more than 3 kg in a month after the twentieth week of gestation often indicates the development of preeclampsia.
- The recommended daily food plan for pregnant women is presented in Table 1-7 (see also www.mypyramid.gov for the MyPyramid plan for guiding nutrition choices).

TABLE 1-7

Daily Food Guide for Pregnancy and Lactation

Food Group	Daily Amount of Food Recommended For Women*	Serving Size
Grains	6- to 8-oz equivalents At least half of grain servings should be whole grains. *Whole grains* are those that contain the entire grain kernel (bran, germ, endosperm) (e.g., whole wheat or cornmeal, oatmeal, and brown rice). *Refined grains* have been milled to remove the bran and germ (e.g., white flour, white bread, degermed cornmeal, white rice, and corn or flour tortillas).	1-oz equivalent = 1 slice bread, 1 cup ready-to-eat cereal, or ½ cup cooked rice or pasta or cooked cereal
Vegetables Vary the vegetables consumed to take advantage of the different nutrients they offer.	2½-3 cups Weekly intake should include at least 3 cups dark green vegetables (e.g., spinach or greens, broccoli, bok choy, romaine lettuce); 2 cups orange vegetables (e.g., carrots; acorn, butternut, or Hubbard squash; sweet potatoes); 3 cups dry beans or peas (e.g., black, navy, or kidney beans; chickpeas; black-eyed peas; split peas; lentils; soybeans; tofu); 3 cups starchy vegetables (corn, green peas, potatoes); and 6½ cups other vegetables (e.g., artichokes, asparagus, bean sprouts, green beans, cauliflower, cucumber, tomatoes, iceberg or head lettuce).	1 cup = 2 cups raw leafy greens; 1 cup other vegetables, raw or cooked; or 1 cup vegetable juice

Food Group	Amount	Notes
Fruits	2 cups	1 cup = 1 cup raw, frozen or canned fruit; 1 cup 100% juice; or ½ cup dried fruit
Milk, yogurt, and cheese (milk group)	3 cups	1 cup = 1 cup milk or yogurt; 1½ oz natural cheese; 2 oz processed cheese (such as American); 2 cups cottage cheese; 1½ cups ice cream (choose fat-free or low-fat most often) Most milk group choices should be fat-free or low-fat.
Meat, poultry, fish, dry beans, eggs, and nuts (meat and beans[†] groups)	5½- to 6½-ounce equivalents	1-oz equivalent = 1 oz (30 g) meat, poultry, or fish; ¼ cup cooked dry beans;[†] 1 egg; 1 Tbsp (15 ml) peanut butter; ½ ounce nuts or seeds Most meat and poultry choices should be lean or low-fat. Fish, nuts, and seeds contain healthy oils, so choose these foods frequently instead of meat or poultry.
Oils	6 tsp (30 ml)	1 tsp = 1 tsp liquid oil (olive, canola, sunflower, safflower, peanut, soybean, cottonseed, etc.) or soft margarine (tub or squeeze bottle); 1 Tbsp mayonnaise or Italian salad dressing; ¾ Tbsp Thousand Island salad dressing; 8 large olives; ⅛ medium avocado; ⅓ oz dry roasted peanuts, mixed nuts, cashews, sunflower seeds[†] Choose oils rather than solid fats. Solid fats are fats that are solid at room temperature, such as butter, shortening, stick margarine, and pork, chicken, or beef fat. Read the label: choose products with no *trans* fats, limit intake of saturated fats, and choose oils high in monounsaturated and polyunsaturated fats.

*These are approximate amounts, based on a relatively sedentary lifestyle, and should be individualized. Intake may have to be increased for women with a more active lifestyle or multiple gestation, those who are underweight before pregnancy, or those exhibiting poor gestational weight gain. †Beans are also part of the vegetable group; avocados are also part of the fruit group, and nuts and seeds are part of the meat and beans group.

- Pregnant women (as well as women who are breastfeeding and young children) should avoid eating fish high in mercury (shark, swordfish, king mackerel, tilefish).
- The artificial sweeteners aspartame (NutraSweet, Equal), acesulfame potassium (Sunette), and sucralose (Splenda) are approved by the U.S. Food and Drug Administration (FDA) for use in pregnancy. However, aspartame should be avoided by women who have phenylketonuria (PKU) because it contains phenylalanine. Stevia (stevioside) is a sweetener sold as a dietary supplement; no acceptable daily intake has been established for stevia.

Special Nutritional Risks in Pregnancy

- Recommended weight gain goals for pregnant adolescents are not different from those of adult women. BMI is calculated as for adult women, rather than by using the adolescent BMI growth charts available from the Centers for Disease Control and Prevention.
- Women expecting twins should gain according to these guidelines:
  - ❏ Underweight BMI, 21 to 28 kg (46 to 62 lb)
  - ❏ Normal BMI, 17 to 25 kg (37 to 54 lb)
  - ❏ Overweight BMI, 14 to 23 kg (31 to 50 lb)
  - ❏ Obese BMI, 11 to 19 kg (25 to 42 lb)
- There is not enough information available to make firm recommendations about optimal weight gain for women with more than two fetuses.
- Excessive weight gained during pregnancy may be difficult to lose after pregnancy, thus contributing to chronic overweight or obesity, an etiologic factor in many chronic diseases, including hypertension, diabetes mellitus, and arteriosclerotic heart disease. The woman who gains 18 kg (40 lb) or more is especially at risk to become overweight or obese.
- Pregnancy is not the time for a weight reduction diet. Dietary restriction results in the catabolism of fat stores, which in turn augments the production of ketones. The long-term effects of mild ketonemia during pregnancy are not known, but ketonuria is associated with the occurrence of preterm labor.
- Severely underweight women are more likely to have preterm labor and to give birth to LBW infants. Both normal-weight and underweight women with inadequate weight gain have an increased risk of giving birth to an infant with IUGR.

- Women with anemia tolerate birth hemorrhage poorly, and iron deficiency in early pregnancy increases the risk of preterm birth. In the United States, anemia is most common among adolescents, African-American women, and women in lower socioeconomic groups. A supplement of 30 mg of ferrous iron daily, starting by 12 weeks of gestation, helps ensure an adequate iron intake.
- Iron should not be taken with certain foods that inhibit its absorption (bran, milk, egg yolks, coffee, tea, or oxalate-containing vegetables such as spinach and Swiss chard). Iron absorption from plant sources is promoted by a diet rich in vitamin C (citrus fruits, melons). However, vitamin C does not increase absorption of iron supplements. Taking iron on an empty stomach also promotes absorption.
- Pregnant women with lactose intolerance may tolerate yogurt, sweet acidophilus milk, buttermilk, cheese, chocolate milk, cocoa, or lactase-treated milk, or they may consume lactase supplements with milk in order to ingest sufficient calcium.
- Women who cannot or will not ingest dairy products need to receive their calcium from other sources (fish, beans, greens, baked products, and certain fruits, such as figs or calcium-enriched orange juice) or take a daily supplement containing 600 mg of elemental calcium. Bone meal is not recommended because it is frequently contaminated with lead, which crosses the placenta to the fetus.
- Calcium supplementation may be recommended for pregnant women with leg cramps caused by a calcium-phosphorus imbalance.
- Sodium is not routinely restricted in pregnancy, and restriction has not proved effective in reducing the rates of preeclampsia. In general, sodium restriction is necessary only if the woman has a medical condition such as renal or liver failure or hypertension that warrants such a restriction. However, excessive sodium intake is unwarranted because it may contribute to development of hypertension in salt-sensitive individuals. An adequate sodium intake for pregnant and lactating women is estimated to be 1.5 g/day.
  - ❏ Women should recognize that table salt is the richest source of sodium. Large amounts of sodium are also found in canned foods, processed foods (especially smoked or cured meats, cold cuts, and corned beef), frozen entrées and meals, baked goods, mixes for casseroles, soups, pickles, condiments, and snacks such as chips and pretzels.

- Pregnant women who smoke need more vitamin C.
- The practice of pica (ingestion of nonfood substances or excessive amounts of low-nutrition-value foods) may cause:
  - More nutritious foods to be displaced from the diet
  - Interference with absorption of nutrients such as iron
  - Ingestion of heavy metals or other toxic substances that can contaminate nonfood items
- Strict vegetarians who eat only plant products (vegans) may have a vitamin B_{12}–deficient diet unless they take a supplement or consume vitamin B_{12}–fortified foods such as soy milk. Vitamin B_{12} deficiency can result in maternal glossitis (inflamed red tongue) and neurologic deficits, maternal-infant megaloblastic anemia, and infant neurodevelopmental delays. All types of vegetarian diets, if not well planned, may be deficient in iron, calcium, and zinc.

CHILDBIRTH AND PERINATAL EDUCATION

The goal of childbirth and perinatal education is to assist individuals and their family members to make informed, safe decisions about pregnancy, birth, and early parenthood. Today perinatal education programs consist of a menu of class series and activities from preconception through the early months of parenting. Expectant parents and their families have different interests and information needs as the pregnancy progresses.

- Early pregnancy ("early bird") classes provide fundamental information, such as:
  - Early fetal development
  - Physiologic and emotional changes of pregnancy
  - Human sexuality
  - Nutritional needs of the mother and fetus
  - Environmental and workplace hazards
  - Exercise
  - Pregnancy warning signs
  - Medications considered safe for use during pregnancy
- Mid-pregnancy classes emphasize the woman's participation in self-management. Classes provide information on:
  - Preparation for breastfeeding and formula feeding
  - Infant care
  - Basic hygiene

- ❑ Common complaints and simple safe remedies
- ❑ Infant health
- ❑ Parenting
- ❑ Updating and refining the birth plan
- ■ Late-pregnancy classes emphasize labor and birth. Historically, popular childbirth methods taught in the United States included the Dick-Read, the Lamaze (psychoprophylaxis), and the Bradley (husband-coached childbirth) methods. Currently, however, most instructors teach a flexible approach, which helps couples learn and master many techniques to use during labor.
- ■ Classes may be designed especially for women and couples with unique learning needs, such as:
  - ❑ Adolescents
  - ❑ First-time mothers older than age 35
  - ❑ Single women
  - ❑ Adoptive parents
  - ❑ Parents of multiples
  - ❑ Women who are vision or hearing impaired
  - ❑ Women planning cesarean birth or vaginal birth after cesarean
  - ❑ Couples with children who need a "refresher" class

PERINATAL CARE CHOICES

Women and their families must make many choices as they plan for pregnancy, birth, and early parenting. Nurses can provide information and resources to help childbearing families make informed decisions. Issues that must be addressed during the perinatal period include:

- ■ Options for pregnancy and birth care providers
  - ❑ Physicians (obstetricians, family medicine physicians)
  - ❑ Nurse-midwives
  - ❑ Direct-entry midwives
  - ❑ Independent (lay) midwives
  - ❑ Doulas
- ■ Birth setting choices
  - ❑ Labor, delivery, recovery (LDR) or labor, delivery, recovery, postpartum (LDRP) birthing rooms
  - ❑ Birth centers
  - ❑ Home birth
- ■ Pain management during labor and birth
- ■ Infant feeding method (breast or bottle)

VARIATIONS IN PRENATAL CARE
Cultural Influences

In every culture certain practices are expected of all women to ensure a good pregnancy outcome. To provide culturally sensitive care, nurses should learn about the varied cultures in the community where they practice. It is not possible, however, to know all there is to know about every culture and subculture or the many lifestyles that exist.

- Some cultural practices that can be assessed include proscriptions (what the woman should not do) and prescriptions (what she should do) about specific diets, special clothing or jewelry, physical activity, sexual activity, and any folk beliefs about what might harm her or the fetus.
- In many cultural groups a physician is deemed appropriate only in times of illness. Because pregnancy is considered a normal process and the woman is in a state of health, the services of a physician are considered inappropriate. Similarly, prenatal care may be considered unnecessary.
- Factors such as lack of money or insurance, lack of transportation, and language barriers may prevent women from diverse cultures from participating in the prenatal care system.
- In many cultures a concern for modesty also is a deterrent to seeking prenatal care. For some women, exposing body parts, especially to a man, is considered a major violation of their modesty.

Age Differences

Women at both ends of the childbearing age spectrum have a higher incidence of poor outcomes; however, age may not be a risk factor in all cases. Both physiologic and psychologic risks should be evaluated.

Adolescents

When adolescents become pregnant and decide to give birth, they are much less likely than older women to receive adequate prenatal care, with many receiving no care at all. These young women also are more likely to smoke and less likely to gain adequate weight during pregnancy. As a result of these and other factors, babies born to adolescents are at greatly increased risk of LBW, of serious and long-term disability, and of dying during the first year of life.

Mature Mothers

Women ages 35 years and older are more likely than are younger primiparas to have LBW infants, premature birth, and multiple births. Infants born to mature mothers are more likely to have chromosomal abnormalities and congenital anomalies. In addition, there is an increased risk of maternal mortality from hemorrhage, infection, embolisms, hypertensive disorders of pregnancy, cardiomyopathy, and strokes.

Multifetal Pregnancy

When the pregnancy involves more than one fetus, both the mother and fetuses are at increased risk for adverse outcomes.

- Risks include preterm labor and birth, anemia, diastasis of the two rectus abdominis muscles, placenta previa, placental abruption, and spontaneous rupture of the membranes before term.
- Congenital malformations are twice as common in monozygotic twins as in singletons, although there is no increase in the incidence of congenital anomalies in dizygotic twins.
- The prenatal visits of these women are scheduled at least every 2 weeks in the second trimester and weekly thereafter. Ultrasound evaluations are scheduled at 18 to 20 weeks and then every 3 to 4 weeks to monitor the fetal growth and amniotic fluid volume.

Selected Pregnancy Complications

EARLY PREGNANCY BLEEDING

Miscarriage (Spontaneous Abortion)

Miscarriage is a pregnancy that ends as a result of natural causes before 20 weeks of gestation. A fetal weight less than 500 g also may be used to define a miscarriage.

Incidence

- Approximately 10% to 15% of all clinically recognized pregnancies end in miscarriage, with the majority (more than 80%) occurring before 12 weeks of gestation.
- At least 50% of all clinically recognized pregnancy losses result from chromosomal abnormalities.

Etiology

Early (Before 12 Weeks of Gestation)

- Endocrine imbalance
- Immunologic factors
- Systemic disorders
- Genetic factors

Late (Between 12 and 20 Weeks of Gestation)

- Advancing maternal age and parity
- Premature dilation of the cervix and other anomalies of the reproductive tract
- Inadequate nutrition
- Tobacco, alcohol, and caffeine use
- Obesity and stressful life events

Types of Miscarriage

Table 2-1 lists types of miscarriage and describes signs and symptoms associated with each type.

TABLE 2-1

Miscarriage: Assessment and Usual Management

Type of Miscarriage	Amount of Bleeding	Uterine Cramping	Passage of Tissue	Cervical Dilation	Management
Threatened	Slight, spotting	Mild	No	No	Bed rest is often ordered, but has not proven to be effective in preventing progression to actual miscarriage. Repetitive transvaginal ultrasounds and assessment of human chorionic gonadotropin (hCG) and progesterone levels may be done to determine if the fetus is still alive and in the uterus. Further treatment depends on whether progression to actual miscarriage occurs.
Inevitable	Moderate	Mild to severe	No	Yes	Bed rest if no pain, fever or bleeding. If rupture of membranes (ROM), bleeding, pain or fever is present, then prompt evacuation of the uterus is accomplished usually by dilation and curettage.
Incomplete	Heavy, profuse	Severe	Yes	Yes, with tissue in cervix	May or may not require additional cervical dilation before curettage. Suction curettage may be performed.

Continued

TABLE 2-1

Miscarriage: Assessment and Usual Management—cont'd

Type of Miscarriage	Amount of Bleeding	Uterine Cramping	Passage of Tissue	Cervical Dilation	Management
Complete	Slight	Mild	Yes	No (cervix has already closed after tissue passed)	No further intervention may be needed if uterine contractions are adequate to prevent hemorrhage and no infection is present. Suction curettage may be performed to ensure no retained fetal or maternal tissue.
Missed	None, spotting	None	No	No	If spontaneous evacuation of the uterus does not occur within 1 month, uterus is emptied by method appropriate to duration of pregnancy. Blood clotting factors are monitored until uterus is empty. Disseminated intravascular coagulation (DIC) and incoagulability of blood with uncontrolled hemorrhage may develop in cases of fetal death after the twelfth week, if products of conception are retained for longer than 5 weeks.

Septic	Varies, usually malodorous	Varies	Varies	Yes, usually	May be treated with dilation and curettage or misoprostol (Cytotec) given orally or vaginally. Immediate evacuation of the uterus by method appropriate to duration of pregnancy. Cervical culture and sensitivity studies are performed, and broad-spectrum antibiotic therapy (e.g., ampicillin) is started. Treatment for septic shock is initiated if necessary.
Recurrent (generally defined as three or more consecutive miscarriages)	Varies	Varies	Yes	Yes, usually	Varies; depends on type. Prophylactic cerclage may be performed if premature cervical dilation is the cause. Tests of value include parental cytogenetic analysis and lupus anticoagulant and anticardiolipin antibody assays on the woman.

hCG: Human chorionic gonadotropin.

Sources: Cunningham, F., Leveno, K., Bloom, S., Hauth, J., Rouse, D., & Spong, C. (2010). *Williams obstetrics* (23rd ed.). New York: McGraw-Hill; Gilbert, E. (2011). *Manual of high risk pregnancy & delivery* (5th ed.). St. Louis: Mosby.

Management

Management depends on the classification of the miscarriage and on signs and symptoms (see Table 2-1).

- Traditionally, threatened miscarriages have been managed expectantly with supportive care. Follow-up treatment depends on whether the threatened miscarriage progresses to actual miscarriage or symptoms subside and the pregnancy remains intact. If bleeding and infection do not occur, expectant management is a reasonable option. In approximately half of all threatened miscarriages managed in this way, the pregnancy continues.

- Medical management is another treatment option if bleeding and infection are not present. Prostaglandin medications (e.g., misoprostol [Cytotec]) may be given orally or vaginally and are usually effective in completing the miscarriage within 7 days. If the products of conception are not passed completely, the woman may be prepared for manual or surgical evacuation of the uterus.

- Surgical management consists of dilation and curettage (D&C), a procedure in which the cervix is dilated and a curette is inserted to scrape the uterine walls and remove uterine contents. Before a D&C is performed, a full history should be obtained and general and pelvic examinations performed. General preoperative and postoperative care is appropriate for the woman requiring surgical intervention for miscarriage.

Postprocedure Care (Applies to Medical and Surgical Management)

- Medications are usually given after the procedure to contract the uterus and control bleeding. See the Medication Guide: Drugs Used to Manage Postpartum Hemorrhage in Appendix B.
- Antibiotics if necessary
- Pain management with analgesics, often antiprostaglandin agents (nonsteroidal antiinflammatory drugs [NSAIDs]).
- $Rh_o(D)$ immunoglobulin for the Rh-negative woman within 72 hours of miscarriage
- Transfusion therapy for shock or anemia
- Care of the fetus/products of conception as per hospital and state protocols

NURSING ALERT   *Procedures for disposition of the fetal remains vary from hospital to hospital and state to state. The nurse should know what the usual procedures are in his or her setting.*

- Discharge teaching (See the Teaching for Self-Management box: Discharge Teaching for the Woman After Early Miscarriage).

Teaching for Self-Management

Discharge Teaching for the Woman After Early Miscarriage

- Clean the perineum after each voiding or bowel movement and change perineal pads often.
- Shower (avoid tub baths) for 2 wk.
- Avoid tampon use, douching, and vaginal intercourse for 2 wk.
- Notify the physician if an elevated temperature or a foul-smelling vaginal discharge develops.
- Eat foods high in iron and protein to promote tissue repair and red blood cell replacement.
- Seek assistance from support groups, clergy, or professional counseling as needed.
- Allow yourself (and your partner) to grieve the loss before becoming pregnant again.

Ectopic Pregnancy

An ectopic pregnancy is a pregnancy in which the fertilized ovum is implanted outside the uterine cavity. The most common site of implantation is the uterine (fallopian) tube, where approximately 95% of ectopic pregnancies occur. Other much less common implantation sites include the abdominal cavity, ovary, and cervix. Ectopic pregnancy is the leading cause of first-trimester maternal mortality and a leading cause of infertility.

Incidence

The reported incidence of ectopic pregnancy rose through 1990 in the United States. Since then, because more cases are managed medically, reliable data on the actual number of ectopic pregnancies have not been available. Improved diagnostic techniques, however, have likely resulted in the identification of more cases.

Etiology

- Tubal infection and damage
- Popularity of contraceptive methods that predispose failures to be ectopic (e.g., the intrauterine device [IUD])
- Use of tubal sterilization methods that increase the chance of ectopic pregnancy
- Increasing use of assisted reproductive techniques
- Increased use of tubal surgery

Signs and Symptoms

- Abdominal pain (occurs in almost every case)
- A period that is delayed 1 to 2 weeks or lighter than usual, or an irregular period
- Abnormal vaginal bleeding (spotting) approximately 6 to 8 weeks after the last normal menstrual period
- If the ectopic pregnancy ruptures, may see the following:
  - Generalized, one sided, or deep lower quadrant acute abdominal pain
  - Referred shoulder pain
  - Signs and symptoms of shock, such as faintness or dizziness
  - Ecchymotic blueness around the umbilicus (Cullen sign)

Diagnosis

- The key to early detection of ectopic pregnancy is having a high index of suspicion for the condition. *Every* woman with complaints of abdominal pain, vaginal spotting or bleeding, and a positive pregnancy test should be screened for ectopic pregnancy.
- Laboratory screening
  - Quantitative beta-human chorionic gonadotropin (β-hCG) levels
  - Serum progesterone levels
- Transvaginal ultrasound
- Only one vaginal examination for adnexal tenderness/fullness
  - Because it is possible to rupture the mass during a bimanual examination, gentleness is critical.

Management

- Surgical management depends on the location and cause of the ectopic pregnancy, the extent of tissue involvement, and the woman's desires regarding future fertility. Options include:
  - Salpingectomy
  - Salpingostomy

- General preoperative and postoperative care is appropriate
  - Preoperative laboratory tests include determination of blood type and Rh factor, complete blood count (CBC), and serum quantitative β-hCG level.
  - Ultrasonography is used to confirm an extrauterine pregnancy.
  - Blood replacement may be necessary.
  - Administer Rh_o(D) immunoglobulin if appropriate.
  - A contraceptive method should be used for at least three menstrual cycles to allow time for the woman's body to heal.
- Medical management involves giving methotrexate to dissolve the tubal pregnancy. Methotrexate is an antimetabolite and folic acid antagonist that destroys rapidly dividing cells.
  - The woman must be hemodynamically stable to be eligible for medical management.
  - The best results following methotrexate therapy are usually obtained if the mass is unruptured and measures less than 3.5 cm in diameter by ultrasound, if no fetal cardiac activity is noted on ultrasound, and if the serum β-hCG level is less than 5000 milli-International Units/ml.
  - The woman must also be willing and able to comply with posttreatment monitoring.
  - See Box 2-1 for information regarding administration, patient and family teaching, and follow-up when ectopic pregnancy is treated with methotrexate.

NURSING ALERT *A woman receiving methotrexate therapy who drinks alcohol and takes vitamins containing folic acid (e.g., prenatal vitamins) increases her risk of experiencing side effects of the drug or exacerbating the ectopic rupture.*

Nursing Considerations

- Encourage expression of feelings related to the pregnancy loss.
- Refer to community resources for grief or infertility support.
- Inform the woman that vaginal intercourse must be avoided until β-hCG levels indicate that the ectopic pregnancy has completely dissolved. This could require abstaining from sexual activity for several months.

Nursing Considerations for Women Undergoing Methotrexate Treatment for Ectopic Pregnancy

ADMINISTRATION
- Obtain woman's height and weight.
- Check to make sure laboratory and diagnostic tests have been completed, including:
  - Complete blood cell count and blood type and Rh-antibody status
  - Liver and renal function tests
  - Serum β-hCG levels (should be <5000 milli-International Units/ml)
  - Transvaginal ultrasound confirming size of mass and absence of fetal cardiac activity
- Administer methotrexate 50 mg/m^2 IM.
- Administer Rh$_0$(D) immunoglobulin (50 mcg to 300 mcg IM as ordered if woman has Rh-negative blood).

PATIENT AND FAMILY TEACHING
- Review how methotrexate works.
- Inform the woman of possible side effects—gas pain, stomatitis, and conjunctivitis are common; rare effects include pleuritis, gastritis, dermatitis, alopecia, enteritis, increased liver enzymes, and bone marrow suppression.
- Advise the woman to:
  - Discontinue folic acid supplements.
  - Avoid "gas-forming" foods.
  - Avoid sun exposure because the drug will make her more photosensitive.
  - Refrain from strenuous activities.
  - Avoid putting anything in her vagina—no tampons, douches, or vaginal intercourse.
  - Report to her health care provider immediately if she has severe abdominal pain that may be a sign of impending or actual tubal rupture.

FOLLOW-UP
- Inform the woman to return to the clinic or office as instructed by her health care provider for measurement of β-hCG level.
- If β-hCG level does not drop appropriately, a second dose of methotrexate may be necessary.
- Advise the woman that she will need to return to the clinic or office for weekly measurements of β-hCG until the level is <15 milli-International Units/ml. Weekly follow-up visits may be required for several months until the desired β-hCG level is reached.

β-hCG, Beta-human chorionic gonadotropin.
Sources: Gilbert, E. (2011). *Manual of high risk pregnancy & delivery* (5th ed.). St. Louis: Mosby; Murray, H., Baakdah, H., Bardell, T., & Tulandi, T. (2005). Diagnosis and treatment of ectopic pregnancy. *Canadian Medical Association Journal, 173*(8), 905-912.

- ❑ There is a small risk that the pelvic pressure associated with vaginal intercourse could rupture the mass. In addition, intercourse will cause pain similar to that experienced with impending or actual tubal rupture, making it difficult to easily identify the source of the pain.
- For future reference, instruct the woman to contact her health care provider immediately if she suspects that she might be pregnant, because of the increased risk for recurrent ectopic pregnancy.

LATE PREGNANCY BLEEDING

Placenta Previa

Placenta previa is the implantation of the placenta in the lower uterine segment such that it completely or partially covers the cervix or is close enough to the cervix to cause bleeding when the cervix dilates or the lower uterine segment effaces.

Types of Placenta Previa

When transvaginal ultrasound is used placenta previa is classified as:
- *Complete:* the placenta totally covers the internal cervical os
- *Marginal:* the edge of the placenta is seen on transvaginal ultrasound to be 2.5 cm or closer to the internal cervical os
- *Low lying:* term used when the exact relationship of the placenta to the internal cervical os has not been determined or when apparent placenta previa is identified in the second trimester

Risk Factors
- History of placenta previa in a previous pregnancy
- History of previous cesarean birth
- History of prior suction curettage
- Advanced maternal age (>35 to 40 years of age)
- Multiparity
- Multiple gestation
- Smoking

Signs and Symptoms
- Painless, bright red vaginal bleeding in the second or third trimester (initially small amount; may stop and recur at any time)
  - ❑ Bleeding is associated with the disruption of placental blood vessels that occurs with stretching and thinning of the lower uterine segment.

❑ Most cases of placenta previa are diagnosed by ultrasound before bleeding occurs.
- Soft, relaxed, nontender uterus with normal tone
- Vital signs may be normal.
- Normal (reassuring) fetal heart rate (FHR) unless a major detachment of the placenta occurs
- Fundal height often greater than expected for gestational age
- Fetal malpresentation common (breech and transverse or oblique lie)

Risks Associated with Placenta Previa

Maternal
- Hemorrhage
- Development of an abnormal placental attachment (e.g., placenta accreta, increta, or percreta)
- Preterm labor
- Hysterectomy
- Surgery-related trauma to structures adjacent to the uterus
- Anesthesia complications
- Blood transfusion reactions
- Anemia
- Thrombophlebitis
- Infection

Fetal
- Preterm birth
- Malpresentation
- Anemia
- Size small for gestational age/intrauterine growth restriction (IUGR)

Diagnosis

All women with painless vaginal bleeding after 20 weeks of gestation should be assumed to have a placenta previa until proven otherwise.
- A transabdominal ultrasound examination should be performed initially followed by a transvaginal scan, unless the transabdominal ultrasound clearly shows that the placenta is not located in the lower uterine segment.
- If ultrasound reveals a normally implanted placenta, a speculum examination is done to rule out local causes of bleeding (e.g., cervicitis, polyps, carcinoma of the cervix), and a coagulation profile is obtained to rule out other causes of bleeding.

Management

The woman will be managed either actively or expectantly, depending on gestational age, amount of bleeding, and fetal condition.

Active Management

Cesarean birth is indicated in all women with ultrasound evidence of placenta previa.

- Immediate cesarean birth in the following situations:
  - ❑ Gestational age of 36 weeks or more
  - ❑ Persistent or excessive bleeding
- Vaginal birth may be attempted in an asymptomatic woman whose placenta lies more than 2 cm from the cervical os.
- Initial/continuing assessment
  - ❑ Gravidity, parity, estimated date of birth (EDB)
  - ❑ Bleeding
  - ❑ Vital signs
  - ❑ Fetal status (continuous electronic fetal monitoring)
- Commonly ordered laboratory studies
  - ❑ CBC
  - ❑ Blood type and Rh factor
  - ❑ Coagulation studies
  - ❑ Type and crossmatch

Expectant Management

- Purpose is to allow the fetus time to mature
- Generally the treatment of choice if:
  - ❑ Less than 36 weeks of gestation
  - ❑ FHR tracing is normal (reassuring)
  - ❑ Bleeding is mild (<250 ml) and stops
  - ❑ Not in labor
- Initial management
  - ❑ Admit to a labor and birth unit for continuous FHR and contraction monitoring.
  - ❑ Initiate large-bore (16- to 18-gauge) IV access.
  - ❑ Initial laboratory tests: hemoglobin, hematocrit, platelet count, coagulation studies
  - ❑ Maintain a "type and screen" sample at all times in the hospital's transfusion services department.
  - ❑ Administer antenatal corticosteroids if the woman is less than 34 weeks of gestation.

- Management after bleeding stops
  - ❑ Bed rest with bathroom privileges and limited activity
  - ❑ Assess bleeding by checking the amount of bleeding on perineal pads, bed pads, and linens.
  - ❑ Monitor for signs of preterm labor.
  - ❑ Ultrasound every 2 to 3 weeks
  - ❑ Fetal surveillance: nonstress test (NST) or biophysical profile (BPP) once or twice weekly
  - ❑ Serial laboratory assessments for decreasing hemoglobin and hematocrit levels and changes in coagulation values
  - ❑ *No* vaginal or rectal examinations
  - ❑ Pelvic rest (nothing inserted in the vagina)
- The woman's condition should always be considered a potential emergency because massive blood loss with resulting hypovolemic shock can occur quickly if bleeding resumes. The possibility always exists that she may require an emergency cesarean birth.
- Criteria for home care
  - ❑ Stable condition with no vaginal bleeding for at least 48 hours before discharge
  - ❑ Willing and able to comply with activity restrictions (bed rest with bathroom privileges and pelvic rest)
  - ❑ Telephone access
  - ❑ Close supervision by family and friends at home
  - ❑ Constant access to transportation
  - ❑ Able to keep all appointments for fetal testing, laboratory assessments, and prenatal care
- Discharge teaching for home care
  - ❑ How to assess uterine activity and bleeding
  - ❑ Pelvic rest and activity limitations
  - ❑ Importance of keeping appointments

Abruptio Placentae (Placental Abruption)

Placental abruption (abruptio placentae) is the detachment of part or all of a normally implanted placenta from the uterus. The separation may be partial, marginal, or complete. Bleeding from the placental site may dissect (separate) the membranes from the decidua basalis and flow out through the vagina (70% to 80%), it may remain concealed (retroplacental hemorrhage) (10% to 20%), or both.

Risk Factors

- Maternal hypertension
- Cocaine use
- External abdominal trauma (motor vehicle accident [MVA] or maternal battering)
- Cigarette smoking
- History of abruption in a previous pregnancy
- Preterm premature rupture of membranes (preterm PROM)
- Presence of inherited or acquired thrombophilias (e.g., factor V Leiden mutation or protein S deficiency)
- Twin (multiple) gestation

Signs and Symptoms

See Table 2-2 for assessment of placental abruption.

- Laboratory signs
  - Positive Apt test (blood in amniotic fluid)
  - Decreased hemoglobin and hematocrit levels
  - Decreased coagulation factor levels
  - Positive Kleihauer-Betke test (to determine the presence of fetal-to-maternal bleeding [transplacental hemorrhage])

Diagnosis

- Placental abruption is primarily a clinical diagnosis. Although ultrasound can be used to rule out placenta previa, it cannot detect all cases of abruption.
  - At least 50% of abruptions cannot be identified on ultrasound.
- The diagnosis of abruption is confirmed after birth by visual inspection of the placenta. Adherent clot on the maternal surface of the placenta and depression of the underlying placental surface are usually present.

Risks Associated with Placental Abruption

Maternal

- Hemorrhage
- Hypovolemic shock
- Hypofibrinogenemia
- Thrombocytopenia
- Infection

TABLE 2-2

Summary of Findings: Placental Abruption

	Grade 1: Mild Separation (10%-20%)	Grade 2: Moderate Separation (20%-50%)	Grade 3: Severe Separation (>50%)
Bleeding (external, vaginal)	Minimal	Absent to moderate	Absent to moderate
Total amount of blood loss	<500 ml	1000-1500 ml	>1500 ml
Color of blood	Dark red	Dark red	Dark red
Shock	Rare; none	Mild shock	Common, often sudden, profound
Coagulopathy	Rare; none	Occasional DIC	Frequent DIC
Uterine tonicity	Normal	Increased, may be localized to one region or diffuse over uterus; uterus fails to relax between contractions	Tetanic, persistent uterine contraction; boardlike uterus
Tenderness (pain)	Usually absent	Present	Agonizing, unremitting uterine pain
Gestational or chronic hypertension	Usual distribution*	Commonly present	Commonly present
Fetal effects	Normal fetal heart rate and pattern	Abnormal fetal heart rate and pattern	Abnormal fetal heart rate and pattern; death can occur

*Usual distribution refers to the usual variations of incidence seen when there is no concurrent problem.

DIC, Disseminated intravascular coagulation.

- Renal failure
- Pituitary necrosis
- Rh isoimmunization in Rh-negative women (rarely occurs)

Fetal/Neonatal

- Fetal death (if more than 50% of the placenta has abrupted)
- Preterm birth
- IUGR
- Neurologic defects
- Cerebral palsy
- Death from sudden infant death syndrome (SIDS)

Management

The woman will be managed either actively or expectantly, depending on the severity of blood loss and fetal maturity and status.

Expectant Management

- May be implemented if the fetus is less than 34 weeks of gestation and the condition of both woman and fetus is stable
- Consists of hospitalization and close observation for signs of bleeding and labor
- Fetal monitoring for appropriate growth
- Regular assessments of fetal well-being (NST, BPP)
- Administration of corticosteroids to accelerate fetal lung maturity

Active Management

- Treatment of choice in the following situations:
  - ❑ Term gestation
  - ❑ Moderate to severe bleeding
  - ❑ Woman or fetus is in jeopardy
- Vaginal birth is usually feasible and especially desirable in cases of fetal death.
- Cesarean birth should be reserved for cases of fetal distress or other obstetric indications.
  - ❑ Surgery should not be attempted when the woman has severe and uncorrected coagulopathy because it may result in uncontrollable bleeding.
- At least one large-bore (16- to 18-gauge) IV line
- Frequent vital signs
- Serial lab tests to monitor hemoglobin, hematocrit, and clotting status

- Continuous electronic fetal monitoring
- Indwelling (Foley) catheter
- Intake and output measurement
- Blood and fluid volume replacement
- Educate woman and family on cause, treatment, and expected outcomes.
- Provide emotional support because the woman and her family may be experiencing fetal loss in addition to the woman's critical illness.

ENDOCRINE AND METABOLIC DISORDERS
Pregestational Diabetes Mellitus

Diabetes mellitus refers to a group of metabolic diseases characterized by hyperglycemia resulting from defects in insulin secretion, insulin action, or both. There are four types of diabetes mellitus: type 1, type 2, other specific types (e.g., diabetes caused by genetic defects in B-cell function or insulin action, disease or injury of the pancreas, or drug-induced diabetes), and gestational diabetes. Type 1 or type 2 diabetes that existed before pregnancy is often referred to as pregestational diabetes. Of the women with pregestational diabetes, the majority (65%) have type 2 diabetes.

Etiology
Type 1 Diabetes

- Pancreatic islet beta-cell destruction
- Autoimmune process
- Unknown cause
- Individuals usually have an absolute insulin deficiency

Type 2 Diabetes

- Specific cause or causes unknown
- Individuals usually have insulin resistance and relative (rather than absolute) insulin deficiency
- Often has a strong genetic predisposition

White's Classification System for Diabetes in Pregnancy

- Developed by Dr. Priscilla White, a physician who worked with pregnant women with diabetes during the 1940s (Table 2-3)
- Based on age at diagnosis, duration of illness, and presence of vascular disease

TABLE 2-3

White's Classification of Diabetes in Pregnancy (Modified)

GESTATIONAL DIABETES

Class A1	Patient has two or more abnormal values on the OGTT with a normal fasting blood sugar. Blood glucose levels are diet controlled.
Class A2	Patient was not known to have diabetes before pregnancy but requires medication for blood glucose control.

PREGESTATIONAL DIABETES

Class B	Onset of disease occurs after age 20 and duration of illness <10 yr
Class C	Onset of disease occurs between 10 and 19 years of age or duration of illness for 10-19 yr or both
Class D	Onset of disease occurs <10 yr of age or duration of illness >20 yr or both
Class F	Patient has developed diabetic nephropathy
Class R	Patient has developed retinitis proliferans
Class T	Patient has had a renal transplant

OGTT, Oral glucose tolerance test.
Sources: Landon, M., Catalano, P., & Gabbe, S. (2007). Diabetes mellitus complicating pregnancy. In S. Gabbe, J. Niebyl, & J. Simpson (Eds.), *Obstetrics: Normal and problem pregnancies* (5th ed.). Philadelphia: Churchill Livingstone; Moore, T., & Catalano, P. (2009). Diabetes in pregnancy. In R. Creasy, R. Resnik, J. Iams, C. Lockwood, & T. Moore (Eds.), *Creasy and Resnik's maternal-fetal medicine: Principles and practice* (6th ed.). Philadelphia: Saunders.

- Has been modified through the years but is still frequently used to assess maternal and fetal risk
  - Women in classes A through C generally have good pregnancy outcomes as long as their blood glucose levels are well controlled.
  - Women in classes D through T usually have poorer pregnancy outcomes because they have already developed the vascular damage that often accompanies long-standing diabetes.

Risks Associated with Pregestational Diabetes

Risks increase with the duration and severity of the diabetic condition. Also pregnancy may contribute to the vascular changes associated with diabetes.

Maternal

- Miscarriage
- Fetal macrosomia
- Cesarean birth
- Operative vaginal birth (forceps or vacuum)
- Preeclampsia
- Chronic hypertension
- Hydramnios (polyhydramnios)
- Preterm labor
- Infection
- Diabetic ketoacidosis
- Hypoglycemia

Fetal/Neonatal

- Intrauterine fetal demise/death (IUFD) (stillbirth)
- Congenital malformations, especially of the cardiovascular system, central nervous system (CNS), and skeletal system
- Macrosomia
- Birth injuries (brachial plexus palsy, facial nerve injury, humerus or clavicle fracture, and cephalhematoma)
- Hypoglycemia

Management

Medical goal of care: Achieving and maintaining constant euglycemia through a combination of diet, insulin, and exercise. The key to an optimal pregnancy outcome is strict maternal glucose control before conception as well as throughout pregnancy. See Table 2-4 for desired blood glucose levels during pregnancy.

Pregnancy

- Assess current health status.
  - ❑ Perform routine prenatal examination.
  - ❑ Determine effects of diabetes on pregnancy:
    - Perform a baseline electrocardiogram to assess cardiovascular status.
    - Evaluate for retinopathy with follow-up as needed by an ophthalmologist each trimester and more often if retinopathy is diagnosed.
  - ❑ Monitor blood pressure.

TABLE 2-4

Target Blood Glucose Levels during Pregnancy

Time of Day	Target Plasma Glucose Level (mg/dl)
Premeal or fasting	>65 but <95
Postmeal (1 hr)	<130-140
Postmeal (2 hr)	<120

Sources: Landon, M., Catalano, P., & Gabbe, S. (2007). Diabetes mellitus complicating pregnancy. In S. Gabbe, J. Niebyl, & J. Simpson (Eds.), *Obstetrics: Normal and problem pregnancies* (5th ed.). Philadelphia: Churchill Livingstone; Moore, T., & Catalano, P. (2009). Diabetes in pregnancy. In R. Creasy, R. Resnik, J. Iams, C. Lockwood, & T. Moore (Eds.), *Creasy and Resnik's maternal-fetal medicine: Principles and practice* (6th ed.). Philadelphia: Saunders.

- ❏ Monitor weight gain.
- ❏ Assess fundal height.
- ■ Laboratory tests
  - ❏ Glycosylated hemoglobin (hemoglobin A_{1c}) (should be ≤6%)
  - ❏ 24-hour urine collection for total protein and creatinine clearance
  - ❏ Urinalysis and culture: initial prenatal visit and throughout the pregnancy
  - ❏ Urine dipstick for ketones
  - ❏ Thyroid function tests
- ■ Diet
  - ❏ Average diet includes 2200 to 2500 calories per day, distributed among three meals and an evening snack or (more commonly) three meals and two or three snacks.
  - ❏ Ideally, 55% of total calories should be carbohydrates.
  - ❏ Simple carbohydrates are limited; complex carbohydrates that are high in fiber content are recommended.
  - ❏ Large bedtime snack (at least 25 g of carbohydrate with some protein) is recommended.
- ■ Exercise
  - ❏ Must be prescribed by the health care provider
  - ❏ Best type of exercise is aerobic exercise with resistance training for at least 30 minutes most days of the week. Non–weight-bearing activities may also be recommended.
  - ❏ Best time for exercise is after meals.

TABLE 2-5

Common Insulin Preparations

Type of Insulin	Examples Generic (Trade) Name	Onset of Action	Peak of Action	Duration of Action
Rapid acting	Lispro (Humalog)	15 min	30-90 min	4-5 hr
	Aspart (NovoLog)	15 min	1-3 hr	3-5 hr
Short acting	Humulin R	30 min	2-4 hr	5-7 hr
	Novolin R	30 min	2.5-5 hr	6-8 hr
Intermediate acting	Humulin NPH	1-2 hr	6-12 hr	18-24 hr
	Novolin N	1.5 hr	4-20 hr	24 hr
	Humulin Lente	1-3 hr	6-12 hr	18-24 hr
	Novolin L	2.5 hr	7-15 hr	22 hr
Long acting	Humulin Ultralente	4-6 hr	8-20 hr	>36 hr
	Glargine (Lantus)	1 hr	None	24 hr

Source: Landon, M., Catalano, P., & Gabbe, S. (2007). Diabetes mellitus complicating pregnancy. In S. Gabbe, J. Niebyl, & J. Simpson (Eds.), *Obstetrics: Normal and problem pregnancies* (5th ed.). Philadelphia: Churchill Livingstone.

- ❏ Regular exercise may be contraindicated in women with diabetes who also have uncontrolled hypertension, advanced retinopathy, or severe autonomic or peripheral neuropathy.
- ■ Insulin
  - ❏ Insulin requirements in general increase as the pregnancy progresses. However, they normally plateau after 35 weeks of gestation and often drop significantly after 38 weeks.
  - ❏ Several types of insulin preparations are available. They differ in onset, peak, and duration of action. See Table 2-5 for further information on common insulin preparations.
  - ❏ Most women are managed with two or three injections per day, although continuous subcutaneous insulin infusion systems (e.g., the insulin pump) are increasingly being used during pregnancy.
- ■ Blood glucose testing
  - ❏ Done several times each day, using a glucose reflectance meter or biosensor monitor
  - ❏ Now considered standard of care for monitoring blood glucose levels during pregnancy

- ❏ Most of the newer reflectance meters are calibrated to provide plasma (rather than whole blood) glucose values. Plasma glucose values are 10% to 15% lower than those measured in whole blood from the same sample.

> **SAFETY ALERT**   *The nurse must be knowledgeable about the specific glucose reflectance meter that the woman uses because target glucose values depend on the type of meter used.*

> **NURSING ALERT**   *Hyperglycemia will most likely be identified in 2-hour postprandial values, because blood glucose levels peak about 2 hours after a meal.*

- ❏ Will be done more frequently following changes in insulin dosage or diet or if nausea, vomiting, diarrhea, or infection occurs
- ■ Fetal assessment
  - ❏ Ultrasounds throughout pregnancy to determine gestational age, monitor fetal growth, estimate fetal weight, and detect hydramnios, macrosomia, and congenital anomalies
  - ❏ Maternal serum alpha-fetoprotein (at 15 to 20 weeks of gestation, ideally between 16 and 18 weeks)
  - ❏ Fetal echocardiography (between 20 and 22 weeks of gestation)
  - ❏ Doppler studies of the umbilical artery
  - ❏ Biophysical testing (NST, contraction stress testing [CST], or BPP) once or twice weekly to evaluate fetal well-being (typically begins around 34 weeks of gestation). This testing should begin around 28 weeks in women who have poor glucose control or significant hypertension.

Intrapartum

- ■ The optimal time for birth is between 38.5 and 40 weeks of gestation, as long as good metabolic control is maintained and parameters of antepartum fetal surveillance remain within normal limits.
- ■ Although vaginal birth is expected for most women with pregestational diabetes, the cesarean rate for these women ranges from 50% to 80%. Suspected macrosomia (estimated fetal weight >4500 g), fetal distress, and induction failures before term contribute to the high rate of cesarean birth in these women.

- Many practitioners schedule elective labor induction between 38 and 40 weeks of gestation.
- Administer IV fluid containing 5% dextrose during active labor to provide the energy (calories) necessary for the woman to accomplish the work and manage the stress of labor and birth.
- Maintain blood glucose levels at less than 140 mg/dl during labor.
  - Measure blood glucose level every hour or so using a bedside monitor.
  - Administer rapid-acting or short-acting insulin by IV drip using a controlled infusion device as needed to maintain blood glucose in the desired range.
- Observe for diabetes-related complications, such as hyperglycemia, ketosis, and ketoacidosis. Treat as needed.
- Observe for normal progression of cervical dilation, fetal descent, and fetal well-being in labor. Failure to progress in labor as expected may indicate a macrosomic infant and cephalopelvic disproportion.
- Often a neonatologist, neonatal nurse practitioner, or pediatrician is present at birth to initiate assessment and neonatal care.

Postpartum

- Insulin requirements decrease substantially during the first 24 hours postpartum. Several days after birth may be required to reestablish carbohydrate homeostasis. Blood glucose levels are monitored regularly, and insulin dosage is adjusted, often using a sliding scale.
- Observe for possible complications, including preeclampsia/eclampsia, hemorrhage, and infection.
- Breastfeeding decreases insulin requirements because of the carbohydrate used in milk production.
- Women with diabetes who breastfeed may be at increased risk for episodes of hypoglycemia, mastitis, and yeast infections of the breast.
- Contraceptive methods
  - *Barrier methods*—Considered safe, inexpensive options that have no inherent risks for women with diabetes. However, they are not as effective as other methods and their use often leads to unplanned pregnancies.

- ❏ *Oral contraceptives*—Use is controversial because of the risk of thromboembolic and vascular complications and the effect on carbohydrate metabolism. In non-smoking women with diabetes who are less than 35 years old and do not have vascular disease, combination low-dose oral contraceptives may be prescribed. Progestin-only oral contraceptives may also be used because they affect carbohydrate metabolism minimally, if at all.
- ❏ *IUD*—May be used without concern for an increased risk of infection.
- ❏ *Long-acting parenteral progestins (e.g., Depo-Provera)*—Opinion is divided. Some health care providers recommend their use, particularly in women who are noncompliant with daily dosing oral contraceptives. Others believe this method may adversely affect diabetic control.
- ❏ *Transdermal (patch) and transvaginal (vaginal ring)*—Particularly effective in women who prefer weekly or every-third-week dosing, respectively. Use of the patch is contraindicated in women who weigh more than 90 kg (198 lb). In addition, women who choose the patch as their contraceptive method should have no risk factors for cardiovascular or thromboembolic disease.
- ❏ *Sterilization*—Often recommended for women who have completed their families, who have poor metabolic control, or who have significant vascular problems.

Nursing Considerations

- ■ Providing the woman with the knowledge, skill, and motivation she needs to achieve and maintain excellent blood glucose control is the primary nursing goal.
- ■ Teaching about diet, insulin administration, exercise, and blood glucose testing is a critical nursing responsibility.
- ■ Pregnant women with diabetes are much more likely to develop hypoglycemia than hyperglycemia. See Table 2-6 for more information on hypoglycemia.

Gestational Diabetes Mellitus

Gestational diabetes mellitus (GDM) is any degree of glucose intolerance with the onset or first recognition occurring during pregnancy. GDM accounts for more than 90% of all cases of diabetes in pregnancy. GDM is likely to recur in future pregnancies, and there is an increased risk for development of overt diabetes in later life.

TABLE 2-6

Hypoglycemia

Causes	Onset	Symptoms	Interventions
HYPOGLYCEMIA (INSULIN SHOCK)			
Excess insulin	Rapid (regular	Irritability	Check blood
Insufficient	insulin)	Hunger	glucose level
food	Gradual (modified	Sweating	when symptoms
(delayed	insulin or oral	Nervousness	first appear.
or missed	hypoglycemic	Personality	Eat or drink 15 g
meals)	agents)	change	fast sugar (simple
Excessive		Weakness	carbohydrate)*
exercise or		Fatigue	immediately.
work		Blurred or	Recheck blood
Indigestion,		double vision	glucose level in
diarrhea,		Dizziness	15 min, and eat or
vomiting		Headache	drink another 15 g
		Pallor; clammy	fast sugar (simple
		skin	carbohydrate)*
		Shallow	if glucose remains
		respirations	low.
		Rapid pulse	Recheck blood
		Laboratory	glucose level in
		values	15 min.
		Urine:	Notify primary
		negative for	health care
		sugar and	provider if no
		acetone	change in glucose
		Blood	level.
		glucose:	If woman is
		≤60 mg/dl	unconscious,
			administer
			50% dextrose
			IV push, 5% to
			10% dextrose in
			water IV drip, or
			1 mg glucagon
			subcutaneously.
			Obtain blood and
			urine specimens
			for laboratory
			testing.

*Examples of 15 g fast sugar (simple carbohydrate): ½ cup (4 oz) unsweetened orange juice; ½ cup (4 oz) regular (not diet) soda; 5 or 6 hard candies; 1 cup (8 oz) skim milk.

Risk Factors for Gestational Diabetes

- Hispanic, Native-American, Asian, and African-American populations
- Maternal age more than 25 years
- Obstetric history of the following:
  - ❏ Previous macrosomic infant
  - ❏ Previous unexplained IUFD
  - ❏ Previous pregnancy with GDM
- Strong immediate family history of type 2 diabetes or GDM
- Obesity (weight >90 kg [198 lb])
- Fasting blood glucose more than 140 mg/dl or random blood glucose more than 200 mg/dl

Screening

All pregnant women not known to have pregestational diabetes should be screened for GDM by history, clinical risk factors, or laboratory screening of blood glucose levels.

Laboratory Screening

- Done on women at high risk for GDM at the first prenatal visit and then repeated at 24 to 28 weeks of gestation if the initial screen is negative.
- Done on other pregnant women at 24 to 28 weeks of gestation, unless the woman is determined by her history and clinical risk factors to be at such low risk for the development of GDM that the test is not cost-effective.
- Usually consists of a 50-g oral glucose load, followed by a plasma glucose determination 1 hour later. The woman need not be fasting.
- A glucose value of 130 to 140 mg/dl or more is considered a positive screen and is followed by a 3-hour (100 g) oral glucose tolerance test.
- The 3-hour oral glucose tolerance test is considered the gold standard for diagnosing GDM. It requires a fasting blood glucose level, which is drawn before giving the 100-g oral glucose load. Blood glucose levels are drawn 1, 2, and 3 hours later. GDM is diagnosed if two or more values are met or exceeded.

Management

Medical goal of care: Achieving and maintaining strict blood glucose control (see Table 2-4)

Pregnancy

- Diet
  - Standard diabetic diet, consisting of 1500 to 2000 calories/day for most women
  - Approximately 50% of total calories should be carbohydrates
- Exercise
  - Found in several studies to improve cardiovascular fitness in women with GDM without improving pregnancy outcome
  - In one study, decreased the need for insulin in overweight women with GDM
- Blood glucose testing
  - Necessary to determine if euglycemia can be maintained by diet and exercise
  - The frequency and timing of blood glucose monitoring should be individualized for each woman. However, a typical schedule for monitoring blood glucose is on rising in the morning, after breakfast, before and after lunch, after dinner, and at bedtime.
- Medication
  - Up to 20% of women with GDM require insulin during the pregnancy to maintain acceptable blood glucose levels, despite compliance with the prescribed diet.
- If fasting plasma glucose levels are greater than 95 mg/dl or 2-hour postprandial levels are greater than 120 mg/dl, then insulin therapy is begun.
  - Glyburide, an oral hypoglycemic agent, rather than insulin is used more frequently in women with GDM for blood glucose control.
    - Because only minimal amounts of glyburide cross the placenta to the fetus, it is a good drug for use during pregnancy.
    - Glyburide should be taken at least 30 minutes (preferably 1 hour) before a meal so that its peak effect covers the 2-hour postprandial blood glucose level.
- Fetal assessment
  - There is no standard recommendation for fetal surveillance in pregnancies complicated by GDM.
  - Limited antepartum fetal testing is performed in women with GDM as long as their fasting and 2-hour postprandial blood glucose levels remain within normal limits and they have no other risk factors.

❏ Women with hypertension, a history of a prior IUFD, or suspected macrosomia or those who require insulin for blood glucose control may have a twice-weekly NST beginning at 32 weeks of gestation.
❏ In general, women with GDM can continue pregnancy until 40 weeks of gestation and the spontaneous onset of labor.

Intrapartum

■ Monitor blood glucose levels hourly to maintain levels at 80 to 120 mg/dl.
❏ Infuse regular insulin intravenously using a controlled infusion device as needed to maintain blood glucose in desired range.
❏ It is usually possible to maintain excellent glucose control in women with class A_1 GDM during labor by simply avoiding dextrose-containing intravenous fluids.
❏ GDM is not an indication for cesarean birth, but this procedure may be necessary in the presence of preeclampsia or macrosomia

Postpartum

■ Most women with GDM return to normal glucose levels after childbirth. However, GDM is likely to recur in future pregnancies, and women with GDM are at significant risk for developing type 2 diabetes within the next 20 years.
■ Assessment for carbohydrate intolerance with a 75-g OGTT should be performed at 6 to 12 weeks postpartum and a random or fasting blood glucose level should be checked each year.
■ Women with a history of GDM, particularly those who are overweight, should be encouraged to make lifestyle changes that include weight loss and exercise to reduce the risk of developing overt diabetes later in life.
■ Children born to women with diabetes are at increased risk for becoming obese in childhood or adolescence.

Hyperemesis Gravidarum

Hyperemesis gravidarum is vomiting during pregnancy that causes weight loss, electrolyte imbalance, nutritional deficiencies, and ketonuria. Hyperemesis gravidarum usually begins during the first trimester of pregnancy. Approximately 10% of women with the disorder continue to have symptoms throughout pregnancy.

Etiology

The etiology remains unclear, although several theories have been proposed:

- May be related to high levels of estrogen or hCG
- May be associated with transient hyperthyroidism during pregnancy
- Gastric dysrhythmias, esophageal reflux, and reduced gastric motility may contribute to the disorder.
- May be associated with psychosocial factors, such as ambivalence toward the pregnancy and increased stress. Conflicting feelings regarding prospective motherhood, body changes, and lifestyle alterations may contribute to episodes of vomiting, particularly if these feelings are excessive or unresolved.

Risk Factors

- Nulliparity
- Increased body weight
- History of migraines
- Multifetal gestation
- Gestational trophoblastic disease
- Fetus with a chromosomal abnormality such as triploidy or trisomy 21
- Female fetus
- Family history of hyperemesis
- Interrelated psychologic component

Signs and Symptoms

- Significant weight loss
- Dehydration
- Inability to keep down even clear liquids
- Electrolyte imbalances

Initial Assessment

- History
  - Frequency, severity, and duration of vomiting episodes
  - Approximate amount and color of emesis
  - Presence of diarrhea, indigestion, and abdominal pain or distention
  - Precipitating factors
  - Pharmacologic or nonpharmacologic treatment instituted
  - Prepregnancy weight/documented weight gain or loss during pregnancy

- Physical exam
  - ❑ Weight
  - ❑ Vital signs
  - ❑ Signs of fluid and electrolyte imbalance
- Lab tests
  - ❑ Determination of ketonuria
  - ❑ Urinalysis
  - ❑ CBC
  - ❑ Electrolytes
  - ❑ Liver enzymes
  - ❑ Bilirubin levels
  - ❑ Thyroid levels
- Psychosocial assessment
  - ❑ Anxiety, fears, and concerns related to the woman's health and the effects on pregnancy outcome
  - ❑ Assess family members for their anxiety and in regard to their role in providing support for the woman.

Management

- IV therapy for correction of fluid and electrolyte imbalances if unable to keep down clear liquids by mouth
- Medications used to treat uncontrolled nausea and vomiting
  - ❑ Pyridoxine (vitamin B_6)
  - ❑ Doxylamine (Unisom)
  - ❑ Promethazine (Phenergan)
  - ❑ Metoclopramide (Reglan)
  - ❑ Prochlorperazine (Compazine)
  - ❑ Ondansetron (Zofran)
  - ❑ Chlorpromazine (Thorazine)
  - ❑ Corticosteroids (methylprednisolone [Medrol] or hydrocortisone)
- Enteral or parenteral nutrition for women who do not respond to other medication therapies
- Once the vomiting has stopped, start with small, frequent feedings by mouth and slowly advance the diet as tolerated.

Nursing Considerations

- Observe for complications such as metabolic acidosis, jaundice, or hemorrhage
- Accurately measure intake and output, especially emesis

Teaching for Self-Management

Diet for Hyperemesis

- Eat frequently, at least every 2-3 hr. Separate liquids from solids and alternate every 2-3 hr.
- Eat a snack at bedtime.
- Eat dry, bland, low-fat, high-protein foods. Cold foods may be better tolerated than those served at a warm temperature.
- In general, eat what sounds good to you, rather than trying to balance your meals.
- Follow the salty and sweet approach; even so-called junk foods are okay.
- Eat protein after sweets.
- Dairy products may stay down more easily than other foods.
- If you vomit even when your stomach is empty, try sucking on a Popsicle.
- Try ginger tea. Peel and finely dice a knuckle-sized piece of ginger and place it in a mug of boiling water. Steep for 5-8 min and add brown sugar to taste.
- Try warm ginger ale (with sugar, not artificial sweetener) or water with a slice of lemon.
- Drink liquids from a cup with a lid.

- Provide oral hygiene, especially while NPO or after an episode of vomiting
- Provide a quiet, restful, odor-free environment
- Dietary instructions (See the Teaching for Self-Management box: Diet for Hyperemesis)

HYPERTENSIVE DISORDERS IN PREGNANCY
Gestational Hypertension

Gestational hypertension is the onset of hypertension without proteinuria after week 20 of pregnancy. It usually develops at or after 37 weeks of gestation. Women with gestational hypertension have no evidence of preexisting hypertension, and their blood pressure (BP) levels return to normal within 6 weeks after giving birth. Gestational hypertension is the most frequent cause of hypertension during pregnancy. The definitions of mild and severe gestational hypertension are the same as the definitions for BP readings for mild and severe preeclampsia (see Table 2-7, maternal effects, BP).

TABLE 2-7

Differentiation Between Mild and Severe Preeclampsia

	Mild Preeclampsia	Severe Preeclampsia
MATERNAL EFFECTS		
Blood pressure (BP)	BP reading ≥140/90 mm Hg × two, at least 4-6 hr apart but within a maximum of a 1-wk period	Rise to ≥160/110 mm Hg on two separate occasions 6 hr apart with pregnant woman on bed rest
Proteinuria		
Qualitative dipstick	≥1+ on dipstick	≥3+ on dipstick
Quantitative 24-hr analysis	Proteinuria of ≥300 mg in a 24-hr specimen	Proteinuria of ≥5 g in a 24-hr specimen
Urine output	Output matching intake, ≥25-30 ml/hr	<400-500 ml/24 hr
Headache	Absent or transient	Persistent or severe
Visual problems	Absent	Blurred, photophobia
Irritability or changes in affect	Transient	May be severe
Epigastric or right upper quadrant pain, nausea, and vomiting	Absent	May be present
Thrombocytopenia	Absent	May be present
Liver function	Normal	May be impaired
Pulmonary edema	Absent	May be present
FETAL EFFECTS		
Placental perfusion	Reduced	Decreased perfusion expressing as IUGR in fetus; abnormal (nonreassuring) fetal status on antepartum testing

IUGR, intrauterine growth restriction.

Sources: American College of Obstetricians and Gynecologists (ACOG). (2002). *Diagnosis and management of preeclampsia and eclampsia.* ACOG Practice Bulletin No. 33. Washington, DC: ACOG; Sibai, B. (2007). Hypertension. In S. Gabbe, J. Niebyl, & J. Simpson (Eds.), *Obstetrics: Normal and problem pregnancies* (5th ed.). Philadelphia: Churchill Livingstone.

BOX 2-2

Risk Factors for Preeclampsia
- First pregnancy or new partner with this pregnancy
- Extremes of maternal age: <19 years or >40 years
- Obesity
- Personal or family history of preeclampsia
- Exposure to abundance of trophoblast tissue
  - ❑ Multifetal gestation
  - ❑ Hydatidiform mole
- Poor outcome in previous pregnancy
  - ❑ Intrauterine growth restriction
  - ❑ Placental abruption
  - ❑ Fetal death
- Preexisting medical or genetic conditions
  - ❑ Chronic hypertension
  - ❑ Renal disease
  - ❑ Type 1 (insulin-dependent) diabetes mellitus
  - ❑ Collagen disease
  - ❑ Thrombophilias
  - ❑ Antiphospholipid antibody syndrome
  - ❑ Protein C, protein S, antithrombin deficiency
- Periodontal disease

Sources: Gilbert, E. (2011). *Manual of high risk pregnancy & delivery* (5th ed.). St. Louis: Mosby; Sibai, B. (2007). Hypertension. In S. Gabbe, J. Niebyl, & J. Simpson (Eds.), *Obstetrics: Normal and problem pregnancies* (5th ed.). Philadelphia: Churchill Livingstone.

Preeclampsia

Preeclampsia is a pregnancy-specific condition in which hypertension and proteinuria develop after 20 weeks of gestation in a previously normotensive woman. Preeclampsia is usually categorized as mild or severe for purposes of management.

Etiology

The etiology of preeclampsia is unknown. Preeclampsia *is* known, however, to be a condition that occurs only during human pregnancies. It is a multisystem, vasospastic disease. Signs and symptoms usually develop only during pregnancy and disappear quickly after birth of the fetus and passage of the placenta.

Risk Factors

Risk factors for preeclampsia are listed in Box 2-2.

Signs and Symptoms

Table 2-7 lists signs and symptoms of mild and severe preeclampsia.

HELLP Syndrome

HELLP syndrome is a laboratory diagnosis for a variant of severe pre-eclampsia that involves hepatic dysfunction, characterized by hemolysis (H), elevated liver enzymes (EL), and low platelets (LP). It is *not* a separate illness. Although no consensus has been reached regarding which laboratory tests should be used to diagnose HELLP syndrome or what values should be considered abnormal, the tests and values listed here are often used to establish the diagnosis.

H	**H**emolysis (burr cells on peripheral smear or total bilirubin level >1.2 mg/dl)
EL	**E**levated **L**iver enzymes (aspartate transaminase [AST] >70 units/L; lactate dehydrogenase [LDH] >600 units/L)
LP	**L**ow **P**latelets (platelet count <100,000/mm³)

- HELLP syndrome is often nonspecific in clinical presentation. It most commonly develops in older, Caucasian, multiparous women.
- Common symptoms include malaise, epigastric or right upper quadrant abdominal pain, nausea, vomiting, and headaches.

NURSING ALERT *An extremely important point to understand is that many women with HELLP syndrome may not have signs or symptoms of severe preeclampsia. For example, although most women have hypertension, BP may be only mildly elevated in 50% of cases. Proteinuria may be absent. As a result, women with HELLP syndrome are often misdiagnosed with a variety of other medical or surgical disorders.*

- Complications reported with HELLP syndrome include pulmonary edema, acute renal failure, disseminated intravascular coagulation (DIC), placental abruption, liver hemorrhage or failure, acute respiratory distress syndrome (ARDS), sepsis, and stroke.

Eclampsia

Eclampsia is the onset of seizure activity or coma in a woman diagnosed with preeclampsia, with no history of a preexisting pathologic condition that can result in seizure activity.

Management

The management of gestational hypertension and preeclampsia varies according to the severity of the disease and the gestational age at diagnosis.

Goals of Care

■ Ensure maternal safety
   ❑ Prevent or control eclamptic seizures
   ❑ Control hypertension
■ Give birth to a healthy newborn as close to term as possible

Mild Gestational Hypertension and Mild Preeclampsia

At or Near Term

■ Labor will most likely be induced. If necessary, cervical ripening will precede induction.

Less Than 36 Weeks of Gestation

The woman should be hospitalized for several days for a thorough evaluation of maternal-fetal status. After the evaluation, a multidisciplinary plan of care is developed with the woman and her family. Women with mild gestational hypertension or mild preeclampsia who are less than 36 weeks of gestation may be discharged with close maternal and fetal surveillance (expectant management).

Expectant Management

Expectant management is usually done at home. If the woman's condition worsens, she will be managed as a person with severe gestational hypertension or severe preeclampsia (see following). If it does not, labor will likely be induced at term.

■ Maternal assessment
   ❑ Weekly lab tests (hematocrit, platelet count, liver function tests, 24-hour urine protein assessment)
   ❑ Urine dipstick protein determination twice weekly by health care provider
   ❑ BP measurement twice weekly by health care provider
   ❑ Daily BP measurement and urine dipstick protein determination by the woman
■ Fetal assessment

- ❑ Daily fetal movement counts
- ❑ NST or BPP once or twice weekly
- ❑ Ultrasound evaluation of amniotic fluid volume and determination of estimated fetal weight at the time of diagnosis and serially thereafter, depending on findings
- Restricted activity
- Nutritious, balanced diet containing no more than 6 g of sodium per day. Limiting excessively salty foods (luncheon meats, pretzels, chips, pickles, and sauerkraut) will likely be necessary to avoid a sodium intake of more than 6 g per day.

Severe Gestational Hypertension and Severe Preeclampsia

Women with severe gestational hypertension are at greater risk for pregnancy complications than are women with mild preeclampsia; therefore, they should be managed as if they have severe preeclampsia.

Antepartum

- Hospitalize immediately for a thorough evaluation of maternal and fetal status.
- Maternal assessment
  - ❑ BP
  - ❑ Urine output
  - ❑ Cerebral status
  - ❑ Presence of epigastric pain, tenderness, signs of labor, or placental abruption
  - ❑ Laboratory tests
    - Platelet count
    - Liver enzymes (AST, alanine aminotransferase [ALT], LDH)
    - Serum creatinine
- Fetal assessment
  - ❑ Continuous FHR monitoring
  - ❑ BPP
  - ❑ Ultrasound assessment of fetal growth and amniotic fluid volume

After the assessment is completed, a plan of care is developed.

- If the pregnancy is 34 weeks of gestation or greater, the woman might give birth promptly, either by cesarean or after labor induction.

BOX 2-3

Care of the Woman with Preeclampsia Receiving Magnesium Sulfate

PATIENT AND FAMILY TEACHING

- Explain technique, rationale, and reactions to expect:
  - ❏ Route and rate
  - ❏ Purpose of "piggyback" infusion
- Reasons for use:
  - ❏ Tailor information to woman's readiness to learn.
  - ❏ Explain that magnesium sulfate is used to prevent disease progression.
  - ❏ Explain that magnesium sulfate is used to prevent seizures, not to decrease blood pressure.
- Reactions to expect from medication:
  - ❏ Initially the woman will appear flushed and feel hot, sedated, nauseated. She may experience burning at the IV site, especially during the bolus.
  - ❏ Sedation will continue.
- Monitoring to anticipate:
  - ❏ Maternal: blood pressure, pulse, respiratory rate, DTRs, level of consciousness, urine output (indwelling catheter), presence of headache, visual disturbances, epigastric pain
  - ❏ Fetal: FHR and activity

ADMINISTRATION

- Verify physician order.
- Place woman in side-lying position.
- Prepare solution and administer with an infusion control device (pump).
- Piggyback a solution of 40 g of magnesium sulfate in 1000 ml lactated Ringer's solution with an infusion control device at the ordered rate: loading dose—initial bolus of 4-6 g over 15-30 min; maintenance dose—2 g/hr, according to unit protocol or specific physician's order.

MATERNAL AND FETAL ASSESSMENTS

Frequency of vital signs and assessments is performed as ordered by the health care provider and per hospital protocol.

- Monitor blood pressure, pulse, and respiratory rate every 15-30 min, depending on woman's condition.
- Monitor FHR and contractions continuously.
- Monitor intake and output, proteinuria, DTRs, presence of headache, visual disturbances, level of consciousness, and epigastric pain at least hourly.

BOX 2-3

Care of the Woman with Preeclampsia Receiving Magnesium Sulfate—cont'd

■ Restrict hourly fluid intake to a total of 100-125 ml/hr; urinary output should be at least 25-30 ml/hr.

REPORTABLE CONDITIONS

■ Blood pressure: systolic ≥160 mm Hg or diastolic ≥110 mm Hg
■ Respiratory rate: ≤12 breaths/min
■ Urinary output <25-30 ml/hr
■ Presence of headache, visual disturbances, decrease in level of consciousness, or epigastric pain
■ Increasing severity or loss of DTRs, increasing edema, proteinuria
■ Any abnormal laboratory values (magnesium level, platelet count, creatinine clearance, levels of uric acid, AST, ALT, prothrombin time, partial thromboplastin time, fibrinogen, fibrin split products)
■ Any other significant change in maternal or fetal status

EMERGENCY MEASURES

■ Keep emergency drugs and intubation equipment immediately available.
■ Keep side rails up.
■ Keep lights dimmed, and maintain a quiet environment.
■ The newborn infant may have depressed respirations and hyporeflexia. Therefore, a neonatal team should attend the birth to provide resuscitation measures if needed.

DOCUMENTATION

■ All of the above

ALT, Alanine aminotransferase; *AST*, aspartate aminotransferase; *DTRs*, deep tendon reflexes; *FHR*, fetal heart rate; *IV*, intravenous.

■ If the pregnancy is less than 34 weeks of gestation, the plan includes:
  ❑ Admission to a tertiary-care center that is able to provide maternal and neonatal intensive care
  ❑ Pharmacologic therapy to prevent seizures and control BP (see Box 2-3 and the Medication Guide: Pharmacologic Control of Hypertension in Pregnancy in Appendix B)
  ❑ Continuous maternal and fetal surveillance for indicators of worsening condition

❏ If the birth can be delayed for 48 hours, corticosteroids (betamethasone) are given to enhance fetal lung maturation.
■ Immediate birth is indicated (regardless of the gestational age) if fetal stress, placental abruption, HELLP syndrome, oliguria, pulmonary edema, eclampsia, or uncontrolled high blood pressure develops.

Intrapartum

■ Bed rest with side rails up in a quiet, darkened environment
■ Continuous FHR and uterine contraction monitoring
■ Monitoring for signs of placental abruption such as hypertonic contractions or vaginal bleeding
■ Monitoring the status of maternal body systems, such as central nervous, cardiovascular, pulmonary, and renal
■ Magnesium sulfate administration to prevent or control convulsions
■ Seizure precautions
   ❏ Suction and oxygen administration equipment tested and ready to use
   ❏ Call button within easy reach
   ❏ Emergency medications readily available
See Box 2-3 for information regarding the care of clients receiving magnesium sulfate.

> **NURSING ALERT** *If magnesium toxicity is suspected, prompt actions are needed to prevent respiratory or cardiac arrest. The magnesium infusion should be discontinued immediately. Calcium gluconate or calcium chloride (antidotes for magnesium sulfate) can be given intravenously.*

> **NURSING ALERT** *High serum levels of magnesium can cause relaxation of smooth muscle, such as the uterus. When administered as a 4- to 6-g loading dose followed by a 1- to 2-g/hr maintenance dose, however, magnesium sulfate has not been shown to significantly affect the need for oxytocin (Pitocin) stimulation of labor. Other than a brief period of uterine muscle relaxation during and immediately after administration of the loading dose, no evidence of decreased uterine contractility has been observed.*

- Antihypertensive medication or medications administered as necessary to maintain BP at less than 160/110 mm Hg. Hydralazine, labetalol, and nifedipine are effective drugs for treating hypertension intrapartum. (See the Medication Guide: Pharmacologic Control of Hypertension in Pregnancy in Appendix B).
  - ❑ In order to maintain uteroplacental perfusion, antihypertensive therapy must not decrease the arterial pressure too much or too rapidly.

Postpartum

- Symptoms of preeclampsia usually resolve within 48 hours. However, approximately 30% of cases of eclampsia and HELLP syndrome occur postpartum. Clinical signs that demonstrate resolution of preeclampsia include diuresis and decreased edema.
- Magnesium sulfate administration is continued after birth for seizure prophylaxis as ordered, usually for 12 to 24 hours.
  - ❑ Assessments for effects and side effects continue until the medication is discontinued (see Box 2-3).
- Women with severe gestational hypertension or severe preeclampsia are frequently discharged from the hospital on an antihypertensive medication. If this is the case, their BP needs to be checked frequently either at home or at the health care provider's office. Often BP returns to normal within a few weeks after birth and antihypertensive medications can be discontinued.

Eclampsia

Eclampsia is usually preceded by premonitory signs and symptoms, including persistent headache, blurred vision, severe epigastric or right upper quadrant abdominal pain, and altered mental status. However, convulsions can appear suddenly and without warning in a seemingly stable woman with only minimal BP elevations.

- Nursing actions during a seizure are directed toward ensuring a patent airway and patient safety. See the Emergency box for more information on caring for women experiencing eclamptic seizures.
- During a seizure the uterus becomes hypercontractile and hypertonic. As a result, the membranes may rupture or the cervix may dilate rapidly, and birth may be imminent.

EMERGENCY

Eclampsia

TONIC-CLONIC CONVULSION SIGNS

- *Stage of invasion:* 2-3 sec, eyes are fixed, twitching of facial muscles occurs
- *Stage of contraction:* 15-20 sec, eyes protrude and are bloodshot, all body muscles in tonic contraction
- *Stage of convulsion:* muscles relax and contract alternately (clonic), respirations are halted and then begin again with long, deep, stertorous inhalation; coma ensues

INTERVENTION

- Keep airway patent: turn head to one side, place pillow under one shoulder or back if possible.
- Call for assistance. Do not leave the bedside.
- Protect with side rails up.
- Observe and record convulsion activity.

AFTER CONVULSION

- Do not leave unattended until fully alert.
- Observe for postconvulsion coma, incontinence.
- Use suction as needed.
- Administer oxygen via nonrebreather face mask at 10 L/min.
- Start IV fluids, and monitor for potential fluid overload.
- Give magnesium sulfate or other anticonvulsant drug as ordered.
- Insert indwelling urinary catheter.
- Monitor blood pressure.
- Monitor fetal and uterine status.
- Expedite laboratory work as ordered to monitor kidney function, liver function, coagulation system, and drug levels.
- Provide hygiene and a quiet environment.
- Support and keep woman and family informed.
- Be prepared for assisting with birth when woman is in stable condition.

- After a seizure the FHR tracing may demonstrate bradycardia, late decelerations, minimal baseline variability, or any combination. These findings usually resolve within a few minutes after the seizure ends and the woman's hypoxia is corrected.

NURSING ALERT *Immediately after a seizure the woman may be very confused and can be combative. Restraints may be necessary temporarily. Several hours may be needed for the woman to regain her usual level of mental functioning.*

■ After stabilization of the woman and fetus, a decision will be made regarding timing and method of birth. Eclampsia alone is not an indication for immediate cesarean birth. The route of birth (induction of labor versus cesarean birth) depends on maternal and fetal condition, fetal gestational age, and the cervical Bishop score.

Nursing Considerations

■ Accurate blood pressure measurement is essential. Box 2-4 explains how to correctly measure blood pressure.
■ Because magnesium sulfate potentiates the action of narcotics, CNS depressants, and calcium channel blockers, these drugs should be administered with caution.

> **SAFETY ALERT** *Magnesium sulfate is considered a high-alert medication because it can cause client harm when administered incorrectly. Measures to improve the safe use of this medication include developing detailed policies, procedures, protocols, and standing orders, as well as thorough assessment and documentation. Do not abbreviate magnesium sulfate as MgSO₄ anywhere in the medical record.*

Chronic Hypertension

Chronic hypertension is defined as hypertension that is present before the pregnancy or develops before 20 weeks of gestation. Hypertension initially diagnosed during pregnancy that persists longer than 6 to 12 weeks postpartum is also classified as chronic hypertension. Hypertension is defined as a BP reading $\geq 140/90$ mm Hg, on two separate occasions at least 4 to 6 hours apart but within a maximum of a 1-week period.

Pregnancy Risks Associated with Chronic Hypertension

■ Placental abruption
■ Superimposed preeclampsia, as evidenced by the following:
  ❑ In women with hypertension before 20 weeks of gestation, new-onset proteinuria (≥ 0.5 g protein in a 24-hour collection)
  ❑ In women with both hypertension and proteinuria before 20 weeks of gestation, a significant increase in hypertension, plus one of the following:
    ■ New onset of symptoms
    ■ Thrombocytopenia
    ■ Elevated liver enzymes

BOX 2-4

Blood Pressure Measurement

- Use correct cuff size; cuff should cover approximately 80% of the upper arm or be 1.5 times the length of the upper arm.
- Measure blood pressure (BP) after the woman sits for 5 min.
- Instruct the woman to refrain from tobacco or caffeine use 30 min before BP measurement.
- Measure BP with the woman sitting or semireclining with her feet flat, not dangling.
- The arm should be supported on a desk at the level of the heart.
- Measurements with an automated device should be checked with a manual device.
- Diastolic pressure should be recorded at Korotkoff phase V (disappearance of sound).
- If the BP is elevated, have the woman rest for 5-10 min and then retake it.
- BP may vary by >10 mm Hg with each arm; record the higher reading.
- Take the average of two readings at least 1 min apart.

- Increased perinatal mortality
- Fetal growth restriction
- Preterm birth

Management

- Preconception counseling to assess the cause and severity of the hypertension and the presence of any target organ (e.g., heart, eye, and kidney) damage
- Encourage preconception lifestyle changes to minimize the risks associated with chronic hypertension in pregnancy:
  - ❏ Weight loss if indicated
  - ❏ Smoking and alcohol cessation
  - ❏ Participation in aerobic exercise
  - ❏ Diet that includes a maximum of 2.4 g sodium per day
- Based on the history and physical findings, women with chronic hypertension are classified as either high or low risk for pregnancy complications.
- Women with low risk chronic hypertension may not require any antihypertensive medication at all during pregnancy. As long as they remain low risk, their pregnancies may continue until 40 weeks of gestation.

- Management of women with high risk chronic hypertension includes:
  - Antihypertensive medication such as methyldopa, labetalol, or nifedipine (see the Medication Guide: Pharmacologic Control of Hypertension in Pregnancy in Appendix B)
  - Frequent maternal and fetal assessment during pregnancy. Method and timing of birth depends on the maternal and fetal status.
  - Close monitoring postpartum for complications such as pulmonary edema, renal failure, heart failure, and encephalopathy.
- Women with chronic hypertension may breastfeed if they desire. All antihypertensive medications are present to some degree in breast milk. Levels of methyldopa in breast milk appear to be low and are considered safe. Labetalol also has a low concentration in breast milk. Little is known about the transfer of calcium channel blockers, such as nifedipine, in breast milk, but no apparent side effects have been noted in infants.

MEDICAL-SURGICAL PROBLEMS
Cardiovascular Disorders

During a normal pregnancy the maternal cardiovascular system undergoes many changes that place a physiologic strain on the heart. The major cardiovascular changes that occur during a normal pregnancy and that affect the woman with cardiac disease are increased intravascular volume, decreased systemic vascular resistance, cardiac output changes occurring during labor and birth, and the intravascular volume changes that occur just after childbirth. The strain is present during pregnancy and continues for a few weeks after birth. The normal heart can compensate for the increased workload so that pregnancy, labor, and birth are generally well tolerated, but the diseased heart is hemodynamically challenged.

Etiology of Selected Cardiovascular Disorders in Pregnant Women

- Congenital cardiac diseases
  - Atrial septal defect

- ☐ Coarctation of the aorta
- ☐ Tetralogy of Fallot
- ■ Acquired cardiac diseases
  - ☐ Mitral valve prolapse
  - ☐ Mitral stenosis
  - ☐ Aortic stenosis
  - ☐ Myocardial infarction
- ■ Other cardiac diseases and conditions
  - ☐ Peripartum cardiomyopathy
  - ☐ Infective endocarditis
  - ☐ Eisenmenger syndrome
  - ☐ Marfan syndrome
  - ☐ Heart transplantation

The degree of disability experienced by the woman with cardiovascular disease is often more important in the treatment and prognosis during pregnancy than the diagnosis of the type of cardiovascular disease. The New York Heart Association functional classification of heart disease is a widely accepted standard.

New York Heart Association Functional Classification of Organic Heart Disease

- ■ Class I: asymptomatic without limitation of physical activity
- ■ Class II: symptomatic with slight limitation of activity
- ■ Class III: symptomatic with marked limitation of activity
- ■ Class IV: symptomatic with inability to carry on any physical activity without discomfort

A woman's functional classification may change as the normal cardiovascular changes of pregnancy place increasing demands on her heart. Therefore, the woman's functional classification is determined at 3 months and again at 7 or 8 months of gestation.

Pregnancy Risks Associated with Cardiovascular Disease

- ■ Miscarriage
- ■ IUFD
- ■ IUGR
- ■ Congenital heart disease in the fetus

Management

- Preconception counseling, including the significant other and other family members, is recommended to help the woman understand her peripartum risks.

Pregnancy

- Goal: to minimize stress on the heart, which is greatest between 28 and 32 weeks of gestation, as the hemodynamic changes of pregnancy reach their maximum
- Continuously monitor for objective signs of cardiac decompensation (see the Signs of Potential Complications box).
- Teach subjective symptoms of cardiac decompensation that are listed in the Signs of Potential Complications box.
- Encourage rest (8 to 10 hours of sleep every day with 30-minute rest periods after meals).
- Limit activity (housework, shopping, exercise) to the amount recommended for the functional classification of the woman's heart disease.
  - ❏ Instruct to immediately stop any activity that causes even minor signs and symptoms of cardiac decompensation.

Signs of Potential Complications

Cardiac Decompensation

PREGNANT WOMAN: SUBJECTIVE SYMPTOMS
- Increasing fatigue or difficulty breathing, or both, with her usual activities
- Feeling of smothering
- Frequent cough
- Palpitations; feeling that her heart is "racing"
- Generalized edema: swelling of face, feet, legs, fingers (e.g., rings do not fit anymore)

NURSE: OBJECTIVE SIGNS
- Irregular, weak, rapid pulse (≥100 beats/min)
- Progressive, generalized edema
- Crackles at base of lungs after two inspirations and exhalations that do not clear after coughing
- Orthopnea; increasing dyspnea

- ❑ Women with class II heart disease will likely be admitted to the hospital near term (or earlier, if signs of cardiac overload or dysrhythmia develop) for evaluation and treatment.
- ❑ Women with class III heart disease need bed rest for much of each day.
- ■ Treat infections promptly.
- ■ Nutrition counseling
  - ❑ Iron and folic acid supplementation
  - ❑ High protein intake
  - ❑ Adequate calories for weight gain
  - ❑ Monitor potassium intake, especially if the woman is taking diuretics.
- ■ Measures to avoid constipation, which might result in straining during defecation (Valsalva maneuver)
  - ❑ Increase intake of fluids and fiber.
  - ❑ Prescribed stool softener
- ■ Teach the importance of daily weighing. A sudden weight gain indicates fluid retention.
- ■ Possible anticoagulant therapy (heparin or low-molecular-weight heparin [Lovenox])
  - ❑ Teach self-injection techniques.
  - ❑ Teach to avoid foods high in vitamin K, such as raw, dark green, and leafy vegetables.
  - ❑ Monitor prothrombin time (e.g., international normalized ratio [INR]).
- ■ Tests for fetal maturity and well-being and placental sufficiency
- ■ Other therapy as indicated for the woman's specific cardiac problem
  - ❑ If surgery to correct a cardiac lesion is necessary during pregnancy, it should be postponed until the third trimester if possible, when the risk to the fetus is considerably decreased.

Intrapartum

- ■ Goal: to promote cardiac function
- ■ Assess for signs of cardiac decompensation
- ■ Minimize anxiety.
- ■ Maintain a calm atmosphere.
  - ❑ Keep woman/family informed of labor progress.

- ❑ Provide anticipatory guidance about events that will probably occur.
- ❑ Promote comfort.
- ■ Support cardiac function.
    - ❑ Keep the woman's head and shoulders elevated.
    - ❑ Use pillows to support body parts.
    - ❑ Side-lying position is recommended to facilitate hemodynamics during labor.
- ■ Relieve discomfort with medication and supportive care; epidural anesthesia provides better pain relief than narcotics and causes fewer alterations in hemodynamics.
- ■ Vaginal birth recommended if there are no obstetric problems
    - ❑ Avoid the use of stirrups.
    - ❑ Open-glottis pushing is recommended.
    - ❑ Avoid use of the Valsalva maneuver during pushing.
    - ❑ Episiotomy, vacuum extraction, or outlet forceps may be used to shorten the second stage of labor, thereby decreasing the workload on the heart.
- ■ Cesarean birth is not routinely recommended because there are risks of dramatic fluid shifts, sustained hemodynamic changes, and increased blood loss.
- ■ Antibiotic prophylaxis (penicillin or vancomycin) to protect against bacterial endocarditis may be ordered in labor and during the immediate postpartum period.

Postpartum

- ■ Goal: to monitor for cardiac decompensation

NURSING ALERT *The immediate postbirth period is hazardous for a woman whose heart function is compromised. Cardiac output increases rapidly as extravascular fluid is remobilized into the vascular compartment. At the moment of birth, intraabdominal pressure is reduced drastically; pressure on veins is removed, the splanchnic vessels engorge, and blood flow to the heart is increased. When blood flow increases to the heart, a reflex bradycardia (slowing of the heart in response to the increased blood flow) may result.*

- ■ The first 24 to 48 hours are the most hemodynamically difficult for the woman.

- Maternal cardiac output is usually stabilized by 2 weeks postpartum.
- Immediate general care
  - Elevate head of bed.
  - Encourage side-lying position.
  - Bed rest, with or without bathroom privileges, may be ordered.
  - Progressive ambulation may be permitted as tolerated.
  - Assistance with infant care and breastfeeding will probably be necessary.
- Preparation for discharge
  - Rest and sleep periods, activity, and diet are similar to those recommended during pregnancy.
  - Avoid constipation.
- Contraception
  - In general, for women with congenital heart disease, the complications associated with pregnancy are usually greater than the risks associated with any form of contraception.
  - Surgery to achieve permanent sterilization, however, is often not a safe procedure for women with class III or class IV cardiac disease.
  - Women at particular risk for thromboembolism should avoid combined estrogen-progestin oral contraceptives, but progestin-only pills may be used.
  - Parenteral progestins (e.g., Depo-Provera) are safe and effective for women with cardiac disease.
  - An IUD may be used by some women with congenital heart lesions. Although a theoretic risk exists of developing endocarditis, the actual risk for women using an IUD is probably minimal.

Anemia

Anemia is a common medical disorder of pregnancy, affecting from 20% to 60% of pregnant women. Anemia in pregnancy is defined as hemoglobin less than 11 g/dl in the first and third trimesters and less than 10.5 g/dl in the second trimester. A hemoglobin level of less than 6 to 8 mg/dl is considered severe anemia. Iron deficiency anemia is the most common anemia of pregnancy.

Iron Deficiency Anemia

- Iron deficiency anemia, especially severe anemia, has been associated with preterm birth and low birth weight infants, although whether these poor pregnancy outcomes are caused by iron deficiency anemia is uncertain.

- Generally iron deficiency anemia is preventable or easily treated with iron supplements. Most women with iron deficiency anemia can absorb as much iron as they need by taking one 325-mg tablet of ferrous sulfate twice each day.

- Teach the importance of iron supplementation for treating iron deficiency anemia (see the Teaching for Self-Management box: Iron Supplementation). In addition, teach dietary ways to decrease the GI side effects of iron therapy.

Teaching for Self-Management

Iron Supplementation

- Vitamin C from plant sources (e.g., citrus fruits, tomatoes, melons, and strawberries) increases the absorption of the iron supplement; therefore include these in the diet often.
- Bran, tea, coffee, milk, oxalates (in spinach and Swiss chard), and egg yolk decrease iron absorption. Avoid consuming them at the same time as the supplement.
- Iron is absorbed best if it is taken when the stomach is empty; that is, take it between meals with a beverage other than tea, coffee, or milk.
- Iron can be taken at bedtime if abdominal discomfort occurs when it is taken between meals.
- If an iron dose is missed, take it as soon as it is remembered if that is within 13 hours of the scheduled dose. Do not double up on the dose.
- Keep the supplement in a childproof container and out of the reach of any children in the household.
- The iron may cause stools to be black or dark green.
- Constipation is common with iron supplementation. A diet high in fiber with adequate fluid intake can help reduce constipation.

Urinary Tract Infections

Urinary tract infections (UTIs) are a common medical complication of pregnancy, occurring in approximately 20% of all pregnancies. They are also responsible for 10% of all hospitalizations during pregnancy. UTIs include asymptomatic bacteriuria, cystitis, and pyelonephritis. They are usually caused by coliform organisms that are a normal part of the perineal flora. By far the most common cause of UTIs is *Escherichia coli,* a gram-negative bacterium responsible for 85% of cases.

Asymptomatic Bacteriuria

- Persistent presence of bacteria within the urinary tract of women who have no symptoms. A clean-voided urine specimen containing more than 100,000 organisms per ml is diagnostic. All women should be screened for asymptomatic bacteriuria at their first prenatal visit.
- If asymptomatic bacteriuria is not treated, up to 40% of infected women will subsequently develop symptomatic infection during the pregnancy.
- Asymptomatic bacteriuria has been associated with preterm birth and low birth weight infants.
- Treat with an antibiotic such as amoxicillin, ampicillin, cephalexin (Keflex), ciprofloxacin (Cipro), levofloxacin (Levaquin), nitrofurantoin (Macrodantin), or trimethoprim-sulfamethoxazole (Bactrim DS). Several different regimens, including single dose, 3-day, 7-day, and 10-day treatment may be used.
- A repeat urine culture is usually ordered 1 to 2 weeks after completing antibiotics because approximately 15% of women will not respond to therapy or will have a reinfection.
- Women who have persistent or frequent recurrences of bacteriuria may be placed on suppressive therapy, often nitrofurantoin each night at bedtime, for the remainder of the pregnancy.

Cystitis

- Cystitis (bladder infection) is characterized by dysuria, urgency, and frequency, along with lower abdominal or suprapubic pain. Usually white blood cells, as well as bacteria, are found in the urine. Microscopic or gross hematuria also may be present.
- Typically symptoms are confined to the bladder rather than becoming systemic.

- Cystitis is usually uncomplicated, but it may lead to an ascending UTI if untreated.
- Cystitis is often treated with a 3-day course of antibiotic therapy. Antibiotics often prescribed include amoxicillin, ampicillin, cephalexin, ciprofloxacin, levofloxacin, nitrofurantoin, and trimethoprim-sulfamethoxazole.
- Phenazopyridine (Pyridium), a urinary analgesic, is often prescribed along with an antibiotic for relief of symptoms caused by irritation of the urinary tract.
  - ❏ Women should be taught that phenazopyridine colors urine and tears orange. Therefore, they should be instructed to avoid wearing contact lenses while taking this medication and warned that it will stain underwear.

Pyelonephritis

Pyelonephritis (renal infection) is a common serious medical complication of pregnancy and the second most common nonobstetric reason for hospitalization.

Complications

- Maternal
  - ❏ Anemia
  - ❏ Septicemia
  - ❏ Renal dysfunction
  - ❏ Pulmonary insufficiency
  - ❏ Urosepsis
  - ❏ Sepsis syndrome
  - ❏ Pulmonary injury resembling ARDS
  - ❏ Preterm labor
- Fetal
  - ❏ IUGR
  - ❏ IUFD

Signs and Symptoms

- Abrupt onset of fever, shaking chills, and aching in the lumbar area of the back
- Anorexia
- Nausea and vomiting
- Costovertebral angle tenderness to palpation

Management

- Initial
  - ❏ Admit to the hospital as soon as pyelonephritis is diagnosed.
  - ❏ Collect urine and blood samples for culture and sensitivity testing before beginning antibiotics.
  - ❏ Begin intravenous broad-spectrum antibiotics, such as ampicillin, gentamicin, cefazolin (Ancef), or ceftriaxone (Rocephin).
  - ❏ Monitor closely for the development of sepsis.
  - ❏ Clinical symptoms usually resolve within a couple of days after antibiotic therapy is begun. Most women become afebrile within 72 hours.
- Follow-up
  - ❏ Continue antibiotics for 7 to 14 days after the woman is discharged from the hospital.
  - ❏ Repeat a urine culture 1 to 2 weeks after antibiotic therapy has been completed. Urine cultures should be obtained each trimester for the remainder of the pregnancy.
  - ❏ Many women will be maintained on a prophylactic antibiotic (often nitrofurantoin once or twice daily) for the remainder of the pregnancy.

Substance Abuse

Substance abuse refers to the continued use of substances despite related problems in physical, social, or interpersonal areas. Any use of alcohol or illicit drugs during pregnancy is considered abuse. Substance abuse in women is a complex problem surrounded by multiple individual, familial, and social issues that require many levels of intervention and treatment.

Prevalence

Because many pregnant women are reluctant to reveal their use of substances or to reveal the extent of their use, data on prevalence are highly variable. Approximately 15% of all mothers have a substance abuse problem.

Risk Factors for Substance Abuse

- History of childhood sexual or physical abuse
- Spouse or partner who abuses substances
- Unemployment

- Unmarried status
- Current psychiatric disorder
- Intimate partner violence

Barriers to Treatment

Less than 10% of pregnant women who are substance abusers receive treatment for their addictions, for a variety of reasons:

- Social stigma
- Labeling
- Guilt
- Fear of losing custody of child or children
- Fear of criminal prosecution
- Concurrent needs for obstetric care and child care for other children
- Long waiting lists
- Lack of health insurance

Commonly Abused Substances

Nicotine

Maternal Risks Associated with Cigarette Smoking

- Cardiovascular heart disease
- Cancer (especially lung and cervical)
- Chronic lung disease

Pregnancy-Related Risks Associated with Cigarette Smoking

- Late miscarriage (between 12 and 20 weeks of gestation)
- Placenta previa
- Placental abruption
- Decreased placental perfusion
- Low birth weight

Alcohol

Maternal Risks Associated with Alcohol Use

- Depression
- MVAs
- Suicide
- Alcohol-related liver damage

Pregnancy-Related Risks Associated with Alcohol Use

- Late miscarriage (between 12 and 20 weeks of gestation)
- Fetal alcohol syndrome (FAS)
  - ❑ Most common cause of preventable mental retardation and birth defects
- Alcohol-related birth defects (ARBDs)
- Alcohol-related neurodevelopmental disorders

Cocaine

Maternal Risks Associated with Cocaine Use

- Poor nutrition
- Sexually transmitted infections
- Hepatitis B infection
- Human immunodeficiency virus (HIV) infection
- Increased cardiovascular stress
- Tachycardia
- Hypertension
- Ventricular arrhythmias
- Sudden coronary artery spasm
- Myocardial infarction

Pregnancy-Related Risks Associated with Cocaine Use

- Miscarriage
- IUGR
- Placental abruption
- Preterm labor
- IUFD

Methamphetamines

Maternal Risks Associated with Methamphetamine Use

- Hypertension
- Ectopic heartbeat
- Seizures
- Myocardial infarction
- Stroke
- Death

Pregnancy-Related Risks Associated with Methamphetamine Use

- IUGR with smaller head circumference
- Preterm labor
- Placental abruption

Opiates

Heroin is one of the most commonly abused opiates. Other drugs in this classification include opium, morphine, codeine, and methadone.

Maternal Risks Associated with Heroin Use

- Hepatitis B, C, or D infection
- HIV infection

Pregnancy-Related Risks Associated with Heroin Use

- Miscarriage
- Preeclampsia
- IUGR
- Premature rupture of membranes
- Preterm labor

Methadone

- Used to treat addiction to other opiates, either by aiding withdrawal or providing maintenance at a stable dose.
- Methadone maintenance treatment is the standard of care for pregnant women who are dependent on heroin or other opiates.

Assessment

- *All* pregnant women should be asked screening questions for alcohol and drug abuse during the first prenatal visit. The approximate frequency and amount should be documented for each drug used. Proceed in this order:
  - ❏ Over-the-counter and prescribed medications
  - ❏ Legal drugs, such as caffeine, nicotine, and alcohol
  - ❏ Illicit drugs, such as cocaine, methamphetamines, and heroin
- Well-known screens for alcohol abuse include:
  - ❏ CAGE questionnaire
  - ❏ Brief Michigan Alcoholism Screening Test (MAST)
  - ❏ 4Ps-Plus (designed specifically to identify pregnant women who need in-depth assessment)

- Also screen for the following:
  - ❑ Physical and sexual abuse
  - ❑ History of psychiatric illness
- Urine toxicology screening or analysis of hair may also be performed.

LEGAL TIP Drug Testing During Pregnancy

Federal law provides no requirement for a health care provider to test either the pregnant woman or the newborn for the presence of drugs. However, nurses need to know the practices of the states in which they are working. In some states a woman whose urine drug screen test is positive at the time of labor and birth must be referred to child protective services. If the mother is not in a drug treatment program or is judged unable to provide care, the infant may be placed in foster care. In 2001 the U.S. Supreme Court ruled that in all states, testing for drug use without the pregnant woman's permission is unlawful.

Management

- Comprehensive physical examination
- Laboratory testing
  - ❑ CBC
  - ❑ Syphilis testing (RPR)
  - ❑ Hepatitis B and C serology
  - ❑ HIV
  - ❑ Tuberculosis
  - ❑ Urine toxicologic testing for suspected drugs used or drugs commonly abused in the community
  - ❑ Liver function tests if alcohol abuse is suspected
- Fetal assessment
  - ❑ Ultrasound to determine gestational age and estimated fetal weight
  - ❑ NST
- Client education
  - ❑ Clearly communicate the consequences of perinatal drug use. Provide information about specific effects on pregnancy, the fetus, and the newborn for each drug used.
  - ❑ Recommend abstinence as the safest course of action, unless the woman is abusing opiates.
- Substance abuse treatment will be individualized for each woman, depending on the type of drug used and the frequency and amount of use.

❏ Treatment programs should include a cognitive-behavioral approach and mostly female staff.

- If possible, enroll the woman in a culturally sensitive, interdisciplinary, comprehensive drug treatment program that also addresses the following:
  - ❏ Stigmatization issues
  - ❏ High probability of past or present sexual and physical abuse
  - ❏ Lack of social support
  - ❏ Need for social services and child care
  - ❏ Need for transportation
  - ❏ Family support services
  - ❏ Medical (particularly women's health) and mental health services
  - ❏ Child development services
  - ❏ Family planning
  - ❏ Respite care
  - ❏ Life skills management
  - ❏ Pharmacologic services
  - ❏ Self-help groups and stress management
  - ❏ Need for support and education in the mothering role
  - ❏ Relationship counseling
  - ❏ Vocational and legal assistance

Nursing Considerations

- Become knowledgeable about how to screen and identify women who abuse substances while pregnant.
- Realize that substance abuse is an illness and that women who abuse substances deserve to be treated with patience, kindness, consistency, and firmness when necessary. Maintain a nonjudgmental, nonpunitive attitude.
- Determine the woman's readiness for change.
- Plan realistic and short-term goals.
- Promote mother-infant attachment by identifying the woman's strengths and reinforcing positive maternal feelings and behaviors.
- If necessary, involve the state's child protective services agency to investigate the home situation before a known substance abuser is discharged with her baby, to determine that the environment is safe and that someone will be available to meet the infant's needs if the mother proves unable to do so.

BASIC DEFINITIONS

dilation: stretching of the external cervical os from an opening a few millimeters in size to an opening large enough to allow the passage of the fetus; dilation is expressed in centimeters from 0 (closed) to 10 (completely or fully dilated)

effacement: thinning and shortening or obliteration of the cervix that occurs during late pregnancy or labor or both; degree of effacement is expressed in percentages from 0% to 100%

engagement: the entrance of the fetal presenting part into the superior pelvic strait and the beginning of the descent through the pelvic canal; usually the lowest part of the presenting part is at or below the level of the ischial spines

position: relationship of a reference point on the presenting part of the fetus, such as the occiput, sacrum, chin, or scapula, to its location in the front, back, or sides of the maternal pelvis (Fig. 3-1)

presentation: that part of the fetus that first enters the pelvis and lies over the inlet; the three main presentations are cephalic (head first), breech (buttocks or feet first), and shoulder (Fig. 3-2)

station: relationship of the presenting fetal part to an imaginary line drawn between the maternal ischial spines; a measure of the degree of descent of the presenting part of the fetus through the birth canal; the placement of the presenting part is measured in centimeters above or below the ischial spines (Fig. 3-3)

uterine resting tone: the tension in the uterine muscle between contractions; relaxation of the uterus

Stages of Labor

Stage 1 labor: begins with the onset of regular uterine contractions and ends with complete or full cervical effacement and dilation. The first stage of labor consists of three phases:

- Latent—through 3 cm of dilation
- Active—4 to 7 cm of dilation
- Transition—8 to 10 cm of dilation

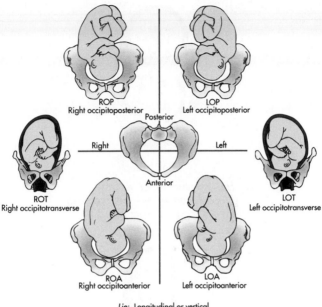

ROP
Right occipitoposterior

LOP
Left occipitoposterior

Posterior

Right

Left

Anterior

ROT
Right occipitotransverse

LOT
Left occipitotransverse

ROA
Right occipitoanterior

LOA
Left occipitoanterior

Lie: Longitudinal or vertical
Presentation: Vertex
Reference point: Occiput

Fig. 3-1 Examples of fetal positions while in vertex presentation.

The length of the first stage of labor varies greatly but is usually shorter as parity increases. Full dilation may occur in less than 1 hour in some multiparous pregnancies. In first-time pregnancy, complete dilation of the cervix can take up to 20 hours.

Stage 2 labor: begins with complete or full cervical dilation (10 cm) and complete effacement (100%) and ends with the baby's birth. The second stage of labor consists of two phases:

- Latent—a period of rest and relative calm at the beginning of the second stage, sometimes referred to as "laboring down," as the fetus passively descends through the birth canal
- Descent—time of active pushing, characterized by strong urges to bear down when the presenting part of the fetus presses on the stretch receptors of the pelvic floor

The second stage of labor lasts an average of 20 minutes for a multiparous woman and 50 minutes for a nulliparous woman.

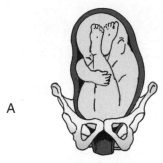

A

Frank breech

Lie: Longitudinal or vertical
Presentation: Breech (incomplete)
Presenting part: Sacrum

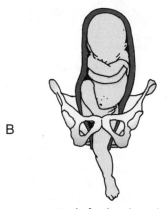

B

Single footling breech

Lie: Longitudinal or vertical
Presentation: Breech (incomplete)
Presenting part: Foot

Fig. 3-2 Fetal presentations. **A** and **B,** Breech (sacral) presentation.

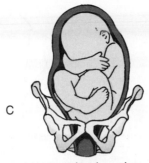

Complete breech

Lie: Longitudinal or vertical
Presentation: Breech (sacrum and feet presenting)
Presenting part: Sacrum (with feet)

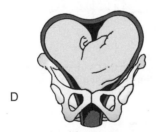

Shoulder presentation

Lie: Transverse or horizontal
Presentation: Shoulder
Presenting part: Scapula

Fig. 3-2, cont'd Fetal presentations. **C,** Breech (sacral) presentation. **D,** Shoulder presentation.

Stage 3 labor: lasts from birth of the baby until the placenta is expelled. The placenta is usually expelled within 10 to 15 minutes after the birth of the baby. If the third stage has not been completed within 30 minutes, the placenta is considered to be retained and interventions to hasten its separation and expulsion are usually instituted.

Stage 4 labor: the first 1 to 2 hours after birth. It is the period of immediate recovery, when homeostasis is reestablished. It is an important period of observation for complications, such as abnormal bleeding.

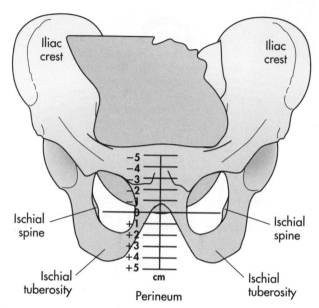

Fig. 3-3 Stations of presenting part, or degree of descent. The lowermost portion of the presenting part is at the level of the ischial spines, station 0.

This is also the time during which the newborn becomes acquainted with the mother as well as other family members

MANAGEMENT OF THE FIRST STAGE OF LABOR

Admission to the Labor and Birth Unit

- On arrival in the labor and birth unit, perform a screening assessment to determine the health status of the woman and her fetus and the progress of her labor.
- Use the agency's triage and/or admission forms (may be paper or electronic) as a guide for obtaining important assessment information. These forms usually address:
  - ❑ Chief complaint: "Why did you come at this time?"
  - ❑ Expected date of birth
  - ❑ Vital signs

- ❏ Contraction status (time of onset, frequency, duration, intensity, resting tone)
- ❏ Fetal heart rate (FHR) and pattern
- ❏ Presence and character of vaginal discharge or show
- ❏ Status of amniotic membranes (ruptured or intact); if ruptured, document time of rupture and characteristics of fluid (e.g., amount, color, unusual odor). See the Procedure box for information regarding tests to confirm membrane rupture.
- ❏ Presence of risk factors, such as vaginal bleeding, decreased or absent fetal movement, and preterm gestation
- ❏ Level of pain
- ❏ Presence of psychosocial or cultural factors that could affect the care provided during labor and birth
- ■ Vaginal examination to determine cervical effacement, dilation, and fetal station
- ■ Perform basic laboratory and diagnostic tests according to hospital protocol. These commonly include the following:
  - ❏ Urine testing for protein, glucose, ketones, leukocytes, and nitrites (done in the hospital laboratory, not in the labor and birth unit)
  - ❏ Blood type and Rh status
  - ❏ Hematocrit or hemoglobin
  - ❏ Rapid group B streptococci (GBS) test (if third-trimester test results are not available)
  - ❏ Rapid human immunodeficiency virus (HIV) test (if third-trimester test results are not available)
- ■ Review the prenatal record to determine the following:
  - ❏ Obstetric history
  - ❏ Problems during the current pregnancy
  - ❏ Laboratory and/or diagnostic test results
  - ❏ Fetal assessment test results
  - ❏ Type of childbirth preparation
- ■ Determine if the woman is in true labor. See Box 3-1 for differences in true and false labor.
- ■ Communicate assessment information to the woman's health care provider so that a decision can be made regarding admission to the labor and birth unit.

Common Characteristics of the First Stage of Labor

Common appearance and behavior of women during each phase of the first stage of labor are listed in Box 3-2.

Procedure

Tests for Rupture of Membranes

NITRAZINE TEST FOR pH
- Explain procedure to the woman or couple.

Procedure
- Wash hands.
- Use a cotton-tipped applicator impregnated with Nitrazine dye for determining pH (differentiates amniotic fluid, which is slightly alkaline, from urine and purulent material [pus], which are acidic).
- Dip the applicator deep into the vagina to pick up fluid (procedure may be performed during speculum examination).

Read Results
- Membranes probably intact: identifies vaginal and most body fluids that are acidic

Yellow	pH 5.0
Olive-yellow	pH 5.5
Olive-green	pH 6.0

- Membranes probably ruptured: identifies amniotic fluid that is alkaline

Blue-green	pH 6.5
Blue-gray	pH 7.0
Deep blue	pH 7.5

- Realize that false results are possible because of presence of bloody show, insufficient amniotic fluid, or semen.
- Provide pericare as needed.
- Remove gloves and wash hands

Document Results
- Results are positive or negative.

TEST FOR FERNING OR FERN PATTERN
- Explain procedure to woman or couple.
- Wash hands, apply sterile gloves, obtain specimen of fluid (usually during sterile speculum examination).
- Spread a drop of fluid from the vagina onto a clean glass slide with a sterile cotton-tipped applicator.
- Allow fluid to dry.
- Examine the slide under a microscope and observe for appearance of ferning (a frondlike crystalline pattern) (do not confuse with cervical mucus test, when high levels of estrogen cause the ferning).

Procedure—cont'd

- Observe for absence of ferning (alerts staff to possibility that amount of specimen was inadequate or that specimen was urine, vaginal discharge, or blood).
- Provide pericare as needed.
- Remove gloves and wash hands.

Document Results
- Results are positive or negative.

BOX 3-1

Differences in True and False Labor

TRUE LABOR
- Contractions
  - Occur regularly, become stronger, last longer, and occur closer together
  - Become more intense with walking
  - Usually felt in lower back, radiating to lower portion of abdomen
  - Continue despite use of comfort measures
- Cervix (by vaginal examination)
  - Shows progressive change (softening, effacement, and dilation signaled by the appearance of bloody show)
  - Moves to an increasingly anterior position
- Fetus
  - Presenting part usually becomes engaged in the pelvis, resulting in increased ease of breathing; at the same time the presenting part presses downward and compresses the bladder, resulting in urinary frequency

FALSE LABOR
- Contractions
  - Occur irregularly or become regular only temporarily
  - Often stop with walking or position change
  - Can be felt in the back or abdomen above the navel
  - Often can be stopped through the use of comfort measures
- Cervix (by vaginal examination)
  - May be soft but there is no significant change in effacement or dilation or evidence of bloody show
  - Is often in a posterior position
- Fetus
  - Presenting part is usually not engaged in the pelvis

BOX 3-2

Common Characteristics of First-Stage Labor

LATENT PHASE (dilation of cervix 0-3 cm; contractions 30-45 sec long, 5-30 min apart, mild to moderate intensity; duration of phase about 6-8 hr)

- Excited
- Thoughts center on self, labor, and baby
- Fairly confident
- Some apprehension
- Pain controlled fairly well
- Able to talk and ambulate through contractions
- Alert, follows directions readily
- Open to instructions

ACTIVE PHASE (dilation of cervix 4-7 cm; contractions 40-70 sec long, 3-5 min apart, moderate to strong intensity; duration of phase about 3-6 hr)

- Becomes more serious, more quiet, doubtful of control of pain, more apprehensive
- Desires companionship and encouragement
- Attention more inwardly directed
- Fatigue evidenced
- Malar (cheeks) flush
- Has some difficulty following directions but accepts coaching
- Describes increasing discomfort

TRANSITION PHASE (dilation of cervix 8-10 cm; contractions 45-90 sec long, 2-3 min apart, strong intensity; duration of phase about 20-40 min)

- Pain described as severe, with backache common
- May voice frustration, fear of loss of control, and irritability
- Expresses doubt about ability to continue
- Vague in communications
- Experiences amnesia between contractions
- Writhing with contractions
- Nausea and vomiting, especially if hyperventilating
- Hyperesthesia
- Circumoral pallor, perspiration on forehead and upper lip
- Shaking tremor of thighs
- Describes feeling of need to defecate, pressure on anus

Nursing Care in the First Stage of Labor

Nursing care for women during the first stage of labor is described in Box 3-3.

FETAL ASSESSMENT DURING LABOR

Because labor is a period of physiologic stress for the fetus, frequent monitoring of fetal status is part of the nursing care during labor. The goals of intrapartum FHR monitoring are to identify and differentiate

---

BOX 3-3

Nursing Care in First-Stage Labor

ASSESSMENT

- Latent phase
  - Perform every 30 to 60 min: maternal blood pressure, pulse, and respirations
  - Perform every 30 to 60 min, depending on risk status: fetal heart rate (FHR) and pattern, uterine activity, vaginal show
  - Assess temperature every 4 hours until membranes rupture, then every 2 hr
  - Perform vaginal examination as needed to identify progress
  - Observe every 30 min: changes in maternal appearance, mood, affect degree of pain, energy level, and condition of partner/coach
- Active phase
  - Perform every 30 min: maternal blood pressure, pulse, and respirations
  - Perform every 15 to 30 min, depending on risk status: FHR and pattern, uterine activity, vaginal show
  - Assess temperature every 4 hr until membranes rupture, then every 2 hr
  - Perform vaginal examination as needed to identify progress
  - Observe every 15 min: changes in maternal appearance, mood, affect degree of pain, energy level, and condition of partner/coach
- Transition phase
  - Perform every 15 to 30 min: maternal blood pressure, pulse, and respirations
  - Perform every 15 to 30 min, depending on risk status: FHR and pattern
  - Assess every 10 to 15 min: uterine activity, vaginal show
  - Assess temperature every 4 hr until membranes rupture, then every 2 hr

---

Continued

BOX 3-3

Nursing Care in First-Stage Labor—cont'd

- ❏ Perform vaginal examination as needed to identify progress
- ❏ Observe every 5 min: changes in maternal appearance, mood, affect degree of pain, energy level, and condition of partner/coach

INTERVENTIONS
- ■ Latent phase
  - ❏ Review birth plan
  - ❏ Discuss process of labor and what to expect
  - ❏ Keep woman/couple informed regarding progress
  - ❏ Demonstrate breathing and relaxation techniques and comfort measures as needed
  - ❏ Create a calm, relaxing, safe environment
  - ❏ Offer fluids as desired and ordered to maintain hydration; initiate intravenous fluids if ordered
  - ❏ Assist with activity and position changes, emphasizing upright positions and movement
  - ❏ Encourage voiding every 2 hr
- ■ Active phase
  - ❏ Inform woman/couple regarding progress
  - ❏ Encourage and assist with nonpharmacologic measures to enhance progress and relieve discomfort
  - ❏ Provide pharmacologic measures for pain relief as ordered by the primary health care provider and as requested by the woman
  - ❏ Offer fluids as desired and ordered to maintain hydration; initiate intravenous fluids if ordered
  - ❏ Assist with activity and position changes, emphasizing upright positions and movement
  - ❏ Help to rest and relax between contractions
  - ❏ Encourage voiding every 2 hr
  - ❏ Assist with hygienic measures: oral care, perineal cleansing
  - ❏ Provide emotional support and encouragement; provide positive reinforcement of her efforts
- ■ Transition phase
  - ❏ Inform woman/couple regarding progress
  - ❏ Encourage and assist with nonpharmacologic measures to enhance progress and relieve discomfort
  - ❏ Provide pharmacologic measures for pain relief as ordered by the primary health care provider and as requested by the woman

---

BOX 3-3

Nursing Care in First-Stage Labor—cont'd

- ❑ Offer fluids as desired and ordered to maintain hydration; initiate intravenous fluids if ordered
- ❑ Assist with activity and position changes, emphasizing upright positions and movement
- ❑ Help to rest and relax between contractions
- ❑ Encourage voiding every 2 hr
- ❑ Assist with hygienic measures: oral care, perineal cleansing
- ❑ Provide emotional support and encouragement; provide positive reinforcement of her efforts

---

the normal (reassuring) patterns from the abnormal (nonreassuring) patterns, which can be indicative of fetal compromise. Fetal well-being during labor can be assessed by the response of the FHR to uterine contractions.

Monitoring Techniques

Intermittent Auscultation (IA)

- Uses listening to fetal heart sounds at periodic intervals to assess the FHR
- IA can be performed with a Pinard stethoscope, a Doppler ultrasound device, an ultrasound stethoscope, or a DeLee-Hillis fetoscope.
- Advantages: easy to use, inexpensive, and less invasive than electronic fetal monitoring. It is often more comfortable for the woman and gives her more freedom of movement.
- Disadvantages: may be difficult to perform in women who are obese. Because IA is intermittent, significant events may occur during a time when the FHR is not being auscultated. Also IA does not provide a permanent documented visual record of the FHR.
- The recommended optimal frequency for IA in low risk women during labor has not been determined. Auscultation frequencies that are often suggested are every 15 to 30 minutes in the active phase of the first stage of labor and every 5 to 15 minutes in the second stage of labor.
- Box 3-4 describes how to perform IA.

BOX 3-4

Procedure for Intermittent Auscultation of the Fetal Heart Rate

1. Palpate the maternal abdomen to identify fetal presentation and position.
2. Apply ultrasonic gel to the device if using a Doppler ultrasound. Place the listening device over the area of maximal intensity and clarity of the fetal heart sounds to obtain the clearest and loudest sound, which is easiest to count. This location will usually be over the fetal back. If using the fetoscope, firm pressure may be needed.
3. Count the maternal radial pulse while listening to the fetal heart rate (FHR) to differentiate it from the fetal rate.
4. Palpate the abdomen for the presence or absence of uterine activity (UA) so as to count the FHR between contractions.
5. Count the FHR for 30 to 60 sec between contractions to identify the auscultated rate, best assessed in the absence of UA.
6. Auscultate the FHR before, during, and after a contraction to identify the FHR during the contraction, as a response to the contraction, and to assess for the absence or presence of increases or decreases in FHR.
7. When distinct discrepancies in the FHR are noted during listening periods, auscultate for a longer period during, after, and between contractions to identify significant changes that may indicate the need for another mode of FHR monitoring.

Source: Tucker, S., Miller, L., & Miller, D. (2009). *Mosby's pocket guide to fetal monitoring: A multidisciplinary approach* (6th ed.). St. Louis: Mosby.

NURSING ALERT   *When the FHR is auscultated and documented, it is inappropriate to use the descriptive terms associated with electronic fetal monitoring (e.g., moderate variability, variable deceleration) because most of the terms are visual descriptions of the patterns produced on the monitor tracing. Terms that are numerically defined, however, such as bradycardia and tachycardia, can be used. Fetal heart rate when auscultated should be described as a baseline number or range, and as having a regular or irregular rhythm. The presence or absence of accelerations or decelerations both during and after contractions should also be noted.*

Uterine Activity (UA) Assessment

■ UA is assessed by palpation. The examiner should keep his or her fingertips placed over the fundus before, during, and after contractions.

- Contraction intensity is usually described as mild, moderate, or strong.
- Contraction frequency is measured in minutes, from the beginning of one contraction to the beginning of the next contraction.
- Contraction duration is measured in seconds, from the beginning to the end of the contraction.
- To evaluate uterine resting tone, or relaxation between contractions, the examiner should keep his or her hand on the fundus after the contraction is over. Resting tone between contractions is usually described as soft or relaxed.

Electronic Fetal Monitoring (EFM)

There are two modes of electronic FHR and contraction monitoring: external and internal. See Table 3-1 for differences in these monitoring modes.

Standardized Definitions for FHR Monitoring

Baseline Patterns

Baseline FHR: average FHR during a 10-minute period that excludes periodic and episodic changes and periods of marked variability; the normal range at term is 110 to 160 beats/min. Baseline FHR is recorded as a single number, not a range.

Bradycardia: baseline FHR less than 110 beats/min and lasting for 10 minutes or longer

Tachycardia: baseline FHR more than 160 beats/min and lasting for 10 minutes or longer

Causes, clinical significance, and nursing interventions for tachycardia and bradycardia are listed in Table 3-2.

FHR variability: normal irregularity of fetal cardiac rhythm or fluctuations from the baseline FHR of two cycles or more; the four possible categories of variability are absent, minimal, moderate, and marked. Figure 3-4 shows the four possible categories of variability.

Periodic and Episodic Patterns

Acceleration: a visually apparent, abrupt (onset to peak <30 seconds) increase in FHR above the baseline rate; the increase is 15 beats/min or greater and lasts 15 seconds or more, with the return to baseline less than 2 minutes from the beginning of the

TABLE 3-1

External and Internal Modes of Monitoring

EXTERNAL MODE	INTERNAL MODE
FETAL HEART RATE	
Ultrasound transducer: High-frequency sound waves reflect mechanical action of the fetal heart. Noninvasive. Does not require rupture of membranes or cervical dilation. Used during both the antepartum and intrapartum periods.	Spiral electrode: Converts the fetal ECG as obtained from the presenting part to the FHR via a cardiotachometer. Can be used only when membranes are ruptured and the cervix is sufficiently dilated during the intrapartum period. Electrode penetrates into fetal presenting part by 1.5 mm and must be attached securely to ensure a good signal.
UTERINE ACTIVITY	
Tocotransducer: Monitors frequency and duration of contractions by means of a pressure-sensing device applied to the maternal abdomen. Used during both the antepartum and intrapartum periods.	Intrauterine pressure catheter (IUPC): Monitors the frequency, duration, and intensity of contractions. The two types of IUPCs are a fluid-filled system and a solid catheter. Both measure intrauterine pressure at the catheter tip and convert the pressure into millimeters of mercury on the uterine activity panel of the strip chart. Both can be used only when membranes are ruptured and the cervix is sufficiently dilated during the intrapartum period.

ECG, Electrocardiogram; *FHR,* fetal heart rate.

acceleration; an acceleration lasting more than 10 minutes is considered a baseline change

Figure 3-5 shows an example of accelerations. Box 3-5 lists causes, clinical significance, and nursing interventions for accelerations.

Deceleration: there are four types of FHR decelerations that may occur in labor: early, late, variable, and prolonged; FHR decelerations

TABLE 3-2

Tachycardia and Bradycardia

TACHYCARDIA	BRADYCARDIA
DEFINITION	
FHR >160 beats/min lasting >10 min	FHR <110 beats/min lasting >10 min
POSSIBLE CAUSES	
Early fetal hypoxemia	Atrioventricular dissociation (heart block)
Fetal cardiac arrhythmias	Structural defects
Maternal fever	Viral infections (e.g., cytomegalovirus)
Infection (including chorioamnionitis)	Medications
Parasympatholytic drugs (atropine, hydroxyzine)	Fetal heart failure
β-Sympathomimetic drugs (terbutaline)	Maternal hypoglycemia
Maternal hyperthyroidism	Maternal hypothermia
Fetal anemia	
Drugs (caffeine, cocaine, methamphetamines)	
CLINICAL SIGNIFICANCE	
Persistent tachycardia in the absence of periodic changes does not appear serious in terms of neonatal outcome (especially true if tachycardia is associated with maternal fever); tachycardia is abnormal when associated with late decelerations, severe variable decelerations, or absent variability.	Baseline bradycardia alone is not specifically related to fetal oxygenation. The clinical significance of bradycardia depends on the underlying cause and the accompanying FHR patterns, including variability, accelerations, or decelerations.
NURSING INTERVENTIONS	
Dependent on cause; reduce maternal fever with antipyretics as ordered and cooling measures; oxygen at 8 or 10 L/min by nonrebreather face mask may be of some value; carry out health care provider's orders based on alleviating cause.	Dependent on cause

FHR, fetal heart rate.

are defined according to their visual relation to the onset and end of a contraction and by their shape.

Early deceleration: a visually apparent gradual (onset to lowest point 30 seconds or more) decrease in and return to the baseline FHR associated with uterine contractions (UCs); generally the onset, nadir, and recovery of the deceleration correspond to the beginning, peak, and end of the contraction.

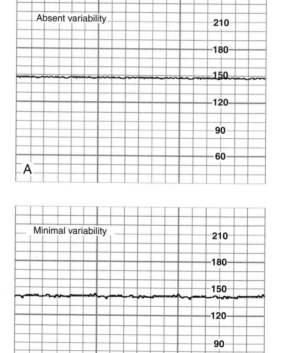

Fig. 3-4 Fetal heart rate variability. **A,** Absent variability; amplitude range undetectable. **B,** Minimal variability; amplitude range detectable up to and including 5 beats/min.

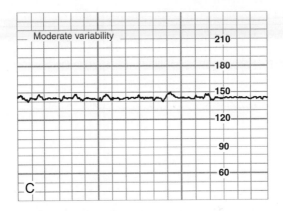

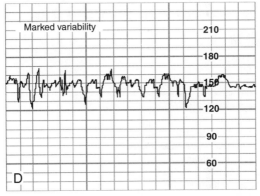

Fig. 3-4 cont'd C, Moderate variability; amplitude range 6 to 25 beats/min. **D,** Marked variability; amplitude range more than 25 beats/min. (From Tucker, S., Miller, L., & Miller, D. [2009]. *Mosby's pocket guide to fetal monitoring: A multidisciplinary approach* [6th ed.]. St. Louis: Mosby.

Figure 3-6 shows an example of early decelerations. Box 3-6 lists causes, clinical significance, and nursing interventions for early decelerations.

Late deceleration: a visually apparent gradual (onset to lowest point 30 seconds or more) decrease in and return to baseline FHR associated with UCs; the deceleration begins after the contraction has started, and the lowest point of the deceleration occurs after

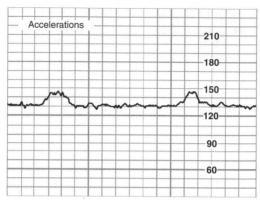

Fig. 3-5 Accelerations. (From Tucker, S., Miller, L., & Miller, D. [2009]. *Mosby's pocket guide to fetal monitoring: A multidisciplinary approach* [6th ed.]. St. Louis: Mosby.

BOX 3-5

Accelerations

CAUSES
- Spontaneous fetal movement
- Vaginal examination
- Electrode application
- Fetal scalp stimulation
- Fetal reaction to external sounds
- Breech presentation
- Occiput posterior position
- Uterine contractions
- Fundal pressure
- Abdominal palpation

CLINICAL SIGNIFICANCE
Normal pattern. Acceleration with fetal movement signifies fetal well-being representing fetal alertness or arousal states.

NURSING INTERVENTIONS
None required

---

the peak of the contraction; the deceleration usually does not return to baseline until after the contraction is over.

Figure 3-7 shows an example of late decelerations. Box 3-7 lists causes, clinical significance, and nursing interventions for late decelerations.

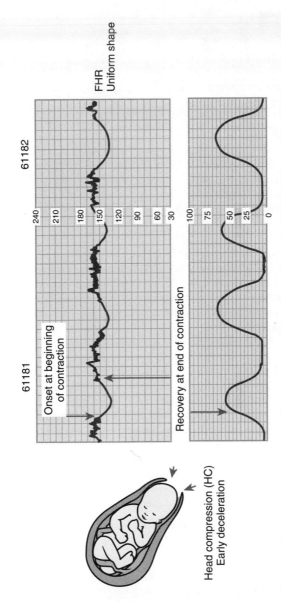

Fig. 3-6 Early decelerations caused by head compression. (From Tucker, S. [2004]. *Pocket guide to fetal monitoring and assessment* [5th ed.]. St. Louis: Mosby.)

BOX 3-6

Early Decelerations

CAUSE
Head compression resulting from the following:
- Uterine contractions
- Vaginal examination
- Fundal pressure
- Placement of internal mode of monitoring

CLINICAL SIGNIFICANCE
Normal pattern. Not associated with fetal hypoxemia, acidemia, or low Apgar scores

NURSING INTERVENTIONS
None required

Variable deceleration: a visually abrupt (onset to lowest point <30 seconds) decrease in FHR below the baseline; the decrease is 15 beats/min or more, lasts at least 15 seconds, and returns to baseline in less than 2 minutes from the time of onset; variable decelerations are not necessarily associated with UCs; they have a U, V, or W shape

Figure 3-8 shows an example of variable decelerations. Box 3-8 lists causes, clinical significance, and nursing interventions for variable decelerations.

Prolonged deceleration: a visually apparent decrease (may be either gradual or abrupt) in FHR of at least 15 beats/min below the baseline and lasting more than 2 minutes but less than 10 minutes; a deceleration lasting more than 10 minutes is considered a baseline change

Figure 3-9 shows an example of prolonged decelerations. Prolonged decelerations indicate a disruption in the fetal oxygen supply. They may be caused by prolonged cord compression, profound uteroplacental insufficiency, or sustained head compression.

Nursing Responsibilities Related to Fetal Monitoring

Assessment of FHR and UA Tracings

- Ensure that the monitor is recording FHR and UA accurately and that the tracing is interpretable.

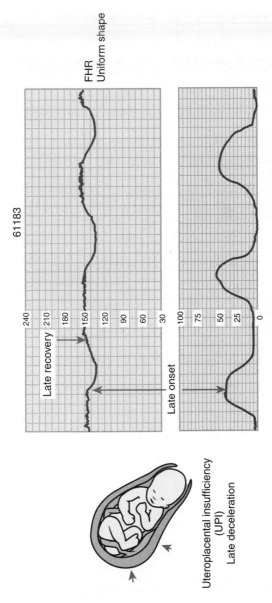

Fig. 3-7 Late decelerations caused by uteroplacental insufficiency. (From Tucker, S. [2004]. *Pocket guide to fetal monitoring and assessment* [5th ed.]. St. Louis: Mosby.)

- Assess the FHR and UA tracings regularly throughout labor.
  - ❑ Assessment should be performed at least every 30 minutes during the first stage of labor and every 15 minutes during the second stage of labor in low risk women. If risk factors are present, assess every 15 minutes in the first stage of labor and every 5 minutes in the second stage of labor.

BOX 3-7

Late Decelerations

CAUSE
Uteroplacental insufficiency caused by the following:
- Uterine tachysystole
- Maternal supine hypotension
- Epidural or spinal anesthesia
- Placenta previa
- Placental abruption
- Hypertensive disorders
- Postmaturity
- Intrauterine growth restriction
- Diabetes mellitus
- Intraamniotic infection

CLINICAL SIGNIFICANCE
Abnormal pattern associated with fetal hypoxemia, acidemia, and low Apgar scores; considered ominous if persistent and uncorrected, especially when associated with fetal tachycardia and loss of variability

NURSING INTERVENTIONS
The usual priority is as follows:
1. Change maternal position (lateral).
2. Correct maternal hypotension by elevating legs.
3. Increase rate of maintenance intravenous solution.
4. Palpate uterus to assess for tachysystole.
5. Discontinue oxytocin if infusing.
6. Administer oxygen at 8-10 L/min by nonrebreather face mask.
7. Notify physician or nurse-midwife.
8. Consider internal monitoring for a more accurate fetal and uterine assessment.
9. Assist with birth (cesarean or vaginal assisted) if pattern cannot be corrected.

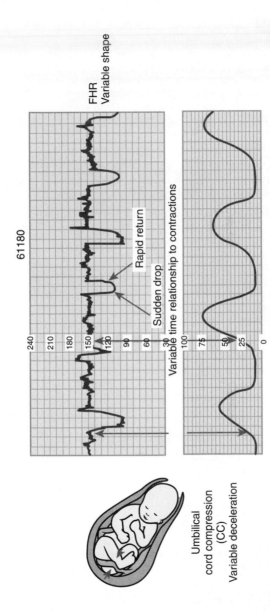

Fig. 3-8 Variable decelerations caused by cord compression. (From Tucker, S. [2004]. *Pocket guide to fetal monitoring and assessment* [5th ed.]. St. Louis: Mosby.)

BOX 3-8

Variable Decelerations

CAUSE
Umbilical cord compression caused by the following:
- Maternal position with cord between fetus and maternal pelvis
- Cord around fetal neck, arm, leg, or other body part
- Short cord
- Knot in cord
- Prolapsed cord

CLINICAL SIGNIFICANCE
Variable decelerations occur in approximately 50% of all labors and usually are transient and correctable.

NURSING INTERVENTIONS
The usual priority is as follows:
1. Change maternal position (side to side, knee-chest).
2. Discontinue oxytocin if infusing.
3. Administer oxygen at 8-10 L/min by nonrebreather face mask.
4. Notify physician or nurse-midwife.
5. Assist with vaginal or speculum examination to assess for cord prolapse.
6. Assist with amnioinfusion if ordered.
7. Assist with birth (vaginal assisted or cesarean) if pattern cannot be corrected.

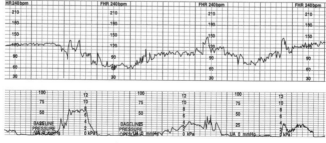

Fig. 3-9 Prolonged decelerations. (From Tucker, S., Miller, L., & Miller, D. [2009]. *Mosby's pocket guide to fetal monitoring: A multidisciplinary approach* [6th ed.]. St. Louis: Mosby.

- FHR tracing assessment
  - ❏ Baseline rate
  - ❏ Baseline variability (absent, minimal, moderate, or marked)
  - ❏ Presence of accelerations
  - ❏ Presence of early, late, variable, or prolonged decelerations
  - ❏ Changes in the FHR pattern over time
- UA tracing assessment
  - ❏ Contraction frequency
  - ❏ Contraction duration
  - ❏ Contraction intensity
  - ❏ Uterine resting tone

Interpretation of FHR and UA Tracings

- Box 3-9 lists a three-tier classification system for FHR tracings with examples of patterns for each category.
  - ❏ Category I FHR tracings are normal. They are strongly predictive of normal fetal acid-base status at the time of observation. These tracings may be followed in a routine manner and do not require any specific action.
  - ❏ Category II FHR tracings are indeterminate. This category includes all tracings that do not meet category I or category III criteria. Category II tracings require continued observation and evaluation.
  - ❏ Category III FHR tracings are abnormal. Immediate evaluation and prompt intervention are required when these patterns are identified.
- Table 3-3 describes normal UA characteristics during labor.
- Montevideo Units (MVUs) are a method of using the intrauterine pressure catheter (IUPC) to evaluate the adequacy of UA for achieving progress in labor.
  - ❏ MVUs are calculated by subtracting the baseline uterine pressure from the peak contraction pressure for each contraction that occurs in a 10 minute window, and then adding together the pressures generated by each contraction that occurs during that period of time.

Management of Abnormal FHR and UA Tracings

- Whenever the FHR or UA tracing is assessed as abnormal, corrective measures must immediately be taken to improve fetal oxygenation.

BOX 3-9

Three-Tier Fetal Heart Rate Classification System

CATEGORY I

Category 1 fetal heart rate (FHR) tracings include all of the following:

- Baseline rate 110-160 beats/min
- Baseline FHR variability: moderate
- Late or variable decelerations: absent
- Early decelerations: either present or absent
- Accelerations: either present or absent

CATEGORY II

Category II FHR tracings include all FHR tracings not categorized as category I or category III. Examples of category II tracings include any of the following:

- Baseline rate
  - Bradycardia not accompanied by absent baseline variability
  - Tachycardia
- Baseline FHR variability
  - Minimal baseline variability
  - Absent baseline variability not accompanied by recurrent decelerations
  - Marked baseline variability
- Accelerations
  - No acceleration produced in response to fetal stimulation
- Periodic or episodic decelerations
  - Recurrent variable decelerations accompanied by minimal or moderate baseline variability
  - Prolonged deceleration (≥ 2 but <10 min)
  - Recurrent late decelerations with moderate baseline variability
  - Variable decelerations with other characteristics, such as slow return to baseline, "overshoots" or "shoulders"

CATEGORY III

Category III FHR tracings include either:

- Absent baseline variability and any of the following:
  - Recurrent late decelerations
  - Recurrent variable decelerations
  - Bradycardia
- Sinusoidal pattern

Source: Macones, G., Hankins, G., Spong, C., Hauth, J., & Moore, T. (2008). The 2008 National Institute of Child Health and Human Development Workshop Report on Electronic Fetal Monitoring: Update on definitions, interpretation, and research guidelines. *Journal of Obstetric, Gynecologic and Neonatal Nursing, 37*(5), 510-515.

TABLE 3-3

Normal Uterine Activity During Labor

CHARACTERISTIC	DESCRIPTION
Frequency	Contraction frequency overall generally ranges from two to five per 10 min during labor, with lower frequencies seen in the first stage of labor and higher frequencies (up to five contractions in 10 min) seen during the second stage of labor.
Duration	Contraction duration remains fairly stable throughout the first and second stages, ranging from 45-80 sec, not generally exceeding 90 sec.
Intensity (peak less resting tone)	Intensity of uterine contractions generally ranges from 25-50 mm Hg in the first stage of labor and may rise to more than 80 mm Hg in second stage. Contractions palpated as "mild" would likely peak at less than 50 mm Hg if measured internally, whereas contractions palpated as "moderate" or greater would likely peak at 50 mm Hg or greater if measured internally.
Resting tone	Average resting tone during labor is 10 mm Hg; if using palpation, should palpate as "soft" (i.e., easily indented, no palpable resistance).
Montevideo units (MVUs)	Ranges from 100-250 MVUs in the first stage, may rise to 300-400 in the second stage. Contraction intensities of 40 mm Hg or more and MVUs of 80-120 are generally sufficient to initiate spontaneous labor. MVUs are used only with internal monitoring of contractions.

Sources: Tucker, S., Miller, L., & Miller, D. (2009). *Mosby's pocket guide to fetal monitoring: A multidisciplinary approach* (6th ed.). St. Louis: Mosby; Macones, G., Hankins, G., Spong, C., Hauth, J., & Moore, T. (2008). The 2008 National Institute of Child Health and Human Development Workshop Report on Electronic Fetal Monitoring: Update on definitions, interpretation, and research guidelines. *Journal of Obstetric, Gynecologic and Neonatal Nursing, 37*(5), 510-515.

- Box 3-10 lists basic interventions as well as interventions for specific problems. (Also see Table 3-2 and Boxes 3-7 and 3-8 for interventions for tachycardia, late decelerations, and variable decelerations.)
- Report abnormal patterns to the primary health care provider.
- Document observations and actions according to the established standard of care.

BOX 3-10

Management of Abnormal Fetal Heart Rate and Uterine Activity Patterns

BASIC INTERVENTIONS
- Administer oxygen by nonrebreather face mask at a rate of 8-10 L/min.
- Assist the woman to a side-lying (lateral) position.
- Increase maternal blood volume by increasing the rate of the primary IV infusion.

INTERVENTIONS FOR SPECIFIC PROBLEMS
- Maternal hypotension
  - ❏ Increase the rate of the primary IV infusion.
  - ❏ Change to lateral or Trendelenburg positioning.
  - ❏ Administer ephedrine or phenylephrine if other measures are unsuccessful in increasing blood pressure.
- Uterine tachysystole
  - ❏ Reduce the dose of or discontinue the dose of any uterine stimulants in use (e.g., oxytocin [Pitocin]).
  - ❏ Administer a uterine relaxant (tocolytic) (e.g., terbutaline [Brethine]).
- Abnormal FHR pattern during the second stage of labor
  - ❏ Use open-glottis pushing.
  - ❏ Use fewer pushing efforts during each contraction.
  - ❏ Make individual pushing efforts shorter.
  - ❏ Push only with every other or every third contraction.
  - ❏ Push only with a perceived urge to push (in women with regional anesthesia).

FHR, Fetal heart rate; *IV,* intravenous.

LEGAL TIP   Fetal Monitoring Standards

Nurses who care for women during childbirth are legally responsible for correctly interpreting FHR patterns, initiating appropriate nursing interventions based on those patterns, and documenting the outcomes of those interventions. Perinatal nurses are responsible for the timely notification of the physician or nurse-midwife in the event of abnormal (nonreassuring) FHR patterns. Perinatal nurses also are responsible for initiating the institutional chain of command should differences in opinion arise among health care providers concerning the interpretation of the FHR pattern and the intervention required.

Other Methods of Assessment

A major shortcoming of EFM is its high rate of false-positive results. Even the most abnormal patterns are poorly predictive of neonatal morbidity. Therefore, other methods of assessment have been developed to evaluate fetal status such as fetal scalp stimulation, vibroacoustic stimulation, and umbilical cord acid-base determination.

Fetal Response to Stimulation

- Methods of stimulation
  - Scalp—digital pressure on the fetal presenting part during a vaginal examination
  - Vibroacoustic—placing an artificial larynx or fetal acoustic stimulation device on the maternal abdomen over the fetal head for 1 to 5 seconds
- Desired result—FHR acceleration of 15 beats for at least 15 seconds
  - If the fetus does not respond to stimulation with an acceleration, fetal compromise is not necessarily indicated; however, further evaluation of fetal well-being is needed.

NURSING ALERT *Fetal stimulation should be performed at times when the FHR is at baseline. Neither fetal scalp stimulation nor vibroacoustic stimulation should be instituted if FHR decelerations or bradycardia is present.*

Umbilical Cord Acid-Base Determination

- Immediately after birth, blood is drawn from the umbilical artery and the umbilical vein and tested for pH, Pco_2, Po_2, and base deficit or base excess.
  - Umbilical arterial values reflect fetal condition, whereas umbilical vein values indicate placental function.
- Normal umbilical artery and vein cord blood values are listed in Table 3-4. Normal findings rule out the presence of acidemia at, or immediately before, birth.
- It is useful in addition to the Apgar score (see Table 7-1) for assessing the immediate condition of the newborn.
- If acidemia is present (e.g., pH <7.20), then the type of acidemia is determined (respiratory, metabolic, or mixed) by analyzing the blood gas values (Table 3-5).

TABLE 3-4

Approximate Normal Values for Cord Blood

CORD BLOOD	pH	CARBON DIOXIDE PRESSURE (P_{CO_2}) (mm Hg)	OXYGEN PRESSURE (P_{O_2}) (mm Hg)	BASE DEFICIT (mmol/L)
Artery	7.2-7.3	45-55	15-25	<12
Vein	7.3-7.4	35-45	25-35	<12

Source: Tucker, S., Miller, L., & Miller, D. (2009). *Mosby's pocket guide to fetal monitoring: A multidisciplinary approach* (6th ed.). St. Louis: Mosby.

TABLE 3-5

Types of Acidemia

BLOOD GASES	RESPIRATORY	METABOLIC	MIXED
pH	<7.20	<7.20	<7.20
Carbon dioxide pressure (P_{CO_2})	Elevated	Normal	Elevated
Base deficit	<12 mmol/L	≥12 mmol/L	≥12 mmol/L

Source: Tucker, S., Miller, L., & Miller, D. (2009). *Mosby's pocket guide to fetal monitoring: A multidisciplinary approach* (6th ed.). St. Louis: Mosby.

Other Interventions

Amnioinfusion and tocolytic therapy are two interventions often used in an attempt to improve abnormal FHR patterns.

Amnioinfusion

- Amnioinfusion is infusion of room-temperature isotonic fluid (usually normal saline or lactated Ringer's solution) into the uterine cavity if the volume of amniotic fluid is low.
- The purpose of amnioinfusion is to relieve intermittent umbilical cord compression that results in variable decelerations and transient fetal hypoxemia by restoring the amniotic fluid volume to a normal or near-normal level.
- Fluid is administered through an intrauterine pressure catheter either by gravity flow or by use of an infusion pump. Usually a bolus of fluid is administered over 20 to 30 minutes, and then the infusion is slowed to a maintenance rate.
- Intensity and frequency of UCs should be continually assessed during the procedure.

- The recorded uterine resting tone during amnioinfusion will appear higher than normal because of resistance to outflow and turbulence at the end of the catheter. Uterine resting tone should not exceed 40 mm Hg during the procedure.
- The amount of fluid return must be estimated and documented during amnioinfusion to prevent overdistention of the uterus. The volume of fluid returned should be approximately the same as the amount infused.

Tocolytic Therapy

- Tocolytic therapy is administering medications that cause relaxation of the uterus by inhibiting UCs
- May be implemented when other interventions to reduce uterine activity, such as position change, hydration, and discontinuance of an oxytocin infusion, have not been effective
- Frequently implemented after a decision for cesarean birth has been made while preparations for surgery are under way
- A commonly used medication in these situations is terbutaline (Brethine), given subcutaneously. (See the Medication Guide: Tocolytic Therapy for Preterm Labor in Appendix B for more information on terbutaline.)

DISCOMFORT DURING LABOR AND BIRTH
Sources of Pain in Labor
Visceral Origin (First Stage of Labor)

- Cervical effacement and dilation
- Distention of the lower uterine segment
- Uterine ischemia
- Referred pain that originates in the uterus and radiates to the abdominal wall, lumbosacral area of the back, iliac crests, gluteal area, thighs, and lower back

Somatic Origin (Second Stage of Labor)

Somatic origin pain is often described as intense, sharp, burning, and well localized.

- Stretching and distention of perineal tissues and the pelvic floor
- Distention and traction on the peritoneum and uterocervical supports during contractions
- Pressure exerted by the presenting part on the bladder and rectum
- Lacerations of soft tissue (cervix, vagina, perineum)

Factors Influencing Pain Response

- Physiology
- Culture
- Anxiety
- Previous experience
- Childbirth preparation
- Comfort and support
- Environment

Selected Measures for Nonpharmacologic Management of Discomfort

Many nonpharmacologic methods for relief of discomfort require practice for best results, although some may be used successfully without the woman or couple having prior knowledge. The analgesic effect of many nonpharmacologic measures is comparable to or even superior to opioids that are administered parenterally. Nonpharmacologic methods are relatively inexpensive and safe with few if any major adverse reactions. They can be used throughout labor but are especially effective for relaxation and pain relief in early labor. Women should be encouraged to try a variety of methods and to seek alternatives, including pharmacologic methods, if the measure being used is no longer effective. Box 3-11 lists several nonpharmacologic methods to encourage relaxation and relieve pain.

Relaxing and Breathing Techniques

- Attention focusing—as the contraction begins the woman focuses on a chosen object and performs a breathing technique to reduce her perception of pain.
- Imagery—the woman focuses her attention on a pleasant scene, a place where she feels relaxed, or an activity she enjoys.
- Breathing techniques—different approaches to childbirth preparation stress various breathing techniques to provide distraction, thereby reducing the perception of pain and helping the woman maintain control throughout contractions. All patterns begin and end with a deep relaxing and cleansing breath. As labor progresses, the woman will need to change to more complex breathing techniques. Box 3-12 lists several paced breathing techniques.

BOX 3-11

Nonpharmacologic Strategies to Encourage Relaxation and Relieve Pain

CUTANEOUS STIMULATION STRATEGIES
- Counterpressure
- Effleurage (light massage)
- Therapeutic touch and massage
- Walking
- Rocking
- Changing positions
- Application of heat or cold
- Transcutaneous electrical nerve stimulation (TENS)
- Acupressure
- Water therapy (showers, whirlpool baths)
- Intradermal water block

SENSORY STIMULATION STRATEGIES
- Aromatherapy
- Breathing techniques
- Music
- Imagery
- Use of focal points

COGNITIVE STRATEGIES
- Childbirth education
- Hypnosis
- Biofeedback

Effleurage and Counterpressure

- Effleurage is light stroking, usually of the abdomen, in rhythm with breathing during contractions.
  - ❑ Used to distract the woman from contraction pain
  - ❑ As labor progresses, hyperesthesia may make effleurage uncomfortable and thus less effective

Counterpressure is steady pressure applied by a support person to the sacral area using a firm object (e.g., tennis ball) or the fist or heel of the hand.

- Helps the woman cope with the sensations of internal pressure and pain in the lower back
- Especially helpful when back pain is caused by pressure of the occiput against spinal nerves when the fetal head is in a posterior position

BOX 3-12

Paced Breathing Techniques

CLEANSING BREATH
- Relaxed breath in through nose and out through mouth. Used at the beginning and end of each contraction.

SLOW-PACED BREATHING
(Approximately 6 to 8 breaths/min)
- Performed at approximately half the normal breathing rate (number of breaths/min divided by 2)
- IN-2-3-4/OUT-2-3-4/IN-2-3-4/OUT-2-3-4...

MODIFIED-PACED BREATHING
(Approximately 32 to 40 breaths/min)
- Performed at about twice the normal breathing rate (number of breaths per minute multiplied by 2)
- IN-OUT/IN-OUT/IN-OUT/IN-OUT...
- For more flexibility and variety, the woman may combine the slow and modified breathing by using the slow breathing for beginnings and ends of contractions and modified breathing for more intense peaks. This technique conserves energy, lessens fatigue, and reduces risk for hyperventilation.

PATTERNED-PACED OR PANT-BLOW BREATHING
(Same rate as modified)
- Enhances concentration
   3:1 Patterned breathing: IN-OUT/IN-OUT/IN-OUT/IN-BLOW (repeat through contraction)
   4:1 Patterned breathing: IN-OUT/IN-OUT/IN-OUT/IN-OUT/IN-BLOW (repeat through contraction)

Sources: Nichols, F. (2000). Paced breathing techniques. In F. Nichols & S. Humenick (Eds.), *Childbirth education: Practice, research, and theory* (2nd ed.). Philadelphia: Saunders; Perinatal Education Associates. (2008). *Breathing*. Available at www.birthsource.com/scripts/article.asp?articleid=211. Accessed September 24, 2010.

- May also be applied bilaterally to the hips or knees to reduce low back pain

Selected Measures for Pharmacologic Management of Discomfort

Pharmacologic measures are often used in addition to nonpharmacologic techniques as labor becomes more active and discomfort and pain intensify. Most women opt for some pharmacologic support in labor.

Epidural anesthesia and analgesia are especially popular in the United States, and their use has been increasing.

The goal of anesthesia and analgesia use during labor is to provide adequate pain relief without increasing maternal or fetal risk or affecting the progress of labor. The type of analgesic or anesthetic chosen is determined in part by the stage of labor and by the method of birth planned.

Systemic Analgesia

- Use is declining although it still remains the major pharmacologic method for relieving the pain of labor when personnel trained in regional (epidural) anesthesia are not available.
- Intravenous (IV) administration is preferable to intramuscular (IM) injection because the medication's onset of action is faster and more predictable; as a result, a higher level of pain relief usually occurs with smaller doses. Also the duration of effect is more predictable.
- IV medication is injected slowly through the port nearest the woman (proximal port) in small doses during a contraction to decrease fetal exposure to the medication. It may be injected over a period of three to five consecutive contractions if needed to complete the dose.
- It is recommended that the administration of systemic opioid analgesics be delayed until labor is well established.

Effects on the Fetus/Newborn

- Analgesics cross the fetal blood-brain barrier more readily than they cross the maternal blood-brain barrier.
- Duration of action will be longer than in the mother because the systemic analgesics used during labor have a significantly longer half-life in the fetus and newborn.
- Fetal/newborn effects can include the following:
  - ❑ Respiratory depression
  - ❑ Decreased alertness
  - ❑ Delayed sucking

Opioid Agonist Analgesics

- Medications in this classification that are commonly prescribed in labor include the following:
  - ❑ Hydromorphone hydrochloride (Dilaudid)

- ❏ Meperidine hydrochloride (Demerol)
    - ○ Meperidine hydrochloride used to be the most commonly used opioid agonist analgesic for women in labor, but is no longer the preferred choice because other medications have fewer side effects. In particular, the accumulation of normeperidine, a toxic metabolite of meperidine, causes prolonged neonatal sedation and neurobehavioral changes that are evident for the first 2 to 3 days of life.
- ❏ Fentanyl (Sublimaze)
- ❏ Sufentanil citrate (Sufenta)
- ■ These medications are effective for relieving severe, persistent, or recurrent pain.
- ■ They have no amnesic effect but create a feeling of well-being or euphoria and enhance the woman's ability to rest between contractions.
- ■ They slow gastric emptying and increase nausea and vomiting.
- ■ Bladder and bowel elimination can be inhibited.
- ■ They should be used cautiously in women with respiratory and cardiovascular disorders.
- ■ Safety precautions should be observed because sedation and dizziness can occur following administration.

SAFETY ALERT *Opioids decrease maternal heart and respiratory rate and blood pressure, thereby affecting fetal oxygenation. Therefore, maternal vital signs and FHR and pattern must be assessed and documented prior to and after administration of opioids for pain relief.*

- ■ Ideally, birth should occur less than 1 hour or more than 4 hours after administration of an opioid agonist analgesic so that neonatal central nervous system (CNS) depression is minimized.
- ■ See the Medication Guide: Opioid Agonist Analgesics in Appendix B.

Opioid Agonist–Antagonist Analgesics

- ■ Medications in this classification that are commonly prescribed during labor include the following:
    - ❏ Butorphanol (Stadol)
    - ❏ Nalbuphine (Nubain)
- ■ These medications provide adequate analgesia without causing significant respiratory depression in the mother or neonate.

- They are less likely to cause nausea and vomiting, but sedation may be as great or greater when compared with opioid agonist analgesics.
- IM, subcutaneous, or IV routes of administration can be used, but the IV route is preferred.

See the Medication Guide: Opioid Agonist–Antagonist Analgesics in Appendix B.

> **NURSING ALERT** *An opioid antagonist should not be given to an opioid-dependent woman because it may precipitate abstinence syndrome (withdrawal symptoms) in both the mother and her newborn.*

Nerve Block Analgesia and Anesthesia

Local anesthetic agents are used to produce regional analgesia (some pain relief and motor block) and anesthesia (complete pain relief and motor block). Local anesthetics work primarily by temporarily interrupting the conduction of nerve impulses, notably pain.

Local Perineal Infiltration Anesthesia

Local anesthetic is injected into the skin and then subcutaneously into the region to be anesthetized.

- Epinephrine is often added to localize and intensify the effect of the anesthesia in a region and to prevent excessive bleeding and systemic absorption by constricting local blood vessels.
- Local anesthetic is often used when an episiotomy is to be performed or when lacerations need to be sutured after birth in a woman who does not have regional anesthesia.
- It rapidly becomes effective.
- Anesthetic effect may be prolonged as needed by repeating injections.

Spinal Anesthesia (Block)

An anesthetic solution alone or in combination with an opioid agonist analgesic is injected through the third, fourth, or fifth lumbar interspace into the subarachnoid space.

- Use of spinal anesthesia (block) for both elective and emergent cesarean births has increased. Low spinal anesthesia (block) may be used for vaginal birth but is not suitable for labor.

- Usually the level of the block will be complete and fixed within 5 to 10 minutes after the anesthetic solution is injected but it can continue to creep upward for 20 minutes or longer. The anesthetic effect will last 1 to 3 hours, depending on the type of agent used.

Advantages

- Ease of administration
- No fetal hypoxia if woman remains normotensive
- Woman remains conscious
- Excellent muscular relaxation
- No excessive blood loss

Disadvantages

- Allergic reaction to the medication or medications used
- Hypotension
- Ineffective breathing pattern
- Increased risk for operative vaginal or cesarean birth
- Bladder and uterine atony after birth
- Postdural puncture headache (spinal headache)

Epidural Anesthesia and Analgesia

A local anesthetic agent, an opioid analgesic, or both is injected into the epidural space, usually between the fourth and fifth lumbar vertebrae. Depending on the type, amount, and number of medications used, an anesthetic or analgesic effect will occur with varying degrees of motor impairment.

- Most effective available pharmacologic pain relief method for labor
- Most commonly used method for relieving pain during labor in the United States. Nearly two thirds of American women in labor choose epidural analgesia.
- Can be used effectively for labor, vaginal birth, and cesarean birth
- Epidural anesthesia in early labor does not increase the rate of cesarean birth and may shorten the duration of labor. Consequently, women in labor must no longer reach a certain level of cervical dilation or fetal station before receiving epidural anesthesia.

NURSING ALERT *Epidural anesthesia effectively relieves the pain caused by uterine contractions. For most women, however, it does not completely remove the pressure sensations that occur as the fetus descends in the pelvis.*

Advantages

- Woman remains alert, is more comfortable and able to participate
- Good relaxation achieved
- Airway reflexes remain intact
- Only partial motor paralysis develops
- Gastric emptying not delayed
- Blood loss not excessive
- The dose, volume, type, and number of medications used can be modified to allow the woman to push, to assume upright positions and even walk, to produce perineal anesthesia, and to permit forceps-assisted, vacuum-assisted, or cesarean birth if required.

Disadvantages

Associated with a number of side effects, including:

- Hypotension (see the Emergency box)
- Local anesthetic toxicity
  - ☐ Lightheadedness
  - ☐ Dizziness
  - ☐ Tinnitus (ringing in the ears)
  - ☐ Metallic taste
  - ☐ Numbness of the tongue and mouth
  - ☐ Bizarre behavior
  - ☐ Slurred speech
  - ☐ Convulsions
  - ☐ Loss of consciousness
- High or total spinal anesthesia
- Fever
- Urinary retention
- Pruritus (itching)
- Limited movement
- Longer second-stage labor
- Increased use of oxytocin
- Increased likelihood of forceps- or vacuum-assisted birth

Combined Spinal-Epidural (CSE) Analgesia

An opioid is injected into the subarachnoid space for rapid pain relief. A catheter is then placed in the epidural space to extend the duration of the analgesia by using a local anesthetic agent alone or in combination

EMERGENCY

Maternal Hypotension with Decreased Placental Perfusion

SIGNS AND SYMPTOMS
- Maternal hypotension (20% decrease from preblock baseline level or ≤100 mm Hg systolic)
- Fetal bradycardia
- Absent or minimal FHR variability

INTERVENTIONS
- Turn woman to lateral position or place pillow or wedge under hip to displace uterus.
- Maintain IV infusion at rate specified, or increase administration as needed per hospital protocol.
- Administer oxygen by nonrebreather face mask at 10 to 12 L/min or per protocol.
- Elevate the woman's legs.
- Notify the primary health care provider, anesthesiologist, or nurse anesthetist.
- Administer IV vasopressor (e.g., ephedrine 5-10 mg or phenylephrine 50-100 mcg) per protocol if previous measures are ineffective.
- Remain with woman; continue to monitor maternal blood pressure and FHR every 5 min until her condition is stable or per primary health care provider's order.

with an opioid agonist analgesic. The CSE technique is an increasingly popular approach that can be used to block pain transmission without compromising motor ability.

Advantages

- More motor function enables the woman to change positions and use upright positions for labor more easily
- Facilitates more effective bearing-down efforts, thereby reducing the risk for forceps- or vacuum-assisted birth

Disadvantages

- Associated with a greater incidence of FHR abnormalities than epidural analgesia alone

Epidural and Intrathecal (Spinal) Opioids

Opioids are injected alone (without local anesthetic agents) into the epidural or subarachnoid space. Commonly used opioids include fentanyl, sufentanil, and preservative-free morphine.

Advantages

- Does not cause maternal hypotension or affect vital signs
- Woman feels contractions but no pain
- Ability to bear down during the second stage of labor is preserved because the pushing reflex is not lost and motor power remains intact
- A more common indication for the administration of epidural or intrathecal analgesics is the relief of postoperative pain. For example, a woman who gives birth by cesarean can receive fentanyl or morphine through a catheter. The catheter may then be removed, and the woman is usually free of pain for 24 hours.
  - ❑ Women receiving epidurally administered morphine after a cesarean birth may ambulate sooner than women who do not. The early ambulation and freedom from pain also facilitate bladder emptying, enhance peristalsis, and prevent clot formation in the lower extremities (e.g., thrombophlebitis).
  - ❑ Women may require additional medication for pain during the first 24 hours after surgery. If so, they will usually be given ketorolac (Toradol), an NSAID, not IV or IM narcotics.

Disadvantages

- For most women, intrathecal opioids alone do not provide adequate analgesia for second-stage labor pain, episiotomy, or birth.
- Side effects: nausea, vomiting, itching, urinary retention, and delayed respiratory depression. These effects are more common when morphine is administered.
- Respiratory depression is a serious concern; for this reason, the woman's respiratory status should be assessed and documented every hour for 24 hours after administration, or as designated by hospital protocol.

Nursing Care of Women Receiving Spinal or Epidural Anesthesia

See Box 3-13.

BOX 3-13

Nursing Care of the Woman Receiving Spinal or Epidural Anesthesia

PRIOR TO THE BLOCK

- Assist the primary health care provider and/or anesthesia care provider with explaining the procedure and obtaining the woman's informed consent.
- Assess maternal vital signs, level of hydration, labor progress, and fetal heart rate (FHR) and pattern.
- Start an intravenous line and infuse a bolus of fluid (Ringer's lactate or normal saline) if ordered (e.g., 500 to 1000 ml 15 to 20 min prior to induction of the anesthesia).
- Obtain laboratory results (hematocrit or hemoglobin level, other tests as necessary).
- Assess the woman's level of pain using a pain scale (from 0 [no pain] to 10 [pain as bad as it could possibly be]).
- Assist the woman to void.

DURING INITIATION OF THE BLOCK

- Assist the woman with assuming and maintaining proper position.
- Verbally guide the woman through the procedure, explaining sounds and sensations as she experiences them.
- Assist the anesthesia care provider with documentation of vital signs, time and amount of medications given, etc.
- Monitor maternal vital signs (especially blood pressure) and FHR as ordered.
- Have oxygen and suction readily available.
- Monitor for signs of local anesthetic toxicity as the test dose of medication is administered.

WHILE THE BLOCK IS IN EFFECT

- Continue to monitor maternal vital signs and FHR as ordered (continuous monitoring of maternal heart rate [electrocardiogram (ECG)] and blood pressure may be ordered to monitor for accidental intravenous injection of medication).
- Continue to assess the woman's level of pain with every check of vital signs using a pain scale (from 0 [no pain] to 10 [pain as bad as it could possibly be]).
- Monitor for bladder distention.
  - ❑ Assist with spontaneous voiding on bedpan or toilet.
  - ❑ Insert urinary catheter if necessary.
- Encourage or assist the woman to change positions from side to side every hour.

BOX 3-13

**Nursing Care of the Woman Receiving Spinal
or Epidural Anesthesia—cont'd**

- Promote safety.
  - ❏ Keep the side rails up on the bed.
  - ❏ Place the telephone and call light within easy reach.
  - ❏ Instruct the woman not to get out of bed without help.
  - ❏ Make sure there is no prolonged pressure on anesthetized body parts.
- Keep the epidural catheter insertion site clean and dry.
- Continue to monitor for anesthetic side effects.

WHILE THE BLOCK IS WEARING OFF AFTER BIRTH
- Assess regularly for the return of sensory and motor function.
- Continue to monitor maternal vital signs as ordered.
- Monitor for bladder distention.
  - ❏ Assist with spontaneous voiding on bedpan or toilet.
  - ❏ Insert urinary catheter if necessary.
- Promote safety.
  - ❏ Keep the side rails up on the bed.
  - ❏ Place the telephone and call light within easy reach.
  - ❏ Instruct the woman not to get out of bed without help.
  - ❏ Make sure there is no prolonged pressure on anesthetized body parts.
- Keep the epidural catheter insertion site clean and dry.
- Continue to monitor for anesthetic side effects.

General Anesthesia

The woman is "put to sleep" and rendered totally unconscious through the administration of several different medications. General anesthesia is rarely used for uncomplicated vaginal birth and is infrequently used for elective cesarean birth.

Indications

- Contraindication to spinal or epidural block
- When rapid birth is necessary, without sufficient time or personnel to perform a block

Major Risks Associated with General Anesthesia

- Difficulty with or inability to intubate
- Aspiration of gastric contents

- Neonatal narcosis because of exposure to the anesthetic agents and CNS depressants administered to the woman

Preoperative Preparations

- Give woman nothing by mouth (e.g., make her NPO)
- Start an IV infusion
- Premedicate according to physician orders
  - ❑ Nonparticulate (clear) oral antacid to neutralize the acidic contents of the stomach (e.g., sodium citrate [Bicitra])
  - ❑ Histamine (H_2)-receptor blocker to decrease the production of gastric acid (e.g., cimetidine [Tagamet] or ranitidine [Zantac])
  - ❑ Medication to accelerate gastric emptying (e.g., metoclopramide [Reglan])
- Preoxygenate with 100% oxygen by nonrebreather face mask for 2 to 3 minutes before anesthesia is given.

Induction Sequence

- Woman is rendered unconscious with IV thiopental, a short-acting barbiturate, or ketamine.
- Succinylcholine, a muscle relaxant, is administered to facilitate passage of an endotracheal tube.
- After the woman is intubated, nitrous oxide and oxygen in a 50-50 mixture are administered.
- Low concentration of a volatile halogenated agent may be administered to increase pain relief and reduce maternal awareness and recall.

MANAGEMENT OF THE SECOND STAGE OF LABOR

The only certain objective sign that the second stage of labor has begun is the inability to feel the cervix during vaginal examination, indicating that the cervix is completely dilated and effaced. The precise moment that this occurs is not easily determined because it depends on when a vaginal examination is performed to validate full dilation and effacement. This makes timing of the actual duration of the second stage difficult.

Common behaviors of women during the second stage of labor are listed in Box 3-14.

BOX 3-14

Common Characteristics of Second-Stage Labor

LATENT PHASE (average duration 10-30 min)

- Spontaneous bearing-down efforts slight to absent, except at peak of strongest contractions
- Quiet; concern over progress
- Experiences sense of relief that transition to second stage is finished
- Feels fatigued and sleepy
- Feels a sense of accomplishment and optimism, because the "worst is over"
- Feels in control

ACTIVE PUSHING (DESCENT) PHASE (average duration varies)

- Increased urge to bear down; becomes stronger as fetus descends to vaginal introitus and reaches perineum
- Grunting sounds or expiratory vocalizations; announces contractions; may scream or swear
- Senses increased urge to push and describes increasing pain; describes ring of fire (burning sensation of acute pain as vagina stretches and fetal head crowns)
- Expresses feeling of powerlessness
- Shows decreased ability to listen or concentrate on anything but giving birth
- Alters respiratory pattern: has short 4- to 5-sec breath holds with regular breaths in between, 5 to 7 times per contraction
- Frequent repositioning
- Often shows excitement immediately after birth of head

Nursing Care in the Second Stage of Labor

Nursing care for women during the second stage of labor is described in Box 3-15.

Assisting with Birth

- Set up the birthing table with sterile instruments and supplies using aseptic technique well before the birth is expected to occur.
  - ❏ The birthing table is usually set up during the transition phase for nulliparous women and during the active phase for multiparous women.
- Prepare for any anticipated problems with the birth, such as meconium-stained amniotic fluid or preterm gestation. Gather

BOX 3-15

Nursing Care in Second-Stage Labor

ASSESSMENT
- Signs that suggest the onset of the second stage
  - ❑ Urge to push or feeling the need to have a bowel movement
  - ❑ Sudden appearance of sweat on upper lip
  - ❑ An episode of vomiting
  - ❑ Increased bloody show
  - ❑ Shaking of extremities
  - ❑ Increased restlessness; verbalization (e.g., "I can't go on")
  - ❑ Involuntary bearing-down efforts
- Physical assessment
  - ❑ Perform every 5 to 30 min: maternal blood pressure, pulse, and respirations
  - ❑ Assess every 5 to 15 min, depending on risk status: fetal heart rate and pattern
  - ❑ Assess every 10 to 15 min: vaginal show, signs of fetal descent, and changes in maternal appearance, mood, affect, energy level and condition of partner/coach
  - ❑ Assess every contraction and bearing-down effort

INTERVENTIONS
- Latent phase
  - ❑ Assist to rest in a position of comfort; encourage relaxation to conserve energy
  - ❑ Promote progress of fetal descent and onset of the urge to bear down by encouraging position changes, pelvic rock, ambulation, showering
- Active pushing (descent) phase
  - ❑ Assist to change position and encourage spontaneous bearing-down efforts
  - ❑ Help to relax and conserve energy between contractions
  - ❑ Provide comfort and pain relief measures as needed
  - ❑ Cleanse perineum promptly if fecal material is expelled
  - ❑ Coach to pant during contractions and to gently push between contractions when head is emerging
  - ❑ Provide emotional support, encouragement, and positive reinforcement of efforts
  - ❑ Keep woman informed regarding progress
  - ❑ Create a calm and quiet environment
  - ❑ Offer mirror to watch birth

supplies and equipment in advance, and make certain that personnel skilled in neonatal resuscitation are present.

■ Estimate the time until the birth will occur, and notify the primary health care provider.

■ Assist the woman to a position of comfort for pushing and giving birth. Encourage nondirected, spontaneous pushing efforts with the woman in an upright or lateral position.

■ Continue to coach and encourage the woman and assess the FHR according to hospital policy until birth is completed.

■ Immediately after the birth, assess and stabilize the newborn. Immediate care includes assigning 1- and 5-minute Apgar scores (see Table 7-1), maintaining a patent airway, supporting respiratory effort, and preventing cold stress.

■ Signs and symptoms of impending birth may occur unexpectedly, requiring immediate action by the nurse. Box 3-16 describes assisting with the vaginal birth of a fetus from a vertex presentation.

MANAGEMENT OF THE THIRD STAGE OF LABOR

The goal in the management of the third stage of labor is the prompt separation and expulsion of the placenta, achieved in the easiest, safest manner.

Nursing Care in the Third Stage of Labor

The major risk for women during the third stage of labor is postpartum hemorrhage caused by uterine atony. Observe for signs of excessive blood loss, such as the following:

■ Alterations in vital signs (increasing pulse rate; decreasing blood pressure)

■ Pallor

■ Lightheadedness

Nursing care for women during the third stage of labor is described in Box 3-17.

MANAGEMENT OF THE FOURTH STAGE OF LABOR

In most centers the mother remains in the labor and birth area during this recovery time. In an institution where labor, delivery, and recovery (LDR) rooms are used, the woman stays in the same room where she

BOX 3-16

Guidelines for Assistance at the Emergency Birth of a Fetus in the Vertex Presentation

1. The woman usually assumes the position most comfortable for her. A lateral position is often recommended to facilitate a controlled birth of the head, thereby minimizing the risk for perineal trauma and neonatal head injury.
2. Reassure the woman that birth is usually uncomplicated in these situations. Use eye-to-eye contact and a calm, relaxed manner. If there is someone else available, such as the partner, that person could help support the woman in the position, assist with coaching, and provide positive reinforcement and praise of her efforts.
3. Wash your hands and put on gloves, if available.
4. Place under woman's buttocks whatever clean material is available.
5. Avoid touching the vaginal area to decrease the possibility of infection.
6. As the head begins to crown, you should perform the following tasks:
   a. Tear the amniotic membranes if they are still intact.
   b. Instruct the woman to pant or pant-blow, thus minimizing the urge to push.
   c. Place the flat side of your hand on the exposed fetal head and apply gentle pressure toward the vagina to prevent the head from "popping out." The mother may participate by placing her hand under yours on the emerging head. Note: Rapid birth of the fetal head must be prevented because a rapid change of pressure within the molded fetal skull follows, which may result in dural or subdural tears. Rapid birth also may cause vaginal or perineal lacerations.
7. After the birth of the head, check for the umbilical cord. If the cord is around the baby's neck, try to slip it over the baby's head or pull it gently to get some slack so that you can slip it over the shoulders.
8. Support the fetal head as external rotation occurs. Then with one hand on each side of the baby's head, exert gentle pressure downward so that the anterior shoulder emerges under the symphysis pubis and acts as a fulcrum; then, as gentle pressure is exerted in the opposite direction, the posterior shoulder, which has passed over the sacrum and coccyx, emerges.

BOX 3-16

Guidelines for Assistance at the Emergency Birth of a Fetus in the Vertex Presentation—cont'd

9. Be alert! Hold the baby securely because the rest of the body may emerge quickly. *The baby will be slippery!*

10. Cradle the baby's head and back in one hand and the buttocks in the other. Keep the baby's head down to drain away the mucus. Use a bulb syringe, if one is available, to remove mucus from the baby's mouth first, then from the nose.

11. Dry the baby quickly to prevent rapid heat loss. Keep the baby at the same level as the mother's uterus until the end of the cord stops pulsating. Note: The baby should be kept at the same level as the mother's uterus to prevent the baby's blood from flowing to or from the placenta and the resultant hypovolemia or hypervolemia. Also, do not "milk" the cord.

12. Place the baby on the mother's abdomen, cover the baby (remember to keep the head warm, too) with the mother's clothing, and have her cuddle the baby. Compliment her (them) on a job well done, and on the baby, if appropriate.

13. Wait for the placenta to separate. Do not tug on the cord. Note: Inappropriate traction may tear the cord, separate the placenta, or invert the uterus. Signs of placental separation include a slight gush of dark blood from the introitus, lengthening of the cord, and change in the uterine contour from a discoid to globular shape.

14. Instruct the mother to push to deliver the separated placenta. Gently ease out the placental membranes using an up-and-down motion until the membranes are removed. If birth occurs outside a hospital setting, to minimize complications, do not cut the cord without proper clamps and a sterile cutting tool. Inspect the placenta for intactness. Place the baby on the placenta and wrap the two together for additional warmth.

15. Check the firmness of the uterus. Gently massage the fundus and demonstrate to the mother how she can massage her own fundus properly.

16. If supplies are available, clean the mother's perineal area and apply a peripad.

17. In addition to gentle massage of the fundus, the following measures can be taken to prevent or minimize hemorrhage:
    a. Put the baby to the mother's breast as soon as possible. Sucking or nuzzling and licking the nipple stimulates the release of oxytocin from the posterior pituitary. Note: If the baby does not or cannot nurse, manually stimulate the mother's nipples.

Continued

BOX 3-16

Guidelines for Assistance at the Emergency Birth of a Fetus in the Vertex Presentation—cont'd

    b. Do not allow the mother's bladder to become distended. Assess the bladder for fullness and encourage her to void if fullness is found.

    c. Expel any clots from the mother's uterus after ensuring that the fundus is firm.

18. Comfort or reassure the mother and her family or friends. Keep the mother and the baby warm. Give her fluids if available and tolerated.

19. If this birth is multifetal, identify the infants in order of birth (using letters A, B, etc.).

20. Make notations regarding the following aspects of the birth:
    a. Fetal presentation and position
    b. Presence of cord around neck (nuchal cord) or other parts and number of times cord encircled part
    c. Color, character, and estimated amount of amniotic fluid, if rupture of membranes occurs immediately before birth
    d. Time of birth
    e. Estimated time of determination of Apgar score (e.g., 1 and 5 min after birth), resuscitation efforts implemented, and ultimate condition of baby
    f. Gender of baby
    g. Time of placental expulsion, as well as the appearance and completeness of the placenta
    h. Maternal condition: affect, behavior, and demeanor, amount of bleeding, and status of uterine tonicity
    i. Any unusual occurrences during the birth (e.g., maternal or paternal response, verbalizations, or gestures in response to birth of baby)

gave birth. In traditional settings, the woman is taken from the delivery room to a separate recovery area for observation.

Nursing Care in the Fourth Stage of Labor

Nursing care during the fourth stage of labor is described in Box 3-18.

Postanesthesia Recovery After Cesarean Birth or Spinal or Epidural Anesthesia for Vaginal Birth

Women who have received general, spinal, or epidural anesthesia must be cleared for transfer from the recovery area by a member of the anesthesia care team.

BOX 3-17

Nursing Care in Third-Stage Labor

ASSESSMENT
- Signs that suggest the onset of the third stage
    - ❏ A firmly contracting fundus
    - ❏ A change in the uterus from a discoid to a globular ovoid shape as the placenta moves into the lower uterine segment
    - ❏ A sudden gush of dark blood from the introitus
    - ❏ Apparent lengthening of the umbilical cord as the placenta descends to the introitus
    - ❏ The finding of vaginal fullness (the placenta) on vaginal or rectal examination or of fetal membranes at the introitus
- Physical assessment
    - ❏ Perform every 15 min: maternal blood pressure, pulse, and respirations
    - ❏ Assess for signs of placental separation and amount of bleeding
    - ❏ Assist with determination of Apgar score at 1 and 5 min after birth (see Table 7-1).
    - ❏ Assess maternal and paternal response to completion of childbirth process and their reaction to the newborn

INTERVENTIONS
- Assist to bear down to facilitate expulsion of the separated placenta.
- Administer an oxytocic medication as ordered to ensure adequate contraction of the uterus thereby preventing hemorrhage.
- Provide nonpharmacologic and pharmacologic comfort and pain relief measures.
- Perform hygienic cleansing measures.
- Keep the woman/couple informed of progress of placental separation and expulsion and of perineal repair if appropriate.
- Explain purpose of medications administered.
- Introduce parents to their baby and facilitate the attachment process by delaying eye prophylaxis; wrap mother and baby together for skin-to-skin contact.
- Provide private time for parents to bond with new baby; help them to create memories.
- Encourage breastfeeding if desired.

Nursing Care in Fourth-Stage Labor

Review prenatal, labor, and birth records for any risk factors. Especially note conditions that could predispose the mother to hemorrhage, such as the following:

- Precipitous labor
- Large baby
- Grand multiparity
- Induced labor

ASSESSMENT
Blood Pressure

- Measure blood pressure every 15 min for the first hour.

Pulse

- Assess rate and regularity. Measure every 15 min for the first hour.

Temperature

- Determine temperature at the beginning of the recovery period and after the first hour of recovery.

Fundus

- Position woman with knees flexed and head flat.
- Just below umbilicus, cup hand and press firmly into abdomen. At the same time, stabilize the uterus at the symphysis with the opposite hand.
- If fundus is firm (and bladder is empty), with uterus in midline, measure its position relative to woman's umbilicus. Lay fingers flat on abdomen under umbilicus. Measure how many fingerbreadths (fb) or centimeters (cm) fit between umbilicus and top of fundus. Fundal height is documented according to agency guidelines. For example, if the fundus is 1 fb or 1 cm above the umbilicus, fundal height may be recorded as either +1, u + 1, or 1/u. If the fundus is 1 fb or 1 cm below the umbilicus, fundal height may be recorded as either -1, u-1, or u/1. If fundus is not firm, massage it gently to contract and expel any clots before measuring distance from umbilicus.
- Place hands appropriately; massage gently only until firm.
- Expel clots. With upper hand, firmly apply pressure downward toward vagina; observe perineum for amount and size of expelled clots.

Bladder

- Assess distention by noting location and firmness of uterine fundus and by observing and palpating bladder. A distended bladder is seen as a suprapubic rounded bulge that is dull to percussion and fluctuates like a water-filled balloon. When the bladder is distended, the uterus is usually boggy in consistency, well above the umbilicus, and to the woman's right side.

BOX 3-18

Nursing Care in Fourth-Stage Labor—cont'd

- Reassess after voiding or catheterization to make sure the bladder is not palpable and the fundus is firm and in the midline

Lochia
- Observe lochia on perineal pads and on linen under the mother's buttocks. Determine amount and color; note size and number of clots; note odor.
- Observe perineum for source of bleeding (e.g., episiotomy, lacerations).

Perineum
- Ask or assist woman to turn onto her side and flex upper leg on hip.
- Lift upper buttock.
- Observe perineum in good lighting.
- Assess episiotomy or laceration repair for redness (erythema), edema, ecchymosis (bruising), drainage, and approximation (REEDA).
- Assess for presence of hemorrhoids.

Interventions
- Perform comfort measures including application of ice to perineum, assist with hygienic measures, and help with position changes and getting out of bed.
- Encourage bladder emptying by assisting to bathroom or providing bedpan. Catheterize as necessary. Measure and record amount of urine output.
- Administer analgesics and oxytocics as ordered by primary health care provider.
- Provide food and fluids as desired.
- Encourage mother and family to hold and touch infant.
- This is an ideal time to initiate breastfeeding; demonstrate how to encourage the baby to latch and how to safely remove the baby from the breast.

NURSING ALERT   *Regardless of her obstetric status, no woman should be discharged from the recovery area until she has completely recovered from the effects of anesthesia.*

- If the woman received general anesthesia:
  - ❏ She should be awake and alert.

- ❏ She should be oriented to time, place, and person.
- ❏ Respiratory rate should be within normal limits.
- ❏ Oxygen saturation should be at least 95%, as measured by a pulse oximeter.
- If the woman received epidural or spinal anesthesia:
  - ❏ She should be able to raise her legs, extended at the knees, off the bed or to flex her knees, place her feet flat on the bed, and raise her buttocks well off the bed.
  - ❏ The numb or tingling, prickly sensation should be entirely gone from her legs.
- Often it takes several hours for these anesthetic effects to disappear.

Selected Childbirth Complications

This section presents information on selected labor and birth complications, including preterm and postterm birth, preterm premature rupture of membranes, infections, dystocia, induction/augmentation of labor, and vaginal birth after cesarean. Assisted births, including cesarean birth and forceps- or vacuum-assisted vaginal births, are also addressed. Finally, information on managing selected emergency situations, meconium-stained amniotic fluid, shoulder dystocia, and prolapsed umbilical cord, is included.

PRETERM LABOR AND BIRTH

Preterm labor is defined as cervical changes and uterine contractions occurring between 20 and 37 weeks of pregnancy. Preterm birth is any birth that occurs before the completion of 37 weeks of pregnancy. About 75% of all preterm births in the United States are termed late preterm births because they occur between 34 and 36 weeks of gestation. The steady increase in the preterm birth rate has been attributed to the rise in the rate of late preterm births, which has increased 25% since 1990.

Etiology

Increasingly, preterm births are being divided into two categories, spontaneous and indicated. Spontaneous preterm births occur following an early initiation of the labor process and comprise nearly 75% of all preterm births in the United States. Box 4-1 lists risk factors for spontaneous preterm labor.

Indicated preterm births, on the other hand, occur as a means to resolve maternal or fetal risk related to continuing the pregnancy. About 25% of all preterm births in the United States are indicated because of medical or obstetric conditions that affect the mother, the fetus, or both. An increase in the number of indicated preterm births accounts for much of the rise in late preterm births. Box 4-2 lists common causes of indicated preterm birth.

BOX 4-1

Risk Factors for Spontaneous Preterm Labor
- Genital tract infection
- Non-Caucasian race
- Multifetal gestation
- Second-trimester bleeding
- Low prepregnancy weight
- History of previous spontaneous preterm birth

Source: Iams, J., Romero, R., & Creasy, R. (2009). Preterm labor and birth. In R. Creasy, R. Resnik, J. Iams, C. Lockwood, & T. Moore (Eds.), *Creasy and Resnik's maternal-fetal medicine: Principles and practice* (6th ed.). Philadelphia: Saunders.

BOX 4-2

Common Causes of Indicated Preterm Birth
- Preeclampsia
- Fetal distress
- Intrauterine growth restriction
- Placental abruption
- Intrauterine fetal demise
- Pregestational and gestational diabetes
- Renal disease
- Rh sensitization
- Congenital malformations

Source: Iams, J., Romero, R., & Creasy, R. (2009). Preterm labor and birth. In R. Creasy, R. Resnik, J. Iams, C. Lockwood, & T. Moore (Eds.), *Creasy and Resnik's maternal-fetal medicine: Principles and practice* (6th ed.). Philadelphia: Saunders.

Predicting Preterm Labor and Birth

- Major risk factors for spontaneous labor and birth include:
  - History of previous preterm birth
  - Multiple gestation
  - Bleeding after the first trimester of pregnancy
  - Low maternal body mass index (BMI)
- Other risk factors for spontaneous labor and birth include
  - Non-Caucasian race
  - Low socioeconomic status
  - Low educational status
  - Living with chronic stress
  - Domestic violence

- ❏ Lack of social support
- ❏ Smoking
- ❏ Substance abuse
- ❏ Physically demanding working conditions
- ❏ Periodontal disease
- ■ At least 50% of all women who ultimately give birth prematurely, however, have no identifiable risk factors.
- ■ Biochemical marker
    - ❏ Fetal fibronectin—Glycoprotein found in plasma and produced during fetal life. Fetal fibronectin normally appears in cervical and vaginal secretions early in pregnancy, and then again in late pregnancy.
    - ❏ The presence of fetal fibronectin during the late second and early third trimesters may be related to placental inflammation, which is thought to be one cause of spontaneous preterm labor. The presence of fetal fibronectin is not very sensitive as a predictor of preterm birth, however. Often the test is used to predict who will *not* go into preterm labor, because preterm labor is very unlikely to occur in women with a negative result.
    - ❏ The test is performed by collecting fluid from the woman's vagina using a swab during a speculum examination.
- ■ Endocervical length
    - ❏ A shortened cervix as determined by ultrasound measurement may precede preterm labor. Changes in cervical length occur before uterine activity, so cervical measurement can identify women in whom the labor process has begun. However, because preterm cervical shortening occurs over a period of weeks, neither digital nor ultrasound cervical examination is very sensitive at predicting imminent preterm birth. Women whose cervical length is more than 30 mm are unlikely to give birth prematurely even if they have symptoms of preterm labor.

Management

Pregnancy

- ■ Teach all pregnant women the early signs and symptoms of preterm labor listed in Box 4-3 and what to do if they occur. (See the Teaching for Self-Management box: What to Do if Symptoms of Preterm Labor Occur.) In particular, education regarding any symptoms of uterine contractions or cramping

BOX 4-3

Signs and Symptoms of Preterm Labor

UTERINE ACTIVITY

- Uterine contractions occurring more frequently than every 10 min persisting for 1 hr or more
- Contractions may be painful or painless

DISCOMFORT

- Lower abdominal cramping similar to gas pains; may be accompanied by diarrhea
- Dull, intermittent low back pain (below the waist)
- Painful, menstrual-like cramps
- Suprapubic pain or pressure
- Pelvic pressure or heaviness; feeling that "baby is pushing down"
- Urinary frequency

VAGINAL DISCHARGE

- Change in character or amount of usual discharge: thicker (mucoid) or thinner (watery), bloody, brown or colorless, increased amount, odor
- Rupture of amniotic membranes

Teaching for Self-Management

What to Do if Symptoms of Preterm Labor Occur

- Empty your bladder.
- Drink two to three glasses of water or juice.
- Lie down on your side for 1 hr.
- Palpate for contractions.
- If symptoms continue, call your health care provider or go to the hospital.
- If symptoms go away, resume light activity, but not what you were doing when the symptoms began.
- If symptoms return, call your health care provider or go to the hospital.
- If any of the following symptoms occur, call your health care provider immediately:
  - ❏ Uterine contractions every 10 min or less for 1 hr or more
  - ❏ Vaginal bleeding
  - ❏ Odorous vaginal discharge
  - ❏ Fluid leaking from the vagina

between 20 and 27 weeks of gestation must emphasize that these symptoms are not just normal discomforts of pregnancy, but rather indications of possible preterm labor.

- If symptoms of preterm labor occur with sexual activity, the woman should be counseled about lifestyle modification until she reaches 37 weeks of gestation.

- Bed rest is frequently prescribed, but there is no evidence in the literature to support the effectiveness of this intervention in reducing preterm birth rates. Therefore, many health care providers now recommend only modified bed rest in which women are usually allowed bathroom privileges for toileting and showering and can be up to the table for meals.

Intrapartum

- The diagnosis of preterm labor requires all of the following:
  - ❑ Gestational age between 20 and 37 weeks
  - ❑ Uterine activity (contractions)
  - ❑ Progressive cervical change (effacement of 80% or greater or cervical dilation of 2 cm or greater)

- If preterm labor is diagnosed, the woman will be admitted to the hospital for tocolytic therapy, medications to suppress uterine activity in an attempt to prevent preterm birth. Research has demonstrated that prolonging the pregnancy 48 hours to several days is the best outcome that can be expected. The purposes of tocolytic therapy are to gain time for administering antenatal corticosteroids and transporting the mother to a facility with a neonatal intensive care unit.

- There is no clear first-line tocolytic drug. Medications commonly used for tocolytic therapy include the following:
  - ❑ Magnesium sulfate
  - ❑ Terbutaline (Brethine)
  - ❑ Nifedipine (Adalat, Procardia)
  - ❑ Indomethacin (Indocin)

See the Medication Guide in Appendix B for information on these medications.

Antenatal glucocorticoids (betamethasone, dexamethasone), given as intramuscular injections to the mother to accelerate fetal lung maturity by stimulating fetal surfactant production, are considered one of the most effective and cost-efficient interventions for preventing neonatal morbidity and mortality associated with preterm labor. Antenatal glucocorticoids have been shown to significantly reduce the incidence of respiratory distress syndrome, intraventricular hemorrhage, necrotizing enterocolitis, and death in neonates, without increasing the risk of infection in mothers or newborns. All women between 24 and 34 weeks of gestation should be given a single course of antenatal glucocorticoids when preterm birth is threatened unless evidence indicates that glucocorticoids will have an adverse effect on the mother or birth is imminent. Because optimal benefit begins 24 hours after the first injection, timely administration is essential. (See the Medication Guide: Antenatal Glucocorticoid Therapy with Betamethasone, Dexamethasone in Appendix B.)

- Management of inevitable preterm birth
  - ❏ Once the cervix dilates to 4 cm or more, preterm birth is likely.
  - ❏ If preterm birth appears inevitable, transfer the woman before birth, if possible, to a facility equipped to care for the infant. Give the first dose of antenatal corticosteroids before transfer.
  - ❏ Monitor for rapid progression to birth. Remember that very tiny preterm infants may pass through a cervix that has not completely dilated.
  - ❏ Gather equipment, supplies, and medications used for neonatal resuscitation in advance and prepare them for immediate use.
  - ❏ Have personnel skilled in neonatal resuscitation present during the birth.
  - ❏ If birth occurs in a hospital that is not prepared to provide continuing care for a preterm neonate, make plans for immediate transfer of the infant to a higher level of care.

Nursing Considerations

- Because at least 50% of all women who give birth prematurely have no identifiable risk factors, *all* pregnant women must be educated about signs and symptoms of preterm labor.
- If the fetal fibronectin test is used, a sample of vaginal fluid for testing must be obtained before a vaginal examination for cervical changes is performed. The lubricant used during the vaginal examination can reduce the accuracy of the fetal fibronectin test. The presence of vaginal bleeding or ruptured membranes, or a history of intercourse within the past 24 hours can also reduce the accuracy of the test results.

PRETERM PREMATURE RUPTURE OF MEMBRANES

Premature rupture of membranes (PROM) is the rupture of the amniotic sac and leakage of amniotic fluid beginning before the onset of labor at any gestational age. In preterm premature rupture of membranes (preterm PROM) rupture of the amniotic sac occurs before 37 weeks of gestation. The woman may complain of either a sudden gush or a slow leak of fluid from the vagina.

Etiology

Preterm PROM most likely results from pathologic weakening of the amniotic membranes caused by inflammation, stress from uterine contractions, or other factors that cause increased intrauterine pressure. Infection of the urogenital tract is a major risk factor associated with preterm PROM.

Risks Associated with Preterm PROM

Maternal

- Infection (chorioamnionitis)
- Placental abruption
- Sepsis
- Death

Fetal

- Intrauterine infection
- Cord prolapse
- Cord compression (related to oligohydramnios)
- Placental abruption
- Pulmonary hypoplasia (when preterm PROM occurs before 20 weeks of gestation)

Management

- Diagnosis is confirmed by a Nitrazine or fern test. The Procedure box: Tests for Rupture of Membranes on page 120 describes these tests in detail. An ultrasound will most likely reveal oligohydramnios or anhydramnios.
- Management decisions are based on gestational age and maternal and fetal condition. The woman may either be admitted to the hospital or be cared for at home with more frequent visits to her health care provider.

- Preterm PROM is often managed expectantly or conservatively if the risks to the fetus and newborn associated with preterm birth are considered to be greater than the risks of infection.
- Conservative management includes the following:
  - ❏ Maternal monitoring for signs of labor, placental abruption, or infectious organisms.
  - ❏ Fetal assessment (daily fetal movement counting, nonstress test, biophysical profile)
  - ❏ Administering antenatal glucocorticoids to women who are less than 34 weeks of gestation because they have been proven to reduce the risk of several neonatal complications
  - ❏ Administering a 7-day course of broad-spectrum antibiotics (e.g., ampicillin, erythromycin) to treat or prevent intrauterine infection

Nursing Considerations

- Whenever preterm PROM is suspected, strict sterile technique should be used in any vaginal examination to avoid introduction of infectious organisms.
- Vigilance for signs of infection is a major part of the nursing care and patient education after preterm PROM. Teach the woman that her genital area must be kept clean and that nothing should be introduced into the vagina.
- Teach the woman to immediately call her health care provider or go to the hospital if she develops fever, uterine contractions, abdominal pain or tenderness, or foul-smelling vaginal discharge.
- Nursing support of the woman and her family is critical. The woman is often anxious about the health of her baby and may fear that she was responsible in some way for the membrane rupture.

POSTTERM PREGNANCY

A postterm pregnancy (also sometimes referred to as a *postdate* or *prolonged pregnancy*) is one that extends beyond the end of week 42 of gestation, or 294 days from the first day of the last menstrual period (LMP). The incidence of postterm pregnancy is estimated to be between 4% and 14% (Resnik & Resnik, 2009). Many pregnancies are misdiagnosed as prolonged because of inaccurate dating.

Etiology

The exact cause of true postterm pregnancy is not known. However, it is clear that the timing of labor is determined by complex interactions among the fetus, the placenta and membranes, the uterine myometrium, and the cervix.

Risk Factors for Postterm Pregnancy

- First pregnancy
- History of previous postterm pregnancy
- Presence of congenital primary fetal adrenal hypoplasia or placental sulfatase deficiency

Clinical Manifestations

- Maternal weight loss (more than 3 lb/wk)
- Decreased uterine size (related to decreased amniotic fluid volume)
- Meconium-stained amniotic fluid
- Advanced bone maturation of the fetal skeleton with an exceptionally hard fetal skull

Maternal Risks

- Perineal injury (related to fetal macrosomia)
- Hemorrhage
- Infection
- Labor induction
- Forceps- or vacuum-assisted birth
- Cesarean birth
- Feelings of depression, frustration, and inadequacy

Fetal Risks

- Abnormal fetal growth
  - ❑ Macrosomia (more than 4000 g) (more likely)
  - ❑ Small for gestational age
- Oligohydramnios
  - ❑ Cord compression
  - ❑ Hypoxemia
- Low Apgar scores
  - ❑ Postmaturity syndrome
  - ❑ Meconium aspiration syndrome

Management

- The management of postterm pregnancy is still controversial. However, because perinatal morbidity and mortality increase greatly after 42 weeks of gestation, pregnancies are usually not allowed to continue after this time.
- In the United States, most physicians induce labor at 41 weeks of gestation. During labor the fetus of a woman with a postterm pregnancy should be continuously monitored electronically for a more accurate assessment of the FHR and pattern.
- An alternative approach for managing postterm pregnancy is to initiate twice-weekly fetal testing at 41 weeks of gestation. The testing generally consists of either a BPP or NST along with an assessment of amniotic fluid volume. In addition, the woman is encouraged to assess fetal activity daily, assess for signs of labor, and keep appointments with her primary health care provider.
- Evidence is insufficient to determine which of the two management approaches described above is better.

Nursing Considerations

The woman and her family should be encouraged to express their feelings (e.g., frustration, anger, impatience, fear) about the prolonged pregnancy and helped to realize that these feelings are normal. At times the emotional and physical strain of a postterm pregnancy may seem overwhelming. Referral to a support group or another supportive resource may be needed.

INFECTIONS

Maternal Group B Streptococci (GBS) Infection

- May be considered part of the normal vaginal flora in women who are not pregnant
- Present in about 20% to 30% of healthy pregnant women

Diagnosis

- Made by screening all pregnant women at 35 to 37 weeks of gestation using a rectovaginal culture

Management

- All women with a positive culture result should receive intravenous antibiotic prophylaxis (IAP) during labor

- Women with an unknown GBS status (i.e., culture was not done or results are unknown) should also receive IAP if any of the following risk factors are present:
  - Less than 37 weeks of gestational age
  - Fever greater than 38.0° C (100.4° F)
  - Ruptured membranes for more than 18 hours
  - History of previous infant with GBS infection
  - GBS-positive urine culture during current pregnancy
- Be aware that some practitioners give IAP during labor to all women with an unknown GBS status, even if none of the risk factors listed above are identified.
- Accurate rapid polymerase chain reaction (PCR) testing is available for use in women who are admitted with an unknown GBS status to give birth.
- Recommended IAP
  - Penicillin G, 5 million units IV loading dose, then 2.5 million units IV every 4 hours during labor, *or*
  - Ampicillin, 2-g loading dose IV followed by 1 g IV every 4 hours during labor
  - Women who are allergic to penicillin may be treated with cefazolin (Ancef), clindamycin (Cleocin), erythromycin, or vancomycin (Vancocin)
- IAP is not necessary before planned cesarean births if the woman is not in labor and the membranes have not ruptured.

Maternal and Newborn Effects

- Most women are asymptomatic. GBS can, however, cause urinary tract infection, chorioamnionitis, or endometritis. Sepsis and meningitis are very rare complications of GBS infection.
- In newborns the major risk is for early-onset infection. The practice of giving prophylactic antibiotics to women in labor who are GBS positive has significantly reduced the incidence and severity of early-onset GBS infection in the newborn.

Chorioamnionitis

- Chorioamnionitis, bacterial infection of the amniotic cavity, is a major cause of complications for mothers and newborns at all gestational ages. Chorioamnionitis is usually caused when organisms that are part of the normal vaginal flora ascend into the amniotic cavity.

- Other terms for this condition include *clinical chorioamnionitis, amnionitis, intrapartum infection, amniotic fluid infection,* and *intraamniotic infection.*

Diagnosis

Chorioamnionitis is usually diagnosed by the clinical findings of maternal fever, maternal and fetal tachycardia, uterine tenderness, and foul-smelling amniotic fluid.

Risk Factors

- Young maternal age
- Low socioeconomic status
- Nulliparity
- Preexisting infections of the lower genital tract
- Associated with an excessively long labor
  - ❑ Prolonged membrane rupture
  - ❑ Multiple vaginal examinations
  - ❑ Use of internal FHR and contraction-monitoring modes

Management

- In order to prevent maternal and neonatal complications, prompt treatment with IV broad-spectrum antibiotics and birth of the fetus are necessary.
- Ampicillin or penicillin and gentamicin are the antibiotics most often used to treat chorioamnionitis during labor.
- After cesarean birth, an antibiotic that provides coverage for anaerobic organisms, such as clindamycin (Cleocin) or metronidazole (Flagyl) should be added.
- Antibiotics can usually be discontinued soon after birth.

Maternal and Newborn Effects

- Maternal
  - ❑ Bacteremia
  - ❑ Dysfunctional labor (increased risk for cesarean birth)
  - ❑ Wound infection or pelvic abscess after cesarean birth
- Newborn
  - ❑ Pneumonia
  - ❑ Bacteremia
  - ❑ Sepsis
  - ❑ Death (more likely in preterm than in term newborns)

❏ Problems with long-term neurologic development, including cerebral palsy

Dysfunctional Labor

Dysfunctional labor (also called dystocia) is defined as a long, difficult, or abnormal labor caused by various conditions associated with the five factors affecting labor. It is the most common indication for cesarean birth. Dysfunctional labor is suspected when there is an alteration in the characteristics of uterine contractions, a lack of progress in the rate of cervical dilation, or a lack of progress in fetal descent and expulsion.

Causes

■ Ineffective uterine contractions or maternal bearing-down efforts (the powers)
■ Alterations in the pelvic structure (the passage)
■ Fetal causes, including abnormal presentation or position, anomalies, excessive size, and number of fetuses (the passenger)
■ Maternal position during labor and birth
■ Psychologic responses of the mother to labor related to past experiences, preparation, culture and heritage, and support system

Management

By reviewing the woman's past labor or labors and observing her physical and psychologic responses to the current labor, factors that might contribute to dysfunctional labor can be identified. Interventions are established for each woman, based on assessment findings. Commonly performed interventions for dysfunctional labor include cervical ripening, induction or augmentation of labor, operative vaginal birth (forceps- or vacuum-assisted birth), and cesarean birth.

Induction/Augmentation of Labor

Induction of labor is the chemical or mechanical initiation of uterine contractions before their spontaneous onset for the purpose of bringing about the birth. Labor may be induced either electively or for indicated reasons. It is likely that the rate of elective inductions is increasing more rapidly than the rate of indicated inductions.

Success rates for induction are higher when the condition of the cervix is favorable or inducible. A rating system such as the Bishop score (Table 4-1) can be used to evaluate inducibility. When the Bishop score totals 8 or more, labor induction is usually successful.

TABLE 4-1

Bishop Score

	SCORE			
	0	1	2	3
Dilation (cm)	0	1-2	3-4	≥5
Effacement (%)	0-30	40-50	60-70	≥80
Station (cm)	−3	−2	−1	+1, +2
Cervical consistency	Firm	Medium	Soft	Soft
Cervix position	Posterior	Midposition	Anterior	Anterior

Cervical Ripening

If the cervix is not "ripe" for induction (e.g., a low Bishop score), chemical, mechanical, physical, or alternative methods may be used to soften and thin it. This treatment usually results in a higher success rate for labor induction.

Chemical Agents

- Prostaglandin E_1: misoprostol (Cytotec)
- Prostaglandin E_2: dinoprostone (Cervidil Insert; Prepidil Gel)
  See the Medication Guides for these medications in Appendix B.

Mechanical Methods

Mechanical methods ripen the cervix by stimulating the release of endogenous prostaglandins and oxytocin.

- Balloon (Foley) catheter inserted into the intracervical canal
- Hydroscopic dilators (laminaria tents; Lamicel)
- Amniotic membrane stripping or sweeping

Alternative Methods

- Ingestion of black cohosh or evening primrose oil

Induction of Labor

Indications

Induction may be indicated for a variety of medical and obstetric reasons (Box 4-4).

Common Methods of Induction

- Amniotomy (artificial rupture of membranes)
- IV oxytocin

- Prostaglandins
- Alternative methods
  - Ingestion of blue cohosh or castor oil
  - Acupuncture

BOX 4-4

Indications and Contraindications for Labor Induction

INDICATIONS
- Hypertensive complications of pregnancy: gestational hypertension, preeclampsia, eclampsia
- Fetal death
- Chorioamnionitis
- Maternal medical conditions: diabetes mellitus, renal disease, cardiopulmonary conditions, chronic hypertension, antiphospholipid syndrome
- Postterm pregnancy, especially when oligohydramnios is present
- Fetal compromise: intrauterine growth restriction, isoimmunization
- Premature rupture of membranes with established fetal maturity

CONTRAINDICATIONS
- Acute, severe fetal distress
- Shoulder presentation (transverse lie)
- Floating fetal presenting part
- Uncontrolled hemorrhage
- Umbilical cord prolapse
- Active genital herpes infection
- Placenta previa
- Previous uterine incision that prohibits a trial of labor

RELATIVE CONTRAINDICATIONS
- Grand multiparity (≥5 pregnancies that ended after 20 wk of gestation)
- Multiple gestation
- Suspected cephalopelvic disproportion
- Breech presentations
- Inability to adequately monitor fetal heart rate or contractions (or both) throughout labor

Sources: Thorp, J. (2009). Clinical aspects of normal and abnormal labor. In R. Creasy, R. Resnik, J. Iams, C. Lockwood, & T. Moore (Eds.), *Creasy and Resnik's maternal-fetal medicine: Principles and practice* (6th ed.). Philadelphia: Saunders; American College of Obstetricians and Gynecologists (ACOG). (2009). Induction of labor. *ACOG Practice Bulletin No. 107.* Washington, DC: ACOG.

Amniotomy

Artificial rupture of membranes (AROM) can be used to induce labor when the cervix is favorable (ripe) or to augment labor if progress begins to slow. Labor usually begins within 12 hours of rupture. The duration of labor can be decreased by up to 2 hours, even without oxytocin administration. The major potential complication of amniotomy is infection.

Management

- The woman should be free of active infection of the genital tract (herpes) and should be human immunodeficiency virus (HIV) negative.
- The presenting part of the fetus should be engaged and well applied to the cervix before amniotomy.
- An amnihook or other sharp instrument is inserted through the vagina and cervix to rupture the membranes.

NURSING ALERT *Nurses should not perform an amniotomy. This procedure should be done by the primary health care provider.*

Nursing Considerations

- The time of rupture and the color, consistency, odor, and amount of the amniotic fluid observed should be documented.
- The FHR is assessed before and immediately after the amniotomy to detect any changes that may indicate cord compression or prolapse.
- The woman's temperature should be assessed at least every 2 hours following amniotomy to detect infection.
- Comfort measures, such as frequently changing the woman's underpads and perineal cleansing, are implemented.

Oxytocin

Oxytocin is a hormone normally produced by the posterior pituitary gland; it stimulates uterine contractions. It may be used either to induce labor or to augment a labor that is progressing slowly because of inadequate uterine contractions. Oxytocin is used in the majority of all births in the United States. It is also the drug most commonly associated with adverse events during childbirth.

Oxytocin use can present risks to the mother and fetus. These risks are primarily dose related, with most problems caused by high doses that are given rapidly. See the Medication Guide: Oxytocin (Pitocin) in Appendix B.

Management

■ The primary health care provider writes the order for the induction or augmentation of labor with oxytocin. The nurse's actions related to assessment and care of a woman whose labor is being induced are guided either by very specific written orders or an evidence-based written hospital protocol.

■ Current protocols are based on research findings related to the pharmacokinetics of oxytocin. The uterus responds to oxytocin within 3 to 5 minutes of IV administration. The half-life of oxytocin (the time required to metabolize and eliminate half the dose) is approximately 10 to 12 minutes. About 40 minutes are required to reach a steady state of oxytocin (the point in time when the rate of oxytocin administered intravenously equals the rate of oxytocin elimination) and for the full effect of a dosage increment to be achieved.

> **NURSING ALERT** *Oxytocin is discontinued immediately and the primary health care provider notified if uterine tachysystole, abnormal (nonreassuring) FHR and pattern, or both occur.*

Nursing Considerations

■ The recommended protocol for administering oxytocin is to begin with a starting dose of 1 milliunit/min and to increase by 1 to 2 milliunits/min no more frequently than every 30 to 60 minutes. This recommendation is based on research findings related to the pharmacokinetics of oxytocin.

■ Safety measures recommended for use of this medication include all of the following:
  ❑ A standard concentration of oxytocin
  ❑ A standard definition of uterine tachysystole that includes neither an abnormal (nonreassuring) FHR pattern nor the woman's perception of pain
  ❑ Standardized treatment of oxytocin-induced uterine tachysystole (see the Emergency box: Uterine Tachysystole with Oxytocin.)

EMERGENCY

Uterine Tachysystole with Oxytocin

SIGNS
- More than five contractions in 10 min
- A series of single contractions lasting more than 2 min
- Contractions of normal duration occurring within 1 min of each other

INTERVENTIONS (WITH NORMAL [REASSURING] FHR)
- Reposition or maintain woman in side-lying position (either side).
- Administer IV fluid bolus with 500 ml of lactated Ringer's solution.
- If uterine activity has not returned to normal after 10 min, decrease the oxytocin dose by at least one half. If uterine activity has not returned to normal after another 10 min, discontinue the oxytocin infusion until fewer than five contractions occur in 10 min.

INTERVENTIONS (WITH ABNORMAL [NONREASSURING] FHR)
- Discontinue oxytocin infusion immediately.
- Reposition or maintain woman in side-lying position (either side).
- Administer IV fluid bolus with 500 ml of lactated Ringer's solution.
- Consider giving oxygen at 10 L/min by nonrebreather face mask if the above interventions do not resolve the abnormal (nonreassuring) FHR and pattern.
- If no response, consider giving 0.25 mg terbutaline subcutaneously.
- Notify primary health care provider of actions taken and maternal and fetal response.

RESUMPTION OF OXYTOCIN AFTER RESOLUTION OF TACHYSYSTOLE
- If the oxytocin infusion has been discontinued for less than 20-30 min, resume at no more than one half the rate that caused the tachysystole.
- If the oxytocin infusion has been discontinued for more than 30-40 min, resume at the initial starting dose.

Sources: Mahlmeister, L. (2008). Best practices in perinatal care: Evidence-based management of oxytocin induction and augmentation of labor. *Journal of Perinatal and Neonatal Nursing, 22*(4), 259-263; Simpson, K., & Knox, G. (2009). Oxytocin as a high-alert medication: Implications for perinatal patient safety. *MCN The American Journal of Maternal/Child Nursing, 34*(1), 8-15.

Augmentation of Labor

Augmentation of labor is the stimulation of uterine contractions after labor has started spontaneously but progress is unsatisfactory. Augmentation is usually implemented for the management of hypotonic uterine dysfunction, resulting in a slowing of the labor process.

Common Methods of Augmentation

- Oxytocin infusion
- Amniotomy
  Noninvasive methods, such as emptying the bladder, ambulation and position changes, relaxation measures, nourishment and hydration, and hydrotherapy, should be attempted before initiating invasive interventions.

Management

The administration procedure and nursing assessment and care measures for augmentation of labor with oxytocin are similar to those used for induction of labor with oxytocin. Less oxytocin may be required to augment labor and achieve spontaneous vaginal birth than to induce labor (see the Medication Guide: Oxytocin [Pitocin] in Appendix B).

OPERATIVE VAGINAL BIRTH

Forceps-Assisted Birth

A forceps-assisted birth is one in which an instrument with two curved blades is used to assist in the birth of the fetal head. There are several types of forceps-assisted births, defined primarily by the station and position of the fetal head in relationship to the maternal pelvis (Table 4-2). The use of forceps during childbirth has been decreasing, replaced by vacuum-assisted or cesarean birth.

Maternal Indications

- Prolonged second-stage labor
- Need to shorten second-stage labor because of maternal exhaustion or maternal cardiopulmonary or cerebrovascular disease

Fetal Indications

- Fetal distress
- Abnormal presentation
- Arrest of rotation
- Delivery of head in a breech presentation

TABLE 4-2

Definitions for Forceps- and Vacuum-Assisted Births

Outlet	Fetal scalp is visible on the perineum without manually separating the labia
Low	Fetal head is at least at the +2 station
Midpelvis	Fetal head is engaged (no higher than 0 station) but above the +2 station

Source: American Academy of Pediatrics (AAP) & American College of Obstetricians and Gynecologists (ACOG). (2007). *Guidelines for perinatal care* (6th ed.). Washington, DC: ACOG.

Preprocedure Requirements

- Completely dilated cervix
- Empty bladder (catheterize just before procedure)
- Engaged presenting part, with vertex presentation desired
- Ruptured membranes
- Maternal pelvis must be assessed as adequate for the estimated fetal head circumference and weight

Management

- Both blades are positioned by the physician and the handles locked.
- Traction is usually applied during contractions.
- If a decrease in fetal heart rate occurs, the forceps are removed and reapplied.
- The mother may be instructed to push during contractions as traction is applied, depending on physician preference.

NURSING ALERT   *Because compression of the cord between the fetal head and the forceps causes a decrease in FHR, the FHR and pattern are assessed, reported, and recorded before and after forceps application.*

- Postbirth assessments
  - ❑ Maternal
    - Vaginal and cervical lacerations
    - Urine retention
    - Hematoma formation in the pelvic soft tissues
- Infant
  - ❑ Bruising or abrasions at the site of the blade applications

❑ Facial palsy resulting from pressure of the blades on the facial nerve
❑ Subdural hematoma

Nursing Considerations

■ Obtain the type of forceps requested by the physician.
■ Patient teaching
  ❑ Explain that the forceps blades fit like two tablespoons around an egg, with the blades coming over the infant's ears.
  ❑ Report to nurse caring for newborn and mother that forceps were used for the birth.

Vacuum-Assisted Birth

A vacuum-assisted birth (vacuum extraction) involves the attachment of a vacuum cup to the fetal head, using negative pressure to assist in the birth of the head. The vacuum is generally not used to assist births before 34 weeks of gestation. Indications for use are the same as those for outlet forceps (see Table 4-2). Advantages of vacuum-assisted birth compared with forceps-assisted birth are the ease with which the vacuum can be placed and the need for less anesthesia. Also it is far easier to learn the skills necessary to safely use the vacuum than to gain a similar level of skill with forceps.

Preprocedure Requirements

■ Completely dilated cervix
■ Ruptured membranes
■ Engaged fetal head
■ Vertex presentation
■ Absence of cephalopelvic disproportion (CPD)

Management

■ The vacuum cup is applied to the fetal head by the primary health care provider.
■ Depending on the type of vacuum used, either the primary health care provider or the nurse will generate the desired amount of negative pressure to create a vacuum.
■ Traction is applied by the primary health care provider.
■ The woman is encouraged to push as traction is applied by the primary health care provider
■ The vacuum cup is released and removed after birth of the head.

Maternal Complications

- Perineal, vaginal, or cervical lacerations
- Soft-tissue hematomas

Fetal Complications

- Cephalhematoma
- Scalp lacerations
- Subdural hematoma
- Hyperbilirubinemia and neonatal jaundice

Nursing Considerations

- Assess FHR frequently during the procedure.
- Encourage the woman to push during contractions.
- If responsible for generating pressure for the vacuum, do not exceed the "green zone" indicated on the pump. Verify with the physician the amount of pressure to be generated.
- Document the number of pulls attempted, maximal pressure used, and any pop-offs that occur.
- Observe the newborn for signs of trauma or infection at the application site and for cerebral irritation, such as poor sucking or listlessness.

CESAREAN BIRTH

Cesarean birth is the birth of a fetus through a transabdominal incision of the uterus. Cesarean births may be either scheduled or unplanned. The incidence of cesarean birth is increasing. Part of the reason for this rise is that a number of common risk factors for cesarean birth are increasing in frequency, especially in developed countries. These factors include fetal macrosomia, advanced maternal age, obesity, gestational diabetes, and multifetal pregnancy. Malpractice concerns are another factor related to the elevated incidence, along with an increase in the number of cesareans done on maternal request.

Indications for Cesarean Birth

Few absolute indications exist for cesarean birth. Most are performed primarily for conditions that might pose a threat to both mother and fetus if vaginal birth occurred. Box 4-5 lists common maternal and fetal indications for cesarean birth.

BOX 4-5

Indications for Cesarean Birth

MATERNAL

- Specific cardiac disease (Marfan syndrome, unstable coronary artery disease)
- Specific respiratory disease (Guillain-Barré syndrome)
- Conditions associated with increased intracranial pressure
- Mechanical obstruction of the lower uterine segment (tumors, fibroids)
- Mechanical vulvar obstruction (condylomata)
- History of previous cesarean birth

FETAL

- Abnormal (nonreassuring) FHR and pattern
- Malpresentation (e.g., breech or transverse lie)
- Active maternal herpes lesions
- Maternal human immunodeficiency virus with a viral load >1000 copies/ml
- Congenital anomalies

MATERNAL-FETAL

- Dystocia (cephalopelvic disproportion, "failure to progress" in labor)
- Placental abruption
- Placenta previa
- Elective cesarean birth

Sources: Duff, P., Sweet, R., & Edwards, R. (2009). Maternal and fetal infections. In R. Creasy, R. Resnik, J. Iams, C. Lockwood, & T. Moore (Eds.), *Creasy and Resnik's maternal-fetal medicine: Principles and practice* (6th ed.). Philadelphia: Saunders; Landon, M. (2007). Cesarean delivery. In S. Gabbe, J. Niebyl, & J. Simpson (Eds.), *Obstetrics: Normal and problem pregnancies* (5th ed.). Philadelphia: Churchill Livingstone; Thorp, J. (2009). Clinical aspects of normal and abnormal labor. In R. Creasy, R. Resnik, J. Iams, C. Lockwood, & T. Moore (Eds.), *Creasy and Resnik's maternal-fetal medicine: Principles and practice* (6th ed.). Philadelphia: Saunders.

Elective Cesarean Birth

Sometimes referred to as cesarean on request or cesarean on demand, an elective cesarean birth refers to a primary cesarean birth without a medical or obstetric indication. Reasons that women request cesarean births include the following:

- Fear of pain in childbirth
- Belief that the surgery will prevent future problems with pelvic support or sexual dysfunction

- Convenience of planning for birth
- Control and choice over when to give birth
- Previous traumatic vaginal birth or psychologic trauma

Maternal Risks

- Aspiration
- Hemorrhage
- Atelectasis
- Endometritis
- Abdominal wound dehiscence or infection
- Urinary tract infection
- Injuries to bowel or bladder
- Anesthetic-related complications
- Economic risk (more expensive than vaginal birth and a longer recovery period is necessary)

Fetal Risks

- Premature birth if gestational age has not been accurately determined
- Fetal injuries (most commonly superficial lacerations)
- Fetal asphyxia if the uterus and placenta are poorly perfused as a result of maternal hypotension caused by regional anesthesia or maternal positioning.

Management

Preoperative

- If this is a scheduled cesarean birth, woman remains NPO (nothing by mouth) for at least 8 hours before surgery
- Informed consent is obtained
- Anesthesia interview
- Intravenous (IV) insertion to maintain hydration and provide an open line for the administration of blood or medications if needed
- Laboratory tests
  - ❑ Complete blood cell count and chemistry
  - ❑ Blood typing and crossmatching
- Maternal vital signs
- Fetal heart rate (FHR) and pattern and contraction monitoring
- Retention (Foley) catheter insertion to keep the bladder empty
- Placement of thromboembolic stockings (TED hose) or sequential compression devices (SCD boots) to prevent blood clots

- Preoperative medications
  - ❏ Medications to prevent aspiration pneumonia
  - ❏ Prophylactic antibiotics to prevent postoperative infection
- Abdominal shave or clipping of pubic hair if ordered
- Removal of contact lenses, dentures, nail polish, and jewelry, according to hospital policy

Intraoperative

- Cesarean birth occurs in an operating room, either in the hospital's surgical unit or in the labor and birth unit.
- If possible, the woman's partner is with her during surgery to provide support and comfort.
- Staff members from the labor and birth unit may scrub and circulate during the surgery, or these functions may be assumed by members of the hospital's surgery staff. In either case, nurses from the labor and birth unit usually provide care for the uncompromised newborn.
- In addition, a pediatrician or nurse team skilled in neonatal resuscitation may be present to provide care for the newborn, because infants born by cesarean are considered to be at risk until there is evidence of physiologic stability after the birth.

Surgical Techniques
Types of Skin Incisions (Fig. 4-1)

- Vertical, extending from near the umbilicus to the mons pubis
- Transverse (Pfannenstiel) in the lower abdomen ("bikini" incision)
  The skin incision (vertical or transverse) does *not* necessarily indicate the type of uterine incision.

Types of Uterine Incisions (Fig. 4-2)
Vertical

- Ideally the vertical incision is contained entirely within the lower uterine segment (see Fig. 4-2, *B*) but can extend into the contractile portion of the uterus (a classic incision [see Fig. 4-2, *C*])
- Indications for a vertical incision
  - ❏ An underdeveloped lower uterine segment
  - ❏ Abnormal fetal presentation (e.g., transverse lie, breech)
  - ❏ Certain fetal anomalies (e.g., massive hydrocephalus)
  - ❏ Anterior placenta previa
- Vaginal birth after cesarean (VBAC) is contraindicated in subsequent pregnancies after a classic uterine incision.

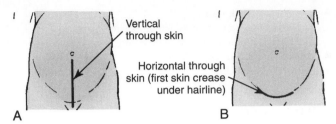

Fig. 4-1 Skin incisions for cesarean birth. **A,** Vertical. **B,** Horizontal (Pfannenstiel).

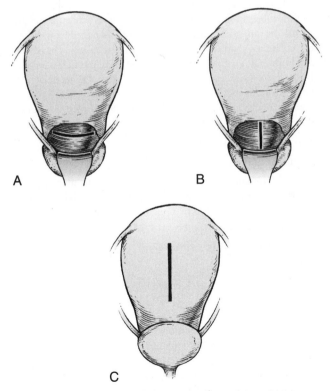

Fig. 4-2 Uterine incisions for cesarean birth. **A,** Low transverse incision. **B,** Low vertical incision. **C,** Classic incision. (From Gabbe, S., Niebyl, J., & Simpson, J. [2007]. *Obstetrics: Normal and problem pregnancies* [5th ed.]. Philadelphia: Churchill Livingstone.)

Low Transverse (see Fig. 4-2, A)

- Performed in more than 90% of all cesarean births
- Compared with the vertical incision, is easier to perform and repair, and is associated with less blood loss. It is also less likely to rupture in subsequent pregnancies.

Postoperative

Immediate Recovery

- Immediately following surgery the mother is transferred to a recovery area. Nursing assessments include degree of recovery from the effects of anesthesia, postoperative and postbirth status, and degree of pain.
- Specific assessments include the following:
  - ❑ Vital signs every 15 minutes for 1 to 2 hours, or until stable
  - ❑ Condition of incisional dressing
  - ❑ Status of uterine fundus and amount of lochia
  - ❑ Intake and output
- If the baby is present, the woman should be given time with him or her to facilitate bonding and attachment. Breastfeeding can be initiated.
- Medications for pain relief should be administered before postoperative pain becomes severe. Common forms of pain relief include the following:
  - ❑ Epidural opioids (if epidural anesthesia was used)
  - ❑ Patient-controlled analgesia (PCA)
  - ❑ IV or intramuscular injections of analgesics
- The woman is ready for discharge from the recovery area once her condition is stable and the effects of anesthesia have worn off (e.g., she is alert, oriented, and able to feel and move extremities).

Postpartum Care

- The woman's physiologic concerns the first few days may be dominated by pain at the incisional site and pain resulting from intestinal gas. For the first 24 hours following surgery, pain relief may be provided by epidural opioids, PCA, or IV or intramuscular injections of analgesics. After this time parenteral medications are generally changed to oral analgesics.
- Commonly ordered analgesics include opioids and nonsteroidal antiinflammatory drugs (NSAIDS) such as the following:
  - ❑ Hydromorphone (Dilaudid)
  - ❑ Meperidine (Demerol)

- ❑ Morphine sulfate
- ❑ Nalbuphine (Nubain)
- ❑ Ketorolac (Toradol)

SAFETY ALERT *When holding her baby or breastfeeding, a woman may become drowsy and even fall asleep because of the sedation that occurs with the use of analgesics. It is important that someone be with her during these times.*

- Other comfort measures include the following:
  - ❑ Position changes
  - ❑ Splinting of the incision with pillows
  - ❑ Breathing and relaxation techniques learned in childbirth classes
- Use of TED hose or SCD boots should be continued as long as the woman remains in bed. They may be removed when she begins ambulating.

SAFETY ALERT *When getting out of bed, the woman should be taught to seek assistance initially especially when an IV and catheter are still in place. Thereafter, when rising from a supine position, she should sit on the side of the bed first to determine if dizziness will occur, then stand at the bedside, and finally ambulate.*

- Management of gas pain
  - ❑ Ambulating
  - ❑ Rocking in a rocking chair
  - ❑ Avoiding gas-forming foods and carbonated beverages
  - ❑ Not drinking liquids through a straw
- The woman may shower after the incisional dressing is removed (usually on the first postoperative day).
- The indwelling (Foley) catheter is generally removed on the first postoperative day.
- Early introduction of solid food is safe. Women who eat early have been found to require less analgesia, and gastrointestinal problems do not occur.
- The woman will usually be discharged by the third postoperative day. Home care may be available for mothers who meet appropriate criteria for discharge and choose to leave sooner than the allowed length of stay.

■ Before discharge the woman must be taught signs of postoperative complications that should be reported immediately to the health care provider. See the Teaching for Self-Management box: Signs of Postoperative Complications After Discharge Following Cesarean Birth.

VAGINAL BIRTH AFTER CESAREAN

Indications for primary cesarean birth, such as dysfunctional labor (dystocia), breech presentation, or fetal distress often are nonrecurring. Therefore, a woman who has had a cesarean birth may subsequently become pregnant, experience no contraindications for labor and birth during the pregnancy, and choose to attempt a VBAC. Box 4-6 lists selection criteria suggested by the American College of

---

Teaching for Self-Management

Signs of Postoperative Complications After Discharge Following Cesarean Birth

Report the following signs to your health care provider:
■ Temperature exceeding 38°C (100.4°F)
■ Urination: dysuria, urgency, cloudy urine
■ Lochia: heavier than a normal menstrual period, clots, odor
■ Cesarean incision (REEDA): *r*edness, *e*dema, *e*cchymosis, *d*rainage, *a*pproximation disrupted (wound separates)
■ Severe, increasing abdominal pain

BOX 4-6

Selection Criteria for Vaginal Birth After Cesarean

■ One previous low-transverse cesarean birth
■ Clinically adequate pelvis
■ No other uterine scars or history of previous rupture
■ Physician immediately available throughout active labor who is capable of monitoring labor and performing an emergency cesarean birth if necessary
■ Availability of anesthesia and personnel for emergency cesarean birth

Source: American College of Obstetricians and Gynecologists (ACOG). (2004). Vaginal birth after a previous cesarean delivery. *ACOG Practice Bulletin No. 54.* Washington, DC: ACOG.

Obstetricians and Gynecologists (ACOG) for identifying candidates for VBAC.

Spontaneous labor with a ripe cervix is more likely to result in a successful VBAC than is labor that has been induced or augmented. Induction or augmentation with oxytocin or prostaglandins increases the risk for uterine rupture, a major concern when a VBAC is attempted. If uterine stimulation is needed, oxytocin is the drug of choice because the risk for rupture is lower than with prostaglandins. Women most likely to have a successful VBAC are those who are less than 35 years of age, whose fetus weighs less than 4000 g, and whose previous cesarean was performed for some reason other than failure of descent in second stage labor.

OBSTETRIC EMERGENCIES
Meconium-Stained Amniotic Fluid

Meconium staining of amniotic fluid occurs when the fetus passes meconium (first stool) at some time before birth. Meconium-stained amniotic fluid is green in color. The consistency of the amniotic fluid is often described as either thin (light) or thick (heavy), depending on the amount of meconium present.

The major risk associated with meconium-stained amniotic fluid is the development of meconium aspiration syndrome (MAS) in the newborn. MAS causes a severe form of aspiration pneumonia that occurs most often in term or postterm infants who have passed meconium in utero. Current thought is that MAS most likely results from a long-standing intrauterine process rather than from aspiration immediately after birth as respirations are initiated.

Management

See the Emergency box: Immediate Management of the Newborn with Meconium-Stained Amniotic Fluid.

NURSING ALERT   *Every birth should be attended by at least one person whose only responsibility is the infant and who is capable of initiating resuscitation. Either that person or someone else who is immediately available should have the skills required to perform a complete resuscitation, including endotracheal suctioning to remove meconium, if necessary.*

EMERGENCY

Immediate Management of the Newborn with Meconium-Stained Amniotic Fluid

BEFORE BIRTH
- Assess amniotic fluid for the presence of meconium after rupture of membranes.
- If the amniotic fluid is meconium stained, gather equipment and supplies before the birth that might be necessary for neonatal resuscitation.
- Have at least one person capable of performing endotracheal intubation on the baby present at the birth.

IMMEDIATELY AFTER BIRTH
- Assess the baby's respiratory efforts, heart rate, and muscle tone.
- Suction only the baby's mouth and nose, using either a bulb syringe or a 12- or 14-French suction catheter if the baby has:
  - ❑ Strong respiratory efforts
  - ❑ Good muscle tone
  - ❑ Heart rate >100 beats/min
- Suction below the vocal cords using an endotracheal tube to remove any meconium present before many spontaneous respirations have occurred or assisted ventilation has been initiated if the baby has:
  - ❑ Depressed respirations
  - ❑ Decreased muscle tone
  - ❑ Heart rate <100 beats/min

Source: American Academy of Pediatrics (AAP) & American Heart Association (AHA). (2006). *Textbook of neonatal resuscitation* (5th ed.). Elk Grove Village, IL: AAP; Dallas, TX: AHA.

Shoulder Dystocia

Shoulder dystocia occurs when the head is born but the anterior shoulder cannot pass under the pubic arch. The incidence of shoulder dystocia has increased in recent years, perhaps because of larger birth weights or simply because more attention is paid to documenting the condition.

Etiology

- Fetopelvic disproportion related to excessive fetal size (>4000 g)
- Maternal pelvic abnormalities
- Maternal diabetes (risk for macrosomia)
- History of shoulder dystocia in a previous birth

In half of all cases of shoulder dystocia, no risk factors are identi-fied. Shoulder dystocia *cannot* be accurately predicted or prevented.

Signs

Signs that could indicate the presence of shoulder dystocia include the following:

- Slowing of the progress of labor
- Formation of a caput succedaneum that increases in size
- When the head emerges, it retracts against the perineum (turtle sign).
- External rotation does not occur.

Associated Risks

Maternal

- Postpartum hemorrhage
- Rectal injuries

Fetal/Neonatal

- Asphyxia (related to delay in completing the birth)
- Brachial plexus injury (Erb palsy) or phrenic nerve injury
- Fracture of the humerus or clavicle

Management

- Immediately call for additional assistance (i.e., extra nurses, anesthesia care provider, and neonatal resuscitation team).
- Suprapubic pressure (Fig. 4-3) can be used to push the anterior shoulder under the symphysis pubis.
- The McRoberts maneuver (Fig. 4-4) in which the woman's legs are flexed apart, with her knees on her abdomen, can be used to decrease the angle of pelvic inclination, freeing the shoulder.
  - Frequently the McRoberts maneuver and suprapubic pressure are used simultaneously.
- Having the woman move to a hands-and-knees position (Gaskin maneuver), a squatting position, or lateral recumbent position has been used to resolve cases of shoulder dystocia.
- Fundal pressure should be avoided as a method of relieving shoulder dystocia. Its use has been associated with neurologic complications.
- The nurse helps the woman assume the position or positions that may facilitate birth of the shoulders, assists the primary health care provider with these maneuvers, and documents the maneuvers.

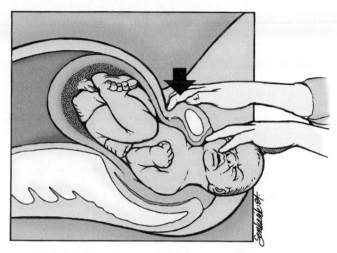

Fig. 4-3 Application of suprapubic pressure. (From Gabbe, S., Niebyl, J., & Simpson, J. [2007]. *Obstetrics: Normal and problem pregnancies* [5th ed.]. Philadelphia: Churchill Livingstone.)

- Following birth, maternal assessment should focus on early detection of hemorrhage and trauma to the soft tissues of the birth canal.
- Newborn assessment should include examination for fracture of the clavicle or humerus as well as brachial plexus injuries and asphyxia.

Prolapsed Umbilical Cord

Prolapse of the umbilical cord (Fig. 4-5) occurs when the cord lies below the presenting part of the fetus. Fetal hypoxia resulting from prolonged cord compression (occlusion of blood flow to and from the fetus for more than 5 minutes) usually results in central nervous system damage or death of the fetus.

Types

- Occult (hidden, not visible)
  - ❑ May occur at any time during labor whether or not the membranes are ruptured
- Frank (visible)
  - ❑ Most often occurs directly after rupture of membranes, when gravity washes the cord in front of the presenting part

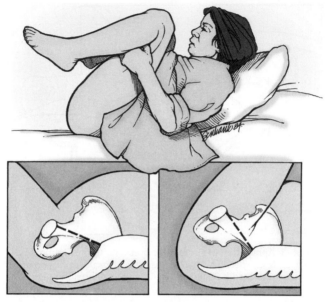

Fig. 4-4 McRoberts maneuver. (From Gabbe, S., Niebyl, J., & Simpson, J. [2007]. *Obstetrics: Normal and problem pregnancies* [5th ed.]. Philadelphia: Churchill Livingstone.)

Contributing Factors

- Long cord (longer than 100 cm)
- Fetal malpresentation (breech or transverse lie)
- Unengaged presenting part
- Small fetus that does not fit snugly into the lower uterine segment

Management

- Prompt recognition and rapid treatment are important to prevent fetal injury or death. See the Emergency box: Prolapsed Umbilical Cord.

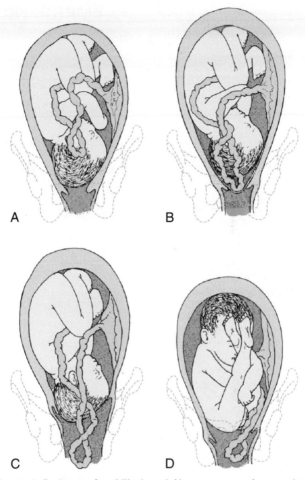

Fig. 4-5 Prolapse of umbilical cord. Note pressure of presenting part on umbilical cord, which endangers fetal circulation. **A,** Occult (hidden) prolapse of cord. **B,** Complete prolapse of cord. Note that membranes are intact. **C,** Cord presenting in front of the fetal head may be seen in vagina. **D,** Frank breech presentation with prolapsed cord.

EMERGENCY

Prolapsed Umbilical Cord

SIGNS

- Variable or prolonged decelerations during uterine contractions
- Woman reports feeling the cord after membranes rupture
- Cord is seen or felt in or protruding from the vagina

INTERVENTIONS

- Call for assistance. Do not leave woman alone.
- Have someone notify the primary health care provider immediately.
- Glove the examining hand quickly and insert two fingers into the vagina to the cervix. With one finger on either side of the cord or both fingers to one side, exert upward pressure against the presenting part to relieve compression of the cord. Do not move your hand! Another person may place a rolled towel under the woman's right or left hip.
- Place woman into an extreme Trendelenburg or a modified Sims position, or a knee-chest position
- If cord is protruding from vagina, wrap loosely in a sterile towel saturated with warm sterile normal saline solution. Do not attempt to replace cord into cervix.
- Administer oxygen to the woman by nonrebreather face mask at 8 to 10 L/min until birth is accomplished.
- Start IV fluids or increase existing drip rate.
- Continue to monitor FHR continuously, by internal fetal scalp electrode, if possible.
- Explain to woman and support person what is happening and the way it is being managed.
- Prepare for immediate vaginal birth if cervix is fully dilated, or cesarean birth if it is not.

SECTION 5

Postpartum

BASIC DEFINITIONS

attachment: The process by which the parent and infant come to love and accept each other

bonding: A process by which parents, over time, form an emotional relationship with their infant

breast engorgement: Swelling of breast tissue caused by increased blood and lymph supply to the breasts as the body produces milk, occurring about 72 to 96 hours after birth

contraception: The intentional prevention of pregnancy during sexual intercourse

involution: Return of the uterus to a nonpregnant state after birth

puerperium: Period between the birth of the newborn and the return of the reproductive organs to their normal nonpregnant state

subinvolution: failure of the uterus to return to a nonpregnant state; the most common causes of subinvolution are retained placental fragments and infection

TRANSFER FROM THE RECOVERY AREA

At the end of the fourth stage of labor the woman changes from an intrapartum to a postpartum status. She can remain in the same room with the same care provider or be transferred to a postpartum room in the same or another nursing unit and change care providers. This is an excellent time to review intrapartum events and plan appropriate postpartum care for her and her newborn.

Information that must be communicated to the postpartum nurse includes the following:

- Name and age of patient
- Identity of the primary health care provider
- Gravidity and parity
- Time of birth
- Duration of labor and time of rupture of membranes

- Whether labor was induced or augmented
- Type of birth (vaginal, operative vaginal [forceps- or vacuum-assisted], cesarean)
- Anesthetic used
- Any medications given
- Intravenous (IV) infusion of any fluids
- Physiologic status since birth
- Description of fundus, lochia, bladder, and perineum
- Laboratory results
  - Blood type and Rh status
  - Group B streptococci status
  - Status of rubella immunity
  - Human immunodeficiency virus (HIV) test result (if positive)
  - Hepatitis B test result (if positive)
  - Syphilis (serology) test result (if positive)
- Other infections identified during pregnancy (i.e., chlamydia, gonorrhea) and whether these were treated before the birth
- Sex and weight of infant
- Any abnormalities noted
- Chosen method of feeding
- Name of pediatric care provider
- Assessment of initial parent-infant interaction

Most of this information is also documented for the nursing staff in the newborn nursery. Other specific information about the newborn that must be communicated to the nursery staff includes the following:

- Mother's correct name and bracelet or other identification numbers
- Apgar scores
- Voiding or stooling since birth
- Whether the infant has nursed or been fed formula since birth
- Nursing interventions that have been completed, such as eye prophylaxis and vitamin K injection

MANAGEMENT OF PHYSICAL NEEDS

Assessment

- Initial postpartum assessment, performed on admission to the postpartum unit (or when woman changes to postpartum status)
- Vital signs including blood pressure
- Emotional status

- Energy level
- Degree of physical discomfort, hunger, thirst
- Intake and output assessment (if IV infusion or a urinary catheter is in place)
- Incisional dressing condition (cesarean birth)
- Ongoing assessment, performed at least once on each shift throughout her hospital stay; the following components should be included in each assessment:
  - ❑ BUBBLE-HE is an acronym for the assessment components.
    - B Breasts (soft, filling, firm; include condition of nipples)
    - U Uterine fundus (location, consistency)
    - B Bowel function (presence or absence of bowel movement)
    - B Bladder function (volume, color)
    - L Lochia
      - Lochia rubra—bright or dark red blood—lasts 3 to 4 days
      - Lochia serosa—pink or brown—lasts up to 2 weeks
      - Lochia alba—thin, yellow to white, can last 4 to 6 weeks
    - E Episiotomy (perineum)
    - H Homans sign (legs)
    - E Emotions

SAFETY ALERT *A perineal pad saturated in 15 minutes or less and pooling of blood under the buttocks are indications of excessive blood loss, requiring immediate assessment, intervention, and notification of the physician or nurse-midwife.*

NURSING ALERT *The nurse always checks under the mother's buttocks as well as on the perineal pad. Blood may flow between the buttocks onto the linens under the mother. Although the amount on the perineal pad is slight, excessive bleeding may go undetected.*

- Signs of potential physiologic complications are listed in the box on p. 208.
- Routine laboratory tests
  - ❑ Hematocrit (on first postpartum day) if ordered
  - ❑ Rubella status (if no results available on admission to the postpartum unit)
  - ❑ Rh status (if no results available on admission to the postpartum unit)

Signs of Potential Complications

Postpartum Physiologic Problems

TEMPERATURE
- More than 38° C after the first 24 hr

PULSE
- Tachycardia or marked bradycardia

BLOOD PRESSURE
- Hypotension or hypertension

ENERGY LEVEL
- Lethargy, extreme fatigue

UTERUS
- Deviated from the midline, boggy consistency, remains above the umbilicus after 24 hr

LOCHIA
- Heavy; bright red bleeding that is not lochia; foul odor

PERINEUM
- Marked discomfort, pronounced edema, not intact, signs of infection

LEGS
- Homans sign positive; painful, reddened area; warmth on posterior aspect of calf

BREASTS
- Pain, cracked and fissured nipples, redness, heat, inverted nipples, palpable mass

APPETITE
- Lack of appetite, nausea or vomiting
- Epigastric pain

ELIMINATION
- Bladder: inability to void, urgency, frequency, dysuria
- Bowel: constipation, diarrhea

REST
- Inability to rest or sleep

NEUROLOGIC
- Headache, blurred vision

General Care
Newborn Safety

- Teach the mother to check the identity of any person who comes to remove the baby from her room. Examples of commonly used infant security systems are:
  - ❏ Picture identification badges worn by hospital staff members
  - ❏ Matching scrubs worn by all unit staff members
  - ❏ Closed-circuit television
  - ❏ Computer monitoring systems
  - ❏ Fingerprint identification pads
- As a rule, the baby is always wheeled in a bassinet, not carried in a staff or family member's or parent's arms, while being transported between the mother's room and the nursery.

Prevention of Infection

- Maintain a clean environment.
- Change bed linens as needed.
- Change disposable pads and draw sheets as needed.
- Have the woman avoid walking barefoot to prevent contamination of bed linens when returning to bed.
- Have all staff members practice conscientious handwashing or use hand sanitizers.
- Practice Standard Precautions.
- Teach the woman proper care of episiotomy and lacerations:
  - ❏ Wash hands thoroughly before and after changing perineal pads.
  - ❏ Wipe from front to back (urethra to anus) after voiding or defecating.
  - ❏ Cleanse the perineum with plain warm water after each voiding.
  - ❏ Change the perineal pad after each time she voids or defecates.

Prevention of Excessive Bleeding

- Maintain good uterine tone.
  - ❏ Massage the fundus until it is firm (teach mother how to massage the fundus).
  - ❏ Administer IV fluids and oxytocic medications (drugs that stimulate contraction of the uterine smooth muscle) as ordered.

- Prevent bladder distention.
  - ❑ Assist the woman to void spontaneously on toilet or bedpan by:
    - ○ Having her listen to running water
    - ○ Placing her hands in warm water
    - ○ Pouring water from a squeeze bottle over her perineum
    - ○ Encouraging her to void in the shower or sitz bath
    - ○ Administering analgesics if ordered to relieve fear of anticipated pain
  - ❑ Catheterize the woman if she is unable to void spontaneously.

Promotion of Comfort and Rest
Comfort

- Nonpharmacologic interventions
  - ❑ Warm or cold applications, topical applications, distraction, imagery, therapeutic touch, relaxation, interaction with the infant, encouraging a side-lying position, sitting on a pillow
- Pharmacologic interventions
  - ❑ Narcotics, nonsteroidal antiinflammatory medications, topical anesthetic ointment or sprays

> **NURSING ALERT** *The nurse should carefully monitor all women receiving opioids because respiratory depression and decreased intestinal motility are side effects.*

Rest

- Comfort measures, such as back rubs
- Medication for sleep as ordered
- Adjust hospital routines when possible to allow for uninterrupted rest.
- Limit visitors.

Promotion of Ambulation and Exercise

- Encourage free movement once anesthesia wears off unless an analgesic has been administered.
- Teach leg exercises to promote circulation in the legs if the woman must remain on bed rest after birth.
- Kegel exercises to strengthen muscle tone of the pubococcygeal muscle are extremely important (see the Teaching for Self-Management box: Kegel Exercises).

Teaching for Self-Management

Kegel Exercises

DESCRIPTION AND RATIONALE

Kegel exercise, or pelvic muscle exercise, is a technique used to strengthen the muscles that support the pelvic floor. This exercise involves regularly tightening (contracting) and relaxing the muscles that support the bladder and urethra. By strengthening these pelvic muscles, a woman can prevent or reduce accidental urine loss.

TECHNIQUE

The woman needs to learn how to target the muscles for training and how to contract them correctly. One suggestion for teaching is to have the woman pretend she is trying to prevent the passage of intestinal gas. Have her use this tightening motion on the muscles around her vagina and the upper pelvis. She should feel these muscles drawing inward and upward. Other suggested techniques are to have the woman pretend she is trying to stop the flow of urine in midstream or to have her think about how her vagina is able to contract around and move up the length of the penis during intercourse.

The woman should avoid straining or bearing-down motions while performing the exercise. She should be taught how bearing down feels by having her take a breath, hold it, and push down with her abdominal muscles as though she were trying to have a bowel movement. Then the woman can be taught how to avoid straining down by exhaling gently and keeping her mouth open each time she contracts her pelvic muscles.

SPECIFIC INSTRUCTIONS

1. Each contraction should be as intense as possible without contracting the abdomen, thighs, or buttocks.
2. Contractions should be held for at least 10 sec. The woman may have to start with as little as 2 sec per contraction until her muscles get stronger.
3. The woman should rest for 10 sec or more between contractions, so that the muscles have time to recover and each contraction can be as strong as the woman can make it.
4. The woman should feel the pulling up over the three muscle layers so that the contraction reaches the highest level of her pelvis.

Continued

Teaching for Self-Management—cont'd

OTHER SUGGESTIONS FOR IMPLEMENTATION

1. At first the woman should set aside about 15 min a day to do the Kegel exercises.

2. The woman may want to put up reminders to do the exercises, such as notes on her bathroom mirror, her refrigerator, her television, or her calendar.

3. Guidelines for practicing Kegel exercises suggest performing between 24 and 100 contractions a day; however, positive results can be achieved with only 24 to 45 a day.

4. The best position for learning how to do Kegel exercises is to lie supine with the knees bent. Another position to use is on the hands and knees. Once the woman learns the proper technique, she can perform the exercises in other positions such as standing or sitting.

Sources: Sampselle, C. (2003). Behavior interventions in young and middle-aged women: Simple interventions to combat a complex problem. *American Journal of Nursing, 103*(Suppl), 9-19; Sampselle, C. (2000). Behavioral interventions for urinary incontinence in women: Evidence for practice. *Journal of Midwifery & Women's Health, 45*(2), 94-103; Sampselle, C., Wyman, J., Thomas, K., Newman, D., Gray, M., Dougherty, M., et al. (2000). Continence for women: A test of AWHONN's evidence-based protocol. *Journal of Obstetric, Gynecologic and Neonatal Nursing, 29*(1), 312-317.

SAFETY ALERT *Have a hospital staff or family member present the first time the woman gets out of bed after birth because she may feel weak, dizzy, faint, or lightheaded.*

Promotion of Healthy Nutrition

- Most women have a good appetite and eat well.
- Cultural dietary preferences must be respected.
- Recommended caloric intake for the moderately active nonlactating postpartum woman is 1800 to 2200 kcal/day.
- Recommended caloric intake for the lactating woman is 2700 kcal/day.

Promotion of Normal Bowel and Bladder Patterns

- Measure the first several voidings to document adequate emptying of the bladder. A volume of at least 150 ml is expected for each voiding.

- Assist the woman to void spontaneously on the toilet or bedpan.
- Teach measures to avoid constipation:
  - Ensure adequate roughage and fluid intake.
  - Encourage exercise.
  - Administer stool softeners and/or laxatives as needed.

Breastfeeding Promotion/ Lactation Suppression

Breastfeeding Promotion

- Newborns without complications should be put to breast within the first hour after birth.
- The baby should remain in direct skin-to-skin contact with the mother until able to breastfeed for the first time.

During the first 3 days of life the breastfed infant receives colostrum, a very concentrated, high-protein fluid containing enzymes, antiinfective agents, hormones, and growth factors. As the baby adjusts to extrauterine life and the digestive tract is cleared of meconium, intake increases from 15 to 30 ml of colostrum per feeding in the first 24 hours to 60 to 90 ml of milk by the end of the first week.

Assisting with Breastfeeding

Positioning

Three of the four basic positions are shown in Figure 5-1.

- Football or clutch hold (under the arm)
  - Often recommended for early feedings because the mother can easily see the baby's mouth as she guides the infant onto the nipple
  - Usually preferred by mothers who gave birth by cesarean
- Cradle
  - Most common breastfeeding position for infants who have learned to latch easily and feed effectively
- Modified cradle or across the lap
  - Works well for early feedings, especially with smaller babies
- Side-lying
  - Allows the mother to rest while breastfeeding
  - Often preferred by women with perineal pain and swelling

Initially it is best to use the position that most easily facilitates latch while allowing maximal comfort for the mother.

Before discharge from the hospital, assist the mother to try all four positions so that she will feel confident in her ability to vary positions at home.

Regardless of the position used, the mother should be comfortable.

- Place infant at the level of the breast, supported by pillows or folded blankets.

- Turn the baby completely onto his or her side and facing the mother, so that the infant is "belly to belly" with the arms "hugging" the breast. The baby's mouth is directly in front of the nipple.

- Mother's hand is used to support the baby's neck and shoulders, not to push on the occiput.

- Baby's body is held in correct alignment, so that ears, shoulders, and hips are in a straight line.

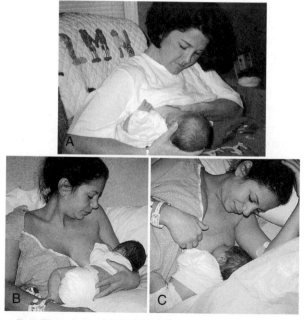

Fig. 5-1 Three breastfeeding positions. **A,** Football hold. **B,** Cradling. **C,** Lying down. (**B** and **C,** Courtesy Marjorie Pyle, RNC, Lifecircle, Costa Mesa, CA.)

Latch

■ To facilitate latch:
  ❏ In preparation for latch during early feedings, have the mother manually express a few drops of colostrum or milk and spread it over the nipple.
■ The latch process is shown in Figure 5-2.
  ❏ Mother supports her breast in one hand with the thumb on top and four fingers underneath at the back edge of the areola. The breast is compressed slightly.
  ❏ With the baby held close to the breast and the mouth held directly in front of the nipple, mother tickles the baby's lower lip with the tip of her nipple, stimulating the mouth to open.
  ❏ When the mouth is open wide and the tongue is down, the mother quickly "hugs" the baby to the breast, bringing the baby onto the nipple.
  ❏ In general, with correct latch, the baby's mouth should cover the nipple and an areolar radius of approximately 2 to 3 cm all around the nipple.
  ❏ When latched correctly, the baby's cheeks and chin are touching the breast. Depressing the breast tissue around the baby's nose to create breathing space is not necessary (Fig. 5-3).

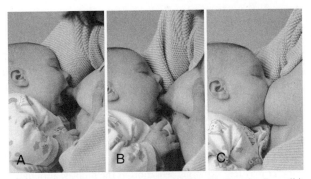

Fig. 5-2 Latch. **A,** Tickle baby's lower lip with the nipple until he or she opens wide. **B,** Once baby's mouth is opened wide, quickly pull baby onto breast. **C,** Baby should have as much areola (dark area around nipple) in his or her mouth as possible, not just the nipple. (Courtesy Medela, Inc., McHenry, IL.)

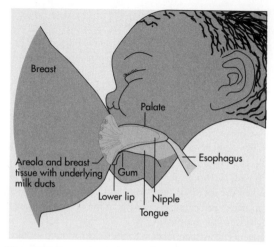

Fig. 5-3 Correct attachment (latch) of infant at breast.

- When the baby is nursing appropriately, the following occur:
  - ❑ Mother reports a firm tugging sensation on her nipples but no pinching or pain.
  - ❑ Baby sucks with cheeks rounded, not dimpled.
  - ❑ Baby's jaw glides smoothly with sucking.
  - ❑ Swallowing is usually audible.
- Any time the signs of adequate latch and sucking are not present, the baby should be taken off the breast and latch attempted again.
- To prevent nipple trauma as the baby is taken off the breast, instruct the mother to break the suction by inserting a finger in the side of the baby's mouth between the gums and leaving it there until the nipple is completely out of the baby's mouth (Fig. 5-4).

Milk Ejection or Let-down

As the baby begins sucking on the nipple, the milk-ejection, or let-down, reflex is stimulated. The following signs indicate that milk ejection has occurred:

- Mother may feel a tingling sensation in the nipples, although many women never feel this.
- Baby's suck changes from quick, shallow sucks to a slower, more drawing, sucking pattern.
- Swallowing is heard as the baby sucks.

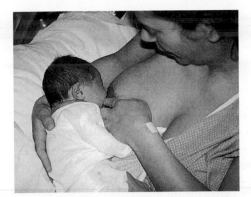

Fig. 5-4 Removing infant from the breast. (Courtesy Marjorie Pyle, RNC, Lifecircle, Costa Mesa, CA.)

- Mother feels uterine cramping and can have increased lochia during and after feedings the first few days after birth.
- Mother feels relaxed or drowsy during feedings.
- The opposite breast may leak.

Frequency of Feedings

- Newborns need to breastfeed 8 to 12 times in a 24-hour period.
- Feeding patterns are variable because each baby is unique.
- Some infants will breastfeed every 2 to 3 hours; others may cluster-feed, feeding every hour or so for three to five feedings and then sleeping for 3 to 4 hours between clusters.
- During the first 24 to 48 hours of life, most babies do not awaken this often to feed.
  - Parents need to awaken the baby to feed at least every 3 hours during the day and at least every 4 hours at night.
- Once the infant is feeding well and gaining weight adequately, demand feeding, in which the infant determines the frequency of feedings, is appropriate.
  - With demand feeding, the infant should still receive at least eight feedings in 24 hours.
- Infants should be fed whenever they exhibit feeding-readiness cues, such as the following:
  - Hand-to-mouth or hand-to-hand movements
  - Sucking motions

❑ Rooting
❑ Mouthing

- Do not wait for the baby to cry to indicate hunger; crying is a late sign of hunger.
- At night babies should be placed in a bassinet close to the mother for convenient breastfeeding.

Duration of Feedings

- Highly variable, because the timing of milk transfer differs for each mother-baby pair
- Average time for feeding is 30 to 40 minutes, or approximately 15 to 20 minutes per breast.
- The first breast offered should be alternated at each feeding to ensure that each breast receives equal stimulation and emptying.
- Rather than teaching mothers to feed for a set number of minutes, teach them to determine when a baby has finished a feeding:
  ❑ Baby's suck and swallow pattern has slowed
  ❑ Breast is softened
  ❑ Baby appears content and may fall asleep or release the nipple

NURSING ALERT *If a baby seems to be feeding effectively and the urine output is adequate but the weight gain is not satisfactory, the mother may be switching to the second breast too soon. The high-lactose, low-fat foremilk can cause the baby to have explosive stools, gas pains, and inconsolable crying. Feeding on the first breast until it softens ensures that the baby receives the higher fat hindmilk, which usually results in increased weight gain.*

Indicators of effective breastfeeding are listed in Box 5-1.

Supplements, Bottles, and Pacifiers

- Unless a medical indication exists, no supplements should be given to breastfeeding infants.
- See Box 5-2 for indications for supplementary feedings.
- Pacifiers are not recommended until breastfeeding is well established, usually after 1 month.
- Consider giving infant a pacifier at nap time or bedtime; a correlation between pacifier use at bedtime and a decreased risk of sudden infant death syndrome (SIDS) has been identified.

BOX 5-1

Indicators of Effective Breastfeeding

MOTHER
- Onset of copious milk production (milk is "in") by day 3 or 4
- Firm tugging sensation on nipple as infant sucks, but no pain
- Uterine contractions and increased vaginal bleeding while feeding (first week or less)
- Feels relaxed and drowsy while feeding
- Increased thirst
- Breasts soften or lighten while feeding
- With milk ejection (let-down), can feel warm rush or tingling in nipples; leaking of milk from opposite breast

INFANT
- Latches without difficulty
- Has bursts of 15 to 20 sucks/swallows at a time
- Swallowing is audible
- Easily releases breast at end of feeding
- Infant appears contented after feeding
- Has at least three substantial bowel movements and six to eight wet diapers every 24 hr after day 4

BOX 5-2

Indications for Supplementary Feedings

INFANT INDICATIONS
- Hypoglycemia
- Dehydration
- Weight loss of 8% to 10% of birth weight associated with delayed lactogenesis
- Delayed passage of bowel movements or meconium continued to day 5
- Poor milk transfer
- Hyperbilirubinemia

MATERNAL INDICATIONS
- Delayed lactogenesis
- Intolerable pain during feedings
- Previous breast surgery

Special Considerations

- To wake a sleepy newborn, do the following:
  - ❏ Lay the baby down and unwrap.
  - ❏ Change the diaper.
  - ❏ Hold the baby upright; turn from side to side.
  - ❏ Talk to the baby with variable pitch.
  - ❏ Massage the chest and back.
  - ❏ Rub the baby's hands and feet.
  - ❏ Sit the baby upright.
- To calm a fussy newborn, do the following:
  - ❏ Swaddle the baby.
  - ❏ Hold the baby close.
  - ❏ Move or rock gently.
  - ❏ Talk soothingly.
  - ❏ Allow baby to suck on a clean finger.
  - ❏ Place baby skin to skin with mother.
- Warning signs of ineffective breastfeeding are in Box 5-3.

Care of the Mother

- Lactating mothers should consume a balanced diet of nutrient-dense foods. Adequate amounts of calcium, minerals, and fat-soluble vitamins are important.
- No specific foods or drinks must be consumed or avoided while breastfeeding.

BOX 5-3

Warning Signs of Ineffective Breastfeeding

- Baby has fewer than six wet diapers per day after the fourth day of life
- Baby is having fewer than three stools per day after the fourth day of life
- Stools are still meconium (black, tarry) by the fourth day of life
- Mother's nipples are painful throughout feeding
- Mother's nipples are damaged (bruised, cracked, bleeding)
- Milk supply has not increased (no breast fullness) by day 4
- Baby seems to be feeding constantly
- Baby is losing weight after the fourth day of life
- Baby is gaining less than 0.5 oz per day after the fourth day of life
- Baby has not regained birth weight by the tenth day of life.

- Continue taking prenatal vitamins as long as the woman is breastfeeding.
- Drink enough fluids to quench thirst.
- Rest as much as possible, especially in the first 1 to 2 weeks after birth. Fatigue and stress can negatively affect milk production and let-down.
- Encourage the mother to sleep when the baby sleeps.

Breast Care

- Normal routine bathing is all that is necessary; avoid washing nipples with soap.
- Breast creams should not be used routinely; modified lanolin with reduced allergens is safe to use on dry or sore nipples.
- A mother with flat or inverted nipples can use a breast pump to pull out the nipple.
- If leakage of milk between feedings occurs, mothers can wear breast pads inside the bra.

Medications and Breastfeeding

- Few drugs are absolutely contraindicated during lactation.
- Caution breastfeeding mothers against taking any medications except those considered essential. Advise mothers to check with their health care provider before taking any medication.
- If the breastfeeding mother is taking a medication that has a questionable effect on the infant, she can take the medication just after nursing the baby or just before the infant is expected to sleep for a long time.
- Smoking can impair milk production and exposes the infant to the risks of secondhand smoke. Nicotine is transferred to the infant in breast milk. Mothers who smoke tobacco while lactating should be advised not to smoke within 2 hours before breastfeeding and never in the same room with the infant.
- Alcohol is concentrated in the milk and is passed on to the infant. Alcohol can also inhibit milk production and let-down.
- Caffeine intake can be associated with reduced iron concentrations in milk and subsequent anemia in the infant. Maternal intake of caffeine can cause infant irritability and poor sleeping patterns. Mothers should limit their intake of caffeine to two servings per day.

SAFETY ALERT   *Herbs and herbal teas can contain pharmacologically active compounds that can have unfavorable effects. The regional poison control center can provide information on the active properties of herbs.*

Common Concerns
Sexual Sensations

- Some women experience rhythmic uterine contractions during breastfeeding. These are disturbing to some mothers who perceive them to resemble orgasm.

Breastfeeding and Contraception

- Breastfeeding confers a period of infertility but is not considered to be an effective method of contraception.
- Lactational amenorrhea method, barrier methods, and intrauterine devices are least likely to affect lactation.
- Hormonal contraceptives can decrease milk supply. Progestin-only kinds are less likely to interfere with milk supply than other hormonal contraceptives.

Breastfeeding During Pregnancy

- Women can conceive and continue breastfeeding throughout pregnancy if no medical contraindications exist.
- The taste and composition of milk are altered during pregnancy.
- When the baby is born, colostrum is produced.
- Nursing a newborn and an older child is called tandem nursing. The mother should always feed the infant first.

Breastfeeding After Breast Surgery

- Surgical procedures can affect the mother's ability to produce milk and to transfer milk to the infant.
- Women who have had augmentation mammoplasty should be able to breastfeed successfully.
- Reduction mammoplasty is more likely to cause problems in lactating successfully.

Breast Engorgement

- Temporary condition that typically occurs 3 to 5 days after birth when the milk "comes in" and lasts about 24 hours

- Prevention
  - ❏ Breastfeed the baby at least every 2 to 3 hours as the milk is coming in.
  - ❏ Encourage the baby to feed at least 15 to 20 minutes on each breast or until one breast softens per feeding.
- Treatment
  - ❏ Feed every 2 hours, massaging the breast as the baby is feeding, softening at least one breast and pumping the other breast as needed to soften it.
  - ❏ Take a warm shower just before feeding or pumping; this may start the milk to leak.
  - ❏ Apply ice packs in a 15-to-20 minutes on, 45 minutes off rotation between feedings. The ice bags should cover both breasts. Large bags of frozen peas or niblet corn make easy packs and can be refrozen.
  - ❏ To reduce swelling, place raw, cool cabbage leaves over the breasts for 15 to 20 minutes.
  - ❏ Take antiinflammatory medications, such as ibuprofen, to decrease pain and swelling.

Sore Nipples

- Prevention
  - ❏ Use correct breastfeeding technique.
- Treatment
  - ❏ Correct the cause by evaluating the latch and baby's position at the breast and repositioning as necessary.
  - ❏ Start the feeding on the least sore side.
  - ❏ Apply ice to the nipple for 2 or 3 minutes to provide a numbing effect that increases comfort with latch.
  - ❏ Express a few drops of colostrum or milk to moisten the nipple and areola before latch.
  - ❏ Purified lanolin ointment and hydrogel dressings or cream can be applied to the nipples.
  - ❏ Wipe the nipples with water to remove the baby's saliva.
  - ❏ A few drops of milk can be expressed, rubbed into the nipple, and allowed to air dry.
  - ❏ Leave nipples open to air as much as possible.
  - ❏ If the mother cannot tolerate breastfeeding, an electric breast pump may be used for 24 to 48 hours to allow the nipples to begin healing before breastfeeding resumes.

> **NURSING ALERT** *Women who are allergic to wool should not use lanolin.*

Lactation Suppression

- Wear a well-fitted support bra or breast binder continuously for at least the first 72 hours after giving birth.
- Avoid all breast stimulation, including running warm water over the breasts, newborn suckling, or pumping of the breasts.
- Manage breast engorgement by doing the following:
  - ❑ Applying ice packs to the breasts, using a 15 minutes on, 45 minutes off schedule
  - ❑ Placing raw, cool cabbage leaves inside the bra for 15 to 20 minutes; replace when wilted
  - ❑ Administering mild analgesics

Heath Promotion
Rubella Vaccination

- Vaccine is given to women who have not had rubella or who are serologically not immune (titer of 1:8 or less or enzyme immunoassay level less than 0.8).
- Rubella vaccine is administered subcutaneously.
- The virus is not communicable in breast milk, so breastfeeding mothers can safely be immunized.

> **SAFETY ALERT** *Because the rubella virus is shed in urine and other body fluids, it should not be given if the mother or other household members are immunocompromised.*

Varicella Vaccination

- Administer before discharge in women who have no immunity.
- A second dose is given at the postpartum follow-up visit (4 to 8 weeks after the first immunization).

Tetanus-Diphtheria-Acellular Pertussis (TDaP) Vaccination

- Administer before discharge from the hospital or as early as possible in the postpartum period to women who have not previously received the vaccine or to women whose most recent tetanus-diphtheria (Td) vaccine was given more than 2 years before the pregnancy. TDaP can be given to breastfeeding women.

LEGAL TIP **Rubella and Varicella Vaccination**
Informed consent for rubella and varicella vaccination in the postpartum period includes information about possible side effects and the risk of teratogenic effects. Women must understand that they must practice contraception to prevent pregnancy for 1 month after being vaccinated.

Prevention of Rh Isoimmunization

- Rh immune globulin is administered either intramuscularly (RhoGAM, Gamulin RH, HypRho-D, Rhophylac) or intravenously (Rhophylac).
- Because Rh immune globulin is usually considered a blood product, precautions similar to those used for transfusing blood are necessary.
- Because Rh immune globulin suppresses the immune response, women who simultaneously receive rubella vaccine should be tested in 3 months to be sure they have developed rubella immunity.

NURSING ALERT *After birth, Rh immune globulin is administered to all Rh-negative, antibody (Coombs')–negative women who give birth to Rh-positive infants. It should never be given to an infant.*

MANAGEMENT OF PSYCHOSOCIAL NEEDS

Areas to be assessed throughout the woman's hospital stay include the following:

- Effect of the birth experience
- Maternal self-image
- Adaptation to parenthood and parent-infant interaction. Box 5-4 lists ways to assess for parental attachment behaviors.
- Family structure and functioning
- Effect of cultural diversity

Transition to Parenthood

Transition to parenthood covers the period from the decision to conceive through the first months after having a child. During this time it is common to feel overwhelmed and insecure and to experience physical and mental fatigue. The transition is an ongoing process as the parents and infant develop and change.

BOX 5-4

Assessing Attachment Behavior
- When the infant is brought to the parents, do they reach out for the infant and call the infant by name? (Recognize that in some cultures, parents may not name the infant in the early newborn period.)
- Do the parents speak about the infant in terms of identification—whom the infant looks like; what appears special about their infant over other infants?
- When parents are holding the infant, what kind of body contact is there—do they feel at ease in changing the infant's position; are fingertips or whole hands used; are there parts of the body they avoid touching or parts of the body they investigate and scrutinize?
- When the infant is awake, what kinds of stimulation do the parents provide—do they talk to the infant, to each other, or to no one; how do they look at the infant—direct visual contact, avoidance of eye contact, or looking at other people or objects?
- How comfortable do the parents appear in terms of caring for the infant? Do they express any concern regarding their ability or disgust for certain activities, such as changing diapers?
- What type of affection do they demonstrate to the newborn, such as smiling, stroking, kissing, or rocking?
- If the infant is fussy, what kinds of comforting techniques do the parents use, such as rocking, swaddling, talking, or stroking?

The early postpartum period is one of emotional and physical vulnerability for many new mothers, who may be psychologically overwhelmed by the reality of parental responsibilities. Common feelings may include:
- Feeling deprived of the supportive care she received from family members and friends during pregnancy
- Regretting the loss of the mother–unborn child relationship
- Having a let-down feeling when labor and birth are complete
- Fatigue after childbirth is compounded by the around-the-clock demands of the new baby

Postpartum Blues or "Baby Blues"
- Experienced by 50% to 80% of women of all ethnic and racial groups
- Characterized by emotional lability, crying easily and for no apparent reason, a let-down feeling, restlessness, fatigue, insomnia, headache, sadness, and anger
- Symptoms are usually mild and short lived

Teaching for Self-Management

Coping with Postpartum Blues

- Remember that the "blues" are normal and both parents may experience them.
- Get plenty of rest; nap when the baby does if possible. Go to bed early, and let friends know when to visit.
- Use relaxation techniques learned in childbirth classes (or ask the nurse to teach you and your partner some techniques).
- Do something for yourself. Take advantage of the time your partner or family members care for the baby—soak in the tub or go for a walk.
- Plan a day out of the house—go to the mall with the baby, being sure to take a stroller or carriage, or go out to eat with friends without the baby. Many communities have churches or other agencies that provide child care programs such as Mothers' Morning Out.
- Talk to your partner about the way you feel—for example, about feeling tied down, how the birth met your expectations, and things that will help you.
- If you are breastfeeding, give yourself and your baby time to learn.
- Seek out and use community resources such as La Leche League or community mental health centers.

Strategies for coping with postpartum blues are in the Teaching for Self-Management box: Coping with Postpartum Blues.

Parental Tasks and Responsibilities

- Reconciling the actual child with the fantasy and dream child by coming to terms with the infant's physical appearance, sex, innate temperament, and physical status
- Becoming adept in caring for the infant, including caregiving activities, noting the communication cues given by the infant to indicate needs and responding appropriately to the infant's needs
- Establishing a place for the newborn within the family group

Factors That Influence the Transition to Parenthood

- Age (especially adolescents and parents older than 35 years)
- Culture
- Socioeconomic level
- Expectations of what the child will be like

Signs of Potential Complications

Listed in the following box are several psychosocial concerns that, at a minimum, warrant ongoing evaluation. Women exhibiting these concerns should be referred to appropriate community resources for further assessment and management.

Signs of Potential Complications

Postpartum Psychosocial Concerns

- Unable or unwilling to discuss labor and birth experience
- Refers to self as ugly and useless
- Excessively preoccupied with self (body image)
- Markedly depressed
- Has difficulty sleeping
- Experiences loss of appetite
- Lacks a support system
- Partner or other family members react negatively to the baby
- Refuses to interact with or care for baby; for example, does not name baby, does not want to hold or feed baby, is upset by vomiting and wet or dirty diapers (cultural appropriateness of actions needs to be considered)
- Expresses disappointment over baby's sex
- Sees baby as messy or unattractive
- Baby reminds mother of family member or person she does not like

DISCHARGE

All health plans are required to allow the new mother and newborn to remain in the hospital for a minimum of 48 hours after a normal vaginal birth and for 96 hours after a cesarean birth unless the attending provider, in consultation with the mother, decides on early discharge. Box 5-5 lists criteria for early discharge for mothers and infants. Hospital stays must be long enough to identify problems and to ensure that the woman is sufficiently recovered and is prepared to care for herself and her baby at home.

LEGAL TIP Early Discharge

Whether or not the woman and her family have chosen early discharge, the nurse and the primary health care provider are held responsible if the woman is discharged before her condition has stabilized within normal limits. If complications occur, the medical and nursing staff could be sued for abandonment.

BOX 5-5

Criteria for Early Discharge

MOTHER
- Uncomplicated pregnancy, labor, vaginal birth, and postpartum course
- No evidence of premature rupture of membranes
- Blood pressure and temperature stable and within normal limits
- Ambulating unassisted
- Voiding adequate amounts without difficulty
- Hemoglobin >10 g
- No significant vaginal bleeding; perineum intact or no more than second-degree episiotomy or laceration repair; uterus is firm
- Received instructions on postpartum self-management

INFANT
- Term infant (38-42 wk) with weight appropriate for gestational age
- Normal findings on physical assessment
- Temperature, respirations, and heart rate within normal limits and stable for the 12 hr preceding discharge
- At least two successful feedings completed (normal sucking and swallowing)
- Urination and stooling have occurred at least once
- No evidence of significant jaundice in the first 24 hr after the birth
- No excessive bleeding at the circumcision site for at least 2 hr
- Screening tests performed according to state regulations; tests to be repeated at follow-up visit if done before the infant is 24 hr old
- Initial hepatitis B vaccine given or scheduled for first follow-up visit
- Laboratory data reviewed: maternal syphilis and hepatitis B status; infant or cord blood type and Coombs' test results if indicated

GENERAL
- No social, family, or environmental risk factors identified
- Family or support person available to assist mother and infant at home
- Follow-up scheduled within 1 wk if discharged before 48 hr after the birth
- Documentation of skill of mother in feeding (breastfeeding or bottle feeding), cord care, skin care, perineal care, infant safety (use of car seat, sleeping positions), and recognizing signs of illness and common infant problems

Source: American Academy of Pediatrics (AAP). (2004). Hospital stay for healthy term infants. *Pediatrics, 113*(5), 1434-1436.

Discharge Teaching Topics

- Maternal and newborn care
- Signs and symptoms of potential physiologic and psychosocial complications (see pp. 208 and 228) and how to obtain assistance quickly if these occur
- Resumption of sexual activity
  - ❏ Sexual activity can be resumed by the second to fourth week after birth when bleeding has stopped and lacerations or the episiotomy has healed.
  - ❏ Extra lubrication with a water-soluble gel, cocoa butter, or a contraceptive cream or jelly may be needed for up to 6 months.
  - ❏ Initially the side-by-side or female-on-top positions may be more comfortable.
  - ❏ Physical reactions to sexual stimulation for the first 3 months after birth will likely be slower and less intense. The strength of the orgasm may be reduced.
  - ❏ Women have reported feeling sexual stimulation and orgasms during breastfeeding.
- Contraception
  - ❏ Many couples resume sexual activity before the traditional 6-week postpartum checkup.
  - ❏ Breastfeeding is not a reliable method of contraception.
  - ❏ Ovulation can occur as soon as 1 month after birth, especially in women who bottle-feed.
- Routinely prescribed medications
  - ❏ Prenatal vitamins
  - ❏ Iron
  - ❏ Stool softeners
  - ❏ Pain medications (analgesics or nonsteroidal antiinflammatory medications)
- Routine mother-baby checkups
  - ❏ Women who experienced uncomplicated vaginal births are commonly scheduled for the traditional 6-week postpartum checkup.
  - ❏ Women who had a cesarean birth may be seen 2 weeks after discharge for a postoperative check.
  - ❏ Most newborns are seen for an initial office or clinic visit within the first week or by 2 weeks of age.

CONTRACEPTION

Contraception is the intentional prevention of pregnancy during sexual intercourse. Birth control is the device and/or practice to decrease the risk of conceiving. Family planning is the conscious decision on when to conceive or avoid pregnancy.

The acronym BRAIDED is useful when obtaining informed consent for a contraceptive method (see the Legal Tip).

> **LEGAL TIP   Informed Consent**
> *B—Benefits: information about advantages and success rates*
> *R—Risks: information about disadvantages and failure rates*
> *A—Alternatives: information about other available methods*
> *I—Inquiries: opportunity to ask questions*
> *D—Decisions: opportunity to decide or to change mind*
> *E—Explanations: information about method and how it is used*
> *D—Documentation: information given and patient's understanding*

METHODS OF CONTRACEPTION

Coitus Interruptus

- Male partner withdraws his penis from the woman's vagina before he ejaculates, It does not protect against sexually transmitted infections (STIs) or HIV infection

Fertility Awareness Methods (FAMs) (Natural Family Planning)

- Three phases of the menstrual cycle are identified
  - ❑ Infertile phase: before ovulation
  - ❑ Fertile phase: about 5 to 7 days around the middle of the cycle, including several days before and after ovulation
  - ❑ Infertile phase: after ovulation
- Ovum can be fertilized no later than 12 to 24 hours after ovulation.
- Techniques to identify high risk, fertile days
  - ❑ Calendar rhythm method
  - ❑ Standard days method—"fixed" number of days of fertility for each cycle (days 8 to 19); CycleBeads necklace can be used to track fertility
  - ❑ Symptoms-based methods
- Techniques require training; consult sources to locate training sites.

Biologic Marker Methods

- Home predictor test kits for ovulation—use either urine or saliva to detect the sudden surge of luteinizing hormone that occurs approximately 12 to 24 hours before ovulation.

Spermicide and Barrier Methods

- Barrier methods are effective as a contraceptive and as a protective measure against the spread of STIs.

Spermicides

- Spermicides act as a chemical barrier and reduce the sperm's mobility.
  - ❏ Nonoxynol-9 is the most commonly used spermicide in the United States.
  - ❏ Intravaginal spermicides include foams, tablets, suppositories, creams, films, and gels.

Advantages

- Sold without a prescription
- Preloaded syringes small enough to carry in purses

Disadvantages

- Women with high risk behaviors should not use nonoxynol-9 spermicide products.
- Effectiveness depends on consistent and accurate use.

SAFETY ALERT   *Frequent use of nonoxynol-9 (more than two times daily) may increase the transmission of HIV and can cause lesions.*

Management

- Insert spermicide high into the vagina so it makes contact with the cervix.
- Spermicide should be inserted at least 15 minutes before, but no longer than 1 hour before sexual intercourse.
- Reapply for each additional act of intercourse.
- Typical failure rate for spermicide alone is about 29%.

Condoms

A male condom is a thin stretchable sheath that covers the penis.

Advantages

- Nonspermicidal latex condoms provide a barrier for STIs and HIV transmission.
- Available over-the counter (OTC) without prescription
- Safe
- No side effects
- Premalignant cervical changes can be prevented or ameliorated in women whose partners use condoms.
- Method of male nonsurgical contraception

Disadvantages

- Latex condoms break down with oil-based lubricants.
- Couple must interrupt lovemaking to apply.
- Sensation may be altered.
- If used improperly, spillage can result in pregnancy.
- Condoms occasionally tear during intercourse.
- Growing number of people have latex allergies
- Typical failure rate is 15%

SAFETY ALERT *Everyone should be questioned about the potential for latex allergy. Latex condom use is contraindicated for people with latex sensitivity.*

Management
Male Condom

- Use a new condom (check expiration date) for each act of sexual intercourse or other acts between partners that involve contact with the penis.
- Place condom after penis is erect and before intimate contact.
- Place condom on head of penis, and unroll it all the way to the base.
- Leave an empty space at the tip, and remove any air remaining in the tip by gently pressing air out toward the base of the penis.
- If a lubricant is desired, use water-based products, such as K-Y lubricating jelly. Do not use petroleum-based products because they can cause the condom to break.
- After ejaculation, carefully withdraw the still-erect penis from the vagina, holding on to the condom rim; remove and discard the condom.

- Store unused condoms in cool, dry place.
- Do not use condoms that are sticky, brittle, or obviously damaged.

Female Condom

The female condom is a lubricated vaginal sheath made of polyurethane with flexible rings at both ends. The closed end is inserted into the vagina and is anchored around the cervix; the open ring covers the labia. The typical failure rate is 21%.

Diaphragm

- The diaphragm is a shallow, dome-shaped latex or silicone device with a flexible rim that covers the cervix.
- Four types of diaphragms are available: coil spring, arcing spring, flat spring, and wide seal rim.
- Available in many sizes; should be the largest size the woman can wear without being aware of its presence.

Advantages

- Protective measure against the spread of STIs
- Avoids use of hormones

Disadvantages

- Reluctance of some women to insert and remove the diaphragm
- Some women (and men) object to the messiness of spermicide
- Possible irritation of tissues related to contact with spermicides
- Not a good option for women with poor vaginal tone
- Typical failure rate is 16%

Management

- Inspect the diaphragm before each use.
- Diaphragm must be used with a spermicidal lubricant to be effective.
- Always empty the bladder before insertion.
- Place 2 teaspoons of contraceptive jelly or cream on the side of the diaphragm that will rest against the cervix, and spread it around to coat the surface and the rim.
- Insert up to 6 hours before intercourse, and leave in place for at least 6 hours after intercourse.
- After each use, wash the diaphragm with warm water and mild soap.

- Store in the plastic case but not near a heat or light source.
- Replace every 2 years.
- Refit for a 20% fluctuation in weight and after childbirth.

Cervical Cap

- Three types of cervical caps are available; two come in varying sizes and one is one-size-fits-all. They are made of rubber or latex-free silicone. The cap fits snugly around the base of the cervix.
- Advantages and disadvantages are similar to those of the diaphragm.

NURSING ALERT   *The nurse should be alert for signs of toxic shock syndrome (TSS) in women who use a diaphragm or cervical cap as a contraceptive method. The most common signs include a sunburn-type rash, diarrhea, dizziness, faintness, weakness, sore throat, aching muscles and joints, sudden high fever, and vomiting.*

Contraceptive Sponge

The vaginal sponge is a small, round polyurethane sponge that contains nonoxynol-9 spermicide. It is designed to fit over the cervix. The concave side fits next to the cervix, and the opposite side has a woven polyester loop to be used for removal of the sponge.

Management

- The sponge must be moistened with water before insertion.
- It provides protection for up to 24 hours and for repeated acts of intercourse.
- Leave it in place for at least 6 hours after the last act of intercourse.
- Wearing it longer than 24 to 30 hours may increase the risk of TSS.

Hormonal Methods

More than 30 different contraceptive formulations are available in the United States, including combined estrogen-progestin medications and progestational agents. Because of the wide variety of preparations available, the woman and the nurse must read the package insert for information about specific products prescribed. The formulations are administered orally, transdermally, vaginally, by implantation, or by injection.

Combined Estrogen-Progestin Contraceptives
Oral Contraceptives

- Regular ingestion of combined oral contraceptive pills (COCs) inhibits ovulation, alters the maturation of the endometrium, and affects the cervical mucus to maintain its thickness.
- Monophasic pills provide fixed dosages of estrogen and progestin, whereas multiphasic pills alter the amount of progestin and sometimes the amount of estrogen during each cycle.
- An extended-cycle oral contraceptive (Seasonale) is taken in 3-month cycles of 12 weeks of active pills and 1 week of inactive pills.

Advantages

- Acceptability, because use is not related directly to the sexual act
- Overall effectiveness rate when taken correctly is almost 100%
- Decreased worries about becoming pregnant, which may lead to improved sexual response
- Convenience of knowing when the next menstrual flow will occur; decreased frequency of menstruation with extended-cycle pills
- Decreased risk of ectopic pregnancy

Disadvantages

- Side effects may include nausea, breast tenderness, fluid retention, chloasma, and irregular bleeding.
- Serious side effects may include stroke, myocardial infarction, thromboembolism, hypertension, gallbladder disease, and liver tumors.

Management

- Take the pill at the same time each day.
- The effectiveness of COCs can be negatively influenced by medications such as ampicillin, anticonvulsants, barbiturates, oxcarbazepine, phenytoin, phenobarbital, felbamate, carbamazepine, primidone, topiramate, griseofulvin, rifampicin, rifabutin, and anti-HIV protease inhibitors such as nelfinavir and amprenavir.

NURSING ALERT *OTC medications, as well as some herbal supplements (such as St. John's wort) can alter the effectiveness of COCs. Women should be asked about their use when COCs are being considered for contraception.*

- Signs of potential complication from COCs include ACHES:
  A—Abdominal pain may indicate a problem with the liver or gallbladder.
  C—Chest pain or shortness of breath may indicate a clot problem.
  H—Headaches (sudden or persistent) may be caused by cardiovascular accident or hypertension.
  E—Eye problems may indicate vascular accident or hypertension.
  S—Severe leg pain may indicate a thromboembolic process.
- COCs do not provide protection from STIs or HIV infection.

Transdermal Contraceptive System

- The contraceptive transdermal patch delivers continuous levels of progesterone and ethinyl estradiol and is available with prescription.
- It is applied to the intact skin of the upper outer arm, upper torso, lower abdomen, or buttocks for 3 weeks. No patches worn for week 4. The patch should not be placed on a breast.
- Withdrawal bleeding occurs during the fourth ("no patch") week.
- Typical failure rate in the first year of use for women weighing less than 198 pounds is less than 8%. The patch should not be used in women who weigh more than 198 pounds.

Vaginal Contraceptive Ring

- The vaginal contraceptive ring is a flexible ring worn in the vagina to deliver continuous levels of estronogestrel and ethinyl estradiol.
- It is worn for 3 weeks, followed by 1 week without the ring, during which time withdrawal bleeding occurs.
- It is available with prescription but does not need to be fitted.
- Typical failure rate during the first year of use is less than 8%.

Progestin-Only Contraceptives

- Progestin-only methods impair fertility by inhibiting ovulation, thickening and decreasing the amount of cervical mucus, thinning the endometrium, and altering cilia in the uterine tubes.

Oral Progestins (Minipill)

- Effectiveness is about 92% in the first year of use but increases if the minipill is taken at the same time every day.
- A common complaint is irregular vaginal bleeding.

Injectable Progestins

- Depot medroxyprogesterone acetate (DMPA or Depo-Provera), 150 mg, is injected intramuscularly into the deltoid or gluteus maximus muscle.
- The injection should be given during the first 5 days of the menstrual cycle and administered every 11 to 13 weeks.

Advantages

- Contraceptive effectiveness comparable to that of COCs
- Long-lasting effects
- Injections required only four times per year
- Lactation unlikely to be impaired

Disadvantages

- Loss of bone mineral density with increasing duration of use
- Weight gain
- Lipid changes
- Increased risk of venous thrombosis and thromboembolism
- Irregular vaginal spotting
- Decreased libido
- Breast changes
- No protection from STIs
- Delay in return to fertility may be as long as 18 months after discontinuing use

SAFETY ALERT   *Women who use DMPA may lose significant bone mineral density with increasing duration of use. It is unknown if this effect is reversible. It is unknown if use of DMPA during adolescence or early adulthood, a critical period of bone accretion, will reduce peak bone mass and increase the risk of osteoporotic fracture in later life. Women who receive DMPA should be counseled about calcium intake and exercise.*

NURSING ALERT   *When administering an intramuscular (IM) injection of progestin (e.g., Depo-Provera), do not massage the site after the injection because this can hasten the absorption and shorten the period of effectiveness.*

Implantable Progestins

- A single rod (Implanon) implanted subdermally is effective for 3 years.
- Advantages and disadvantages are similar to those for other progestins.

Emergency Contraception

- Emergency contraception Plan B is available in one or two doses of levonorgestrel and is available without prescription for women 17 years of age and older.
- Other options include high doses of oral progestins or COCs and insertion of a copper intrauterine device (IUD) available only by prescription.

Management

- Emergency contraception should be taken as soon as possible but within 120 hours of unprotected intercourse or birth control mishap.
- To minimize the effects of nausea the woman should take an OTC antiemetic 1 hour before each dose.
- Women with contraindications for estrogen should take progestin-only emergency contraception.
- If the woman does not begin to menstruate within 21 days after taking emergency contraception, she should be evaluated for pregnancy.
- Risk of pregnancy is reduced by 75% to 89% if the woman takes emergency contraceptive pills.

> **NURSING ALERT** *Emergency contraception will not protect the woman against pregnancy if she engages in unprotected intercourse in the days or weeks that follow treatment. Because ingestion of emergency contraceptive pills may delay ovulation, caution the woman that she needs to establish a reliable form of birth control in order to prevent unintended pregnancy. Information about emergency contraception method options and access to providers are available at www.NOT-2-LATE.com or by calling 1-888-NOT-2-LATE.*

Intrauterine Devices

- An IUD is a small T-shaped device with bendable arms that is inserted by a trained health care provider through the cervix and against the uterine fundus.

- The IUD adversely affects the sperm motility and irritates the lining of the uterus.
- Before IUD insertion the woman should have a negative pregnancy test, treatment for dysplasia if present, cervical cultures to rule out STIs, and a signed consent form.
- Two types of IUDs have been approved by the U.S. Food and Drug Administration (FDA) for use in the United States:
  - ❑ Copper IUD: approved for 10 years of use
  - ❑ Hormonal IUD: approved for 5 years of use

Advantages

- Long-term protection from pregnancy
- Immediate return to fertility when removed

Disadvantages

- Increased risk of pelvic inflammatory disease shortly after placement
- Unintentional expulsion of the device
- Infection
- Possible uterine perforation
- Possible bleeding and cramping the first year after insertion (copper IUD) or irregular spotting (hormonal IUD).

Management

- Women in mutually monogamous relationships are the best candidates.
- Signs of possible complications include PAINS:
  P—Period late, abnormal spotting or bleeding
  A—Abdominal pain, pain with intercourse
  I—Infection exposure, abnormal vaginal bleeding
  N—Not feeling well, fever, or chills
  S—String missing, shorter or longer
- Report any signs of flulike illness or rash.

Sterilization

- Surgical procedures intended to render the person infertile usually involve the occlusion of the passageways for the ova and sperm.
- For the woman, the oviducts (uterine tubes) are occluded; for the man the sperm ducts (vas deferens) are occluded.

Advantages

- Procedures can be safely done on an outpatient basis
- Nonhormonal forms of contraception
- Very low (<1%) failure rate

Disadvantages

- Possible complications of anesthesia, infection, hemorrhage, and trauma to the organs
- Sterilization reversal is costly, difficult, and uncertain
- No protection from STIs

Management

- Offer information about alternatives to sterilization, and obtain informed consent.
- For tubal ligation topics should include the following:
  - ❏ Expect no change in hormones and their influence.
  - ❏ Menstrual periods will be about the same.
  - ❏ Pain at ovulation may be felt but the ovum disintegrates in the abdominal cavity.
  - ❏ It is highly unlikely that the woman will become pregnant.
  - ❏ There should be no change in sexual function.

LEGAL TIP   Sterilization

- *If federal funds are used for sterilization, the person must be age 21 years or older on the day the consent form is signed.*
- *Informed consent must include an explanation of the risks, benefits, and alternatives; a statement that describes sterilization as a permanent, irreversible method of birth control; and a statement that mandates a 30-day waiting period between giving consent and the sterilization.*
- *Informed consent must be in the person's native language, or an interpreter must be provided to read the consent form to the person.*

Selected Postpartum Complications

POSTPARTUM HEMORRHAGE

Postpartum hemorrhage (PPH) is a life-threatening event that can occur with little warning and is often unrecognized until the mother has profound symptoms.

- PPH can be defined as follows:
  - ❑ Loss of more than 500 ml of blood after vaginal birth
  - ❑ Loss of more than 1000 ml of blood after cesarean birth
  - ❑ A 10% change in hematocrit between admission for labor and postpartum or the need for red blood cell transfusion
- *Early, acute,* or *primary PPH:* occurs within 24 hours of birth
- *Late* or *secondary PPH:* occurs more than 24 hours and up to 6 to 12 weeks postpartum

NURSING ALERT *Early discharge increases the potential for acute episodes of PPH to occur outside the hospital or birth center setting. Discharge teaching should emphasize the signs of normal involution, as well as potential complications.*

Risk Factors and Etiology

- Box 6-1 lists predisposing factors for PPH.
- Early postpartum hemorrhage
  - ❑ Uterine atony (marked hypotonia of the uterus)
  - ❑ Incomplete placental separation
  - ❑ Lacerations of the genital tract
- Late postpartum hemorrhage
  - ❑ Subinvolution of the uterus
  - ❑ Endometritis
  - ❑ Retained placental fragments

Uterine Atony

Uterine atony is marked hypotonia of the uterus and is the leading cause of PPH.

BOX 6-1

Predisposing Factors and Causes of Postpartum Hemorrhage

- Uterine atony
- Overdistended uterus
  - ❑ Large fetus
  - ❑ Multiple fetuses
  - ❑ Hydramnios
  - ❑ Distention with clots
- Anesthesia and analgesia
  - ❑ Conduction anesthesia
  - ❑ Previous history of uterine atony
- High parity
- Prolonged labor or oxytocin-induced labor
- Trauma during labor and birth
- Forceps-assisted birth
- Vacuum-assisted birth
- Cesarean birth
- Unrepaired lacerations of the birth canal
- Retained placental fragments
- Ruptured uterus
- Inversion of the uterus
- Placenta accreta, increta, percreta
- Coagulation disorders
- Placental abruption
- Placenta previa
- Manual removal of a retained placenta
- Magnesium sulfate administration during labor or postpartum period
- Chorioamnionitis
- Uterine subinvolution

- It is associated with high parity, hydramnios, a macrosomic fetus, and multifetal gestation. In such conditions the uterus is "overstretched" and contracts poorly after birth.
- Other causes of atony include traumatic birth, use of halogenated anesthesia (e.g., halothane) or magnesium sulfate, rapid or prolonged labor, chorioamnionitis, and use of oxytocin for labor induction or augmentation. PPH in a previous pregnancy is a major risk factor.

Management

- Assess vital signs every 15 minutes during the first hour after birth to identify trends related to blood loss (e.g., tachycardia, tachypnea, decreasing blood pressure) (see Box 6-2 for noninvasive assessments of cardiac output).

NURSING ALERT *Vital signs may not be reliable indicators of shock immediately postpartum because of the physiologic adaptations of this period.*

- Firmly massage the uterine fundus
- Express clots from the uterus.
- Eliminate bladder distention by voiding or catheterization.
- Notify the primary health care provider.
- Administer a continuous IV infusion of 10 to 40 units of oxytocin in 1000 ml of lactated Ringer's or normal saline solution.

BOX 6-2

Noninvasive Assessments of Cardiac Output in Postpartum Women Who Are Bleeding

- Palpation of pulses (rate, quality, equality)
  - ❑ Arterial
- Auscultation
  - ❑ Heart sounds and murmurs
  - ❑ Breath sounds
- Inspection
  - ❑ Skin color, temperature, turgor
  - ❑ Capillary refill
  - ❑ Neck veins
  - ❑ Mucous membranes
- Observation
  - ❑ Level of consciousness
  - ❑ Presence or absence of anxiety, apprehension, restlessness, and disorientation
- Measurement
  - ❑ Blood pressure
  - ❑ Pulse oximetry
  - ❑ Urinary output

- Administer other medications, such as ergonovine (Ergotrate) or methylergonovine (Methergine) or prostaglandin $F_2\alpha$, IM to stimulate uterine contraction according to standing orders or protocol. See Appendix B for the table comparing medications used to manage PPH.
- Administer crystalloid solutions or blood or blood products to restore the woman's intravascular volume.
- Give oxygen 10 to 12 L/min by nonrebreather face mask.
- Obtain laboratory studies including complete blood count (CBC) with platelet count, fibrinogen, fibrin split products, prothrombin time, and partial thromboplastin time.
- If the preceding procedures are ineffective, the bleeding can be managed surgically by vessel ligation (uteroovarian, uterine, or hypogastric), selective arterial embolization, or hysterectomy.
- Provide explanations to the woman and the family about interventions being performed and the need to act quickly.

NURSING ALERT *Use of ergonovine or methylergonovine is contraindicated in the presence of hypertension or cardiovascular disease. Prostaglandin $F_{2\alpha}$ should be used cautiously in women with cardiovascular disease or asthma.*

Lacerations of the Genital Tract

Hemorrhage caused by lacerations of the cervix, vagina, or the perineum should be suspected if bleeding continues despite a firm, contracted uterine fundus. This bleeding can be a slow trickle, oozing, or frank hemorrhage.

- Lacerations of the perineum are the most common of all injuries of the lower portion of the genital tract. They are classified as first, second, third, or fourth degree. An episiotomy can extend to become either a third- or fourth-degree laceration.
- Most cervical lacerations are shallow, and bleeding is minimal. More extensive lacerations can extend into the vaginal vault or into the lower uterine segment.
- Pelvic hematomas may be vulvar, vaginal, or retroperitoneal in origin.
  - ❑ Vulvar hematomas are the most common. Pain is the most common symptom, and most vulvar hematomas are visible.

- ❏ Vaginal hematomas occur in association with a forceps-assisted birth, an episiotomy, or primigravidity. Symptoms include persistent perineal or rectal pain or a feeling of pressure in the vagina.
- ❏ A retroperitoneal hematoma may cause minimal pain, and the initial symptoms may be signs of shock.

Management

After the bleeding has been controlled, the care of the woman with lacerations of the perineum is similar to that for women with episiotomies (analgesia as needed for pain and hot or cold applications as necessary).

- ■ The need for increased roughage in the diet and increased intake of fluids is emphasized.
- ■ Stool softeners may be used to assist the woman in reestablishing bowel habits without straining and putting stress on the suture lines.

> **NURSING ALERT** *To avoid injury to the suture line, do not give a woman with third- or fourth-degree lacerations rectal suppositories or enemas.*

Retained Placenta

- ■ A retained placenta results from partial separation of a normal placenta, entrapment of a partially or completely separated placenta, mismanagement of the third stage of labor, or abnormal adherence of the entire placenta or a portion of it to the uterine wall.
- ■ Placental retention because of poor separation is common in very preterm births (20 to 24 weeks of gestation).

Management

- ■ Manual separation and removal by the primary health care provider
- ■ Adherent retained placenta occurs for unknown reasons. Attempts to remove it in the usual manner are unsuccessful and laceration or perforation of the uterine wall may result.
- ■ Unusual placental adherence may be partial or complete. The following degrees of attachment are recognized:
  - ❏ *Placenta accreta*—slight penetration of myometrium by placental trophoblast

- ❏ *Placenta increta*—deep penetration of myometrium by placenta
- ❏ *Placenta percreta*—perforation of uterus by placenta
- ■ Hysterectomy is indicated in approximately two thirds of women with retained placenta.
- ■ Blood component replacement therapy is often necessary.

Inversion of the Uterus

- ■ Uterine inversion is an emergency situation requiring immediate recognition, replacement of the uterus within the pelvic cavity, and correction of associated clinical conditions.

SAFETY ALERT *The umbilical cord should not be pulled on strongly unless the placenta has definitely separated.*

- ■ Uterine inversion in which the placenta remains attached and the uterus is pulled inside out can be partial or complete.
  - ❏ Complete inversion appears as a large, red, rounded mass that protrudes 20 to 30 cm outside the introitus.
  - ❏ Incomplete inversion cannot be seen but must be felt; a smooth mass can be palpated through the dilated cervix.
- ■ Contributing factors to uterine inversion include:
  - ❏ Fundal implantation of the placenta
  - ❏ Manual extraction of the placenta
  - ❏ Short umbilical cord
  - ❏ Uterine atony
  - ❏ Leiomyomas
  - ❏ Abnormally adherent placental tissue
- ■ Primary presenting signs are hemorrhage, shock, and pain in the absence of an abdominally palpable fundus.

Management

- ■ Medical management includes tocolysis to relax the uterus, repositioning the uterus, giving oxytocin after the uterus is repositioned, treating shock, and initiating broad-spectrum antibiotics.

Subinvolution of the Uterus

Subinvolution is the failure of the uterus to return to a nonpregnant state.

- Recognized causes of subinvolution include retained placental fragments and pelvic infection.
- Signs and symptoms include prolonged lochial discharge, irregular or excessive bleeding, and sometimes hemorrhage.
- A pelvic examination usually reveals a uterus that is larger than normal and that may be boggy.

Management

- Treatment of subinvolution depends on the cause.
- Ergonovine, 0.2 mg every 3 to 4 hours for 24 to 48 hours, and antibiotic therapy are most commonly used.
- If bleeding persists, bimanual compression can be considered by the obstetrician or nurse-midwife.
- If the uterus still does not become firm, manual exploration of the uterine cavity for retained placental fragments is implemented.
- If the preceding procedures are ineffective, the bleeding can be managed surgically by D&C to remove retained placental fragments or to debride the placental site, vessel ligation (uteroovarian, uterine, or hypogastric), selective arterial embolization, or hysterectomy.

Discharge Teaching

Discharge instructions for the woman who has had PPH are similar to those for any postpartum woman.

- Limit her physical activities to conserve her strength if fatigued.
- Increase her dietary iron and protein intake and iron supplementation if necessary.
- Seek assistance with infant care and household activities until she has regained strength.
- Seek consultation for problems with delayed or insufficient lactation and postpartum depression.
- Refer for home care follow-up or to community resources as indicated.

HEMORRHAGIC (HYPOVOLEMIC) SHOCK

Hemorrhage may result in hemorrhagic (hypovolemic) shock. Shock is an emergency situation in which the perfusion of body organs may become severely compromised and death may occur.

- In case of shock:
  - ❏ Pulse is rapid, weak, and irregular
  - ❏ Respirations are rapid and shallow
  - ❏ Blood pressure decreases (late sign)
  - ❏ Central venous pressure is decreased
  - ❏ Skin is cool, pale, and clammy
  - ❏ Urinary output decreases
  - ❏ Level of consciousness ranges from lethargy to coma
  - ❏ Mental status ranges from anxiety to coma

Management

- Restore circulating blood volume.
  - ❏ Rapidly infuse an IV of crystalloid solution given at a rate of 3 ml infused for every 1 ml of estimated blood loss.
  - ❏ Packed red blood cells (RBCs) are usually infused if the woman is still actively bleeding.
- Infuse fresh-frozen plasma if clotting factors and platelet count are below normal values.
- Auscultate breath sounds before beginning fluid volume replacement.
- Treat the cause of the hemorrhage.
- Monitor the pulse, respirations, and blood pressure.
- Assist with the placement of a central venous pressure (CVP) or pulmonary artery (Swan-Ganz) catheter.
- Monitor the pulmonary artery pressure or pulmonary artery wedge pressure as ordered.
- Inspect for oozing at sites of incisions or injections and presence of petechiae or ecchymosis in areas not associated with surgery or trauma (evaluation for DIC).
- Monitor oxygen saturation with a pulse oximeter.

NURSING ALERT *Measurements of oxygen saturation with a pulse oximeter may not be accurate in a woman with hypovolemia or decreased perfusion.*

- Assess level of consciousness (woman may report "seeing stars" or feeling dizzy or nauseated; she can be restless and orthopneic, and confused).
- Continuous electrocardiographic monitoring may be indicated.
- Insert an indwelling catheter with urometer to monitor urinary output (30 ml/hr indicates adequate organ perfusion).

COAGULOPATHIES

- When bleeding is continuous and no identifiable source is found, a coagulopathy may be the cause.
- Causes of coagulopathies can be pregnancy complications such as idiopathic thrombocytopenic purpura or von Willebrand disease and DIC.
- Assess the woman's coagulation status quickly and continually.
- Draw and send blood to the laboratory for clotting studies as ordered.
  - ❑ Abnormal results depend on the cause and can include increased prothrombin time, increased partial thromboplastin time, decreased platelets, decreased fibrinogen level, increased fibrin degradation products, and prolonged bleeding time.

Idiopathic Thrombocytopenic Purpura

Idiopathic or immune thrombocytopenia purpura (ITP) is an autoimmune disorder in which antiplatelet antibodies decrease the life span of the platelets.

- Thrombocytopenia, capillary fragility, and increased bleeding time are diagnostic findings.
- ITP may cause severe hemorrhage after cesarean birth or from cervical or vaginal lacerations.
- The incidence of postpartum uterine bleeding and vaginal hematomas is increased in the presence of ITP.

Management

- Control platelet stability.
- If ITP was diagnosed during pregnancy, the woman likely was treated with corticosteroids or IV immunoglobulin.
- Platelet transfusions are usually given when bleeding is significant.
- A splenectomy may be needed if the ITP does not respond to medical management.

von Willebrand Disease

von Willebrand disease (vWD), a type of hemophilia, is probably the most common of all hereditary bleeding disorders. Although rare, vWD is among the most common congenital clotting defects in U.S. women of childbearing age.

- vWD results from a deficiency or defect in a blood clotting protein called von Willebrand factor (vWF).
- Symptoms include recurrent bleeding episodes such as nosebleeds or after tooth extraction, bruising easily, prolonged bleeding time (the most important test), factor VIII deficiency (mild to moderate), and bleeding from mucous membranes.
- The woman may be at risk for bleeding for up to 4 weeks postpartum.

Management

- Administer desmopressin, which promotes the release of vWF and factor VIII, nasally, intravenously, or orally.
- Transfusion therapy with plasma products that have been treated for viruses and contain factor VIII and vWF (e.g., Humate-P, Alphanate) also can be used.

THROMBOEMBOLIC DISEASE

A thrombosis results from the formation of a blood clot or clots inside a blood vessel and is caused by inflammation (thrombophlebitis) or partial obstruction of the vessel. Three thromboembolic conditions are of concern in the postpartum period:

- *Superficial vein thrombosis:* involvement of the superficial saphenous venous system
- *Deep vein thrombosis:* involvement varies but can extend from the foot to the iliofemoral region
- *Pulmonary embolism:* complication of deep vein thrombosis occurring when part of a blood clot dislodges and is carried to the pulmonary artery, where it occludes the vessel and obstructs blood flow to the lungs

Etiology

- The major causes of thromboembolic disease are venous stasis and hypercoagulation, both of which are present in pregnancy and continue into the postpartum period.
- Other risk factors include operative vaginal birth, cesarean birth, history of venous thrombosis or varicosities, obesity, maternal age older than 35 years, multiparity, infection, immobility, and smoking.

Clinical Manifestations

- Superficial vein thrombosis is the most frequent form of postpartum thrombophlebitis. It is characterized by pain and tenderness in the lower extremity.
  - ❑ Physical examination may reveal redness, warmth, and an enlarged, hardened vein over the site of the thrombosis. It is almost always unilateral.
- Deep vein thrombosis is more common during pregnancy.
  - ❑ Physical examination may reveal redness and warmth, but many women exhibit few if any symptoms.
  - ❑ A positive Homans sign may be present, but further evaluation is needed because the calf pain may be attributed to other causes such as a strained muscle resulting from the birthing position.
- Acute pulmonary embolism is characterized by dyspnea and tachypnea (>20 breaths/min). Other signs and symptoms include apprehension, cough, tachycardia (>100 beats/min), hemoptysis, elevated temperature, syncope, and pleuritic chest pain.
- Physical examination is not a sensitive diagnostic indicator for thrombosis.
- Venography is the most accurate method for diagnosing deep vein thrombosis but it is an invasive procedure associated with serious complications.
- Noninvasive diagnostic methods include real-time and color Doppler ultrasound.

Management

- Superficial vein thrombosis is treated with analgesia (nonsteroidal antiinflammatory agents), rest with elevation of the affected leg, and elastic stockings. Local application of heat also may be used.
- Deep vein thrombosis is initially treated with anticoagulant (usually continuous IV heparin) therapy, bed rest with the affected leg elevated, and analgesia.
  - ❑ After the symptoms have decreased, the woman may be fitted with elastic stockings to use when she is allowed to ambulate.
  - ❑ IV heparin therapy continues for 3 to 5 days or until symptoms resolve.

❑ Oral anticoagulant therapy (warfarin [Coumadin]) is started
   during this time and is continued for approximately 3 months.
■ Pulmonary embolism is treated with continuous IV heparin
   therapy until symptoms have resolved.
   ❑ Intermittent subcutaneous heparin or oral warfarin therapy
      follows and is usually continued for 6 months.

Nursing Interventions

Assessment in the Hospital Setting

■ Inspect and palpate the affected area.
■ Palpate peripheral pulses.
■ Check Homans sign.
■ Measure and compare leg circumferences.
■ Inspect for signs of bleeding.
■ Monitor for signs of pulmonary embolism, including chest pain,
   coughing, dyspnea, and tachypnea; and respiratory status for
   presence of crackles.
■ Monitor laboratory reports for prothrombin or partial
   thromboplastin times.
■ Assess the woman and her family for their level of understanding
   of the diagnosis and their ability to cope during the unexpected
   extended period of recovery.

Interventions

■ Provide explanations and education about the diagnosis and the
   treatment.
■ Assist with personal care as long as the woman is on bed rest.
■ Encourage the family to participate in the care if that is the desire
   of the woman and the family.
■ While the woman is on bed rest, encourage her to change
   positions frequently but not to place her knees in a sharply
   flexed position that could cause pooling of blood in her lower
   extremities. Caution her not to rub the affected area because this
   could cause the clot to dislodge.
■ Once the woman is allowed to ambulate, teach her how to
   prevent venous congestion by putting on elastic stockings before
   getting out of bed.
■ Administer heparin and warfarin as ordered, and notify the
   physician if clotting times are outside the therapeutic level.
■ If the woman is breastfeeding, assure her that neither heparin
   nor warfarin is excreted in significant quantities in breast milk. If

the infant has been discharged, encourage the family to bring the infant for feedings as permitted by hospital policy; the mother also can express milk to be sent home.

■ Pain can be managed with a variety of measures:
   ❑ Position changes, elevating the leg, and application of moist, warm heat may decrease discomfort.
   ❑ Administration of analgesics and antiinflammatory medications may be needed.

NURSING ALERT *Medications containing aspirin are not given to women receiving anticoagulant therapy because aspirin inhibits synthesis of clotting factors and can lead to a prolonged clotting time and increased risk of bleeding.*

■ The woman is usually discharged home with oral anticoagulants and will need explanations about the treatment schedule and possible side effects.
■ If subcutaneous injections are to be given, teach the woman and family how to administer the medication and about site rotation.
■ Give the woman and her family information about safe care practices to prevent bleeding and injury while she is receiving anticoagulant therapy, such as using a soft toothbrush and an electric razor.
■ Provide diet counseling about foods to avoid when on anti-coagulant therapy.
■ Provide information about follow-up with the woman's primary health care provider to monitor clotting times and to make sure the correct dose of anticoagulant therapy is maintained.
■ Instruct the woman to use a reliable method of birth control if taking warfarin, because this medication is considered teratogenic.
■ Oral contraceptives are contraindicated because of the increased risk for thrombosis.

POSTPARTUM INFECTIONS

Postpartum or puerperal infection is any clinical infection of the genital tract that occurs within 28 days after childbirth, miscarriage, or induced abortion.

■ Postpartum infection is defined as a fever of 38° C (100.4° F) or more on 2 successive days of the first 10 postpartum days (not counting the first 24 hours after birth).

- Common postpartum infections include endometritis, wound infections, mastitis, urinary tract infections (UTIs), and respiratory tract infections.
- The most common infecting organisms are the numerous streptococcal and anaerobic organisms.
- *Staphylococcus aureus*, gonococci, coliform bacteria, and clostridia are less common but serious pathogenic organisms that also cause puerperal infection.
- Postpartum infections are more common in women who have concurrent medical or immunosuppressive conditions or who had a cesarean or operative vaginal birth.
- Intrapartal factors, such as prolonged rupture of membranes, prolonged labor, and internal maternal or fetal monitoring, also increase the risk of infection. Factors that predispose the woman to postpartum infection are listed in Box 6-3.

BOX 6-3

Predisposing Factors for Postpartum Infection

PRECONCEPTION OR ANTEPARTAL FACTORS
- History of previous venous thrombosis, urinary tract infection, mastitis, pneumonia
- Diabetes mellitus
- Alcoholism
- Drug abuse
- Immunosuppression
- Anemia
- Malnutrition

INTRAPARTAL FACTORS
- Cesarean birth
- Operative vaginal birth
- Prolonged rupture of membranes
- Chorioamnionitis
- Prolonged labor
- Bladder catheterization
- Internal fetal heart rate or uterine pressure monitoring
- Multiple vaginal examinations after rupture of membranes
- Epidural analgesia/anesthesia
- Retained placental fragments
- Postpartum hemorrhage
- Episiotomy or lacerations
- Hematomas

Prevention

- The most effective and least expensive treatment of postpartum infection is prevention.
  - ❑ Prenatal nutrition to control anemia
  - ❑ Maternal perineal hygiene with thorough handwashing
  - ❑ Strict adherence by all health care personnel to aseptic techniques during childbirth and the postpartum period

Endometritis

Endometritis is the most common type of postpartum infection.

- It usually begins as a localized infection at the placental site but can spread to involve the entire endometrium. Incidence is higher after cesarean birth.
- Assessment for signs of endometritis may reveal the following:
  - ❑ A fever (usually >38° C [100.4° F])
  - ❑ Increased pulse
  - ❑ Chills
  - ❑ Anorexia
  - ❑ Nausea
  - ❑ Fatigue and lethargy
  - ❑ Pelvic pain
  - ❑ Uterine tenderness
  - ❑ Foul-smelling, profuse lochia
  - ❑ Leukocytosis and a markedly increased RBC count and sedimentation rate
  - ❑ Anemia
- Blood cultures or intracervical or intrauterine bacterial cultures (aerobic and anaerobic) should reveal the offending pathogens within 36 to 48 hours.

Management

- Continuing assessment of lochia, vital signs, and changes in the woman's condition during treatment.
- Administration of intravenous broad-spectrum antibiotic therapy (cephalosporins, penicillins, or clindamycin and gentamicin).
  - ❑ Antibiotic therapy is usually discontinued 24 hours after the woman is asymptomatic.
- Supportive care, including hydration, rest, and pain relief.

- Comfort measures depend on the symptoms and may include cool compresses, warm blankets, perineal care, and sitz baths.
- Teaching should include side effects of therapy, prevention of spread of infection, signs and symptoms of worsening condition, and adherence to the treatment plan and the need for follow-up care.
- Women may need to be encouraged or assisted to maintain mother-infant interactions and breastfeeding (if allowed during treatment).

Wound Infections

- Wound infections are common postpartum infections but often develop after the woman is at home. Predisposing factors are similar to those for endometritis.
- Sites of infection include the cesarean incision and the episiotomy or repaired laceration site.
- Signs of wound infection include erythema, edema, warmth, tenderness, seropurulent drainage, and wound separation.
- Fever and pain also may be present.

Management

- Combine antibiotic therapy with wound debridement:
  - ❑ Open and drain wounds.
  - ❑ Assess wound and vital signs frequently and provide wound care.
- Provide comfort measures including sitz baths, warm compresses, and perineal care.
- Teaching includes:
  - ❑ Changing perineal pads front to back
  - ❑ Handwashing before and after perineal care
  - ❑ Self-care measures
  - ❑ Signs of worsening condition to report to the health care provider.
- The woman is usually discharged to home for self-management or home nursing care after treatment is initiated in the inpatient setting.

Urinary Tract Infections

- UTIs occur in 2% to 4% of postpartum women.
- Risk factors include urinary catheterization, frequent pelvic examinations, epidural anesthesia, genital tract injury, history of UTI, and cesarean birth.

- Signs and symptoms include dysuria, frequency and urgency, low-grade fever, urinary retention, hematuria, and pyuria.
- Costovertebral angle (CVA) tenderness or flank pain may indicate an upper UTI.
- Urinalysis results may reveal *Escherichia coli,* although other gram-negative aerobic bacilli also may cause UTIs.

Management

- IV broad-spectrum antibiotic therapy, analgesia, hydration, and rest.
- Postpartum women are usually treated on an outpatient basis.
- Teaching should include:
  - ❑ Instructions on how to monitor temperature, bladder function, and appearance of urine.
  - ❑ Signs of potential complications and the importance of taking all antibiotics as prescribed.
  - ❑ Prevention of UTIs:
    - ○ Proper perineal care
    - ○ Wiping from front to back after urinating or having a bowel movement
    - ○ Increasing fluid intake

Mastitis

- Mastitis, inflammation in the breast, affects approximately 1% to 10% of women soon after childbirth, most of whom are first-time mothers who are breastfeeding. Mastitis almost always is unilateral and develops well after the flow of milk has been established. The infecting organism generally is the hemolytic *Staphylococcus aureus.*
- An infected nipple fissure usually is the initial lesion, but the ductal system is involved next.
- Inflammatory edema and engorgement of the breast obstruct the flow of milk in a lobe; regional and then generalized mastitis follow.
- If treatment is not prompt, mastitis can progress to a breast abscess.
- Symptoms rarely appear before the end of the first postpartum week and are more common in the second to fourth weeks.
  - ❑ Chills, fever, malaise, and local breast tenderness are noted first.

❏ Pain, swelling, redness, and axillary adenopathy may occur.
■ Because mastitis rarely occurs before the postpartum woman is discharged, teaching should include warning signs of mastitis and counseling about preventing cracked nipples.

Management

■ Breast support with a well-fitted bra, local application of heat (or cold), adequate hydration, analgesics, and antibiotic therapy (e.g., dicloxacillin or flucloxacillin).
■ Lactation can be maintained by emptying the breasts every 2 to 4 hours by breastfeeding, manual expression, or breast pump.
■ Almost all instances of acute mastitis can be avoided by proper breastfeeding technique to prevent cracked nipples.
■ Missed feedings, waiting too long between feedings, and abrupt weaning may lead to clogged nipples and mastitis.
■ Cleanliness practiced by all who have contact with the newborn and new mother also reduces the incidence of mastitis.

POSTPARTUM DEPRESSION AND PSYCHOSIS
Postpartum Depression Without Psychotic Features

Postpartum depression (PPD) is an intense and pervasive sadness with severe and labile mood swings and is more serious and persistent than postpartum blues. PPD occurs in 10% to 15% of new mothers.

Risk Factors

■ Prenatal depression
■ Low self-esteem
■ Stress of child care
■ Prenatal anxiety
■ Life stress
■ Lack of social support
■ Marital relationship problems
■ History of depression
■ "Difficult" infant temperament
■ Postpartum blues
■ Single status
■ Low socioeconomic status
■ Unplanned/unwanted pregnancy

Clinical Manifestations

- Feelings of guilt and inadequacy about being a competent and adequate parent
- Odd food cravings (often, sweet desserts) and binges with abnormal appetite and weight gain
- Increased yearning for sleep, sleeping heavily but awakening instantly with any infant noise, and an inability to go back to sleep after infant feedings
- Severe anxiety, panic attacks, and spontaneous crying long after the usual duration of baby blues
- Fear that the offspring will take her place in her partner's affections
- Episodes of irritability that flare up with little provocation
- Rejection of the infant, often caused by abnormal jealousy; obsessive thoughts about harming the baby

Management

- Treatment options include antidepressants, antianxiety agents (shorter acting), mood stabilizers, antipsychotics, and electroconvulsive therapy (ECT).
- Alternative therapies, such as herbs, dietary supplements, massage, aromatherapy, bright light therapy, and acupuncture, may be helpful.
- Supportive treatment alone is not efficacious for major postpartum depression.
  - Encourage woman to take time for herself, rest and relax, ask friends and family for help as needed.
  - Exercise, proper nutrition, and adequate sleep contribute to symptom alleviation.
- Support groups and marital counseling may be helpful. For some women, hospitalization is necessary.

Postpartum Depression with Psychotic Features

Postpartum psychosis is most commonly associated with a diagnosis of bipolar disorder.

Clinical Manifestations

- Symptoms often begin within days after the birth, usually within 2 weeks postpartum.
- Complaints of fatigue, insomnia, and restlessness

- Episodes of tearfulness and emotional lability
- Complaints regarding the inability to move, stand, or work
- Suspiciousness, confusion, incoherence, irrational statements, and obsessive concerns about the baby's health and welfare
- Delusions and hallucinations
  - ❑ When delusions are present, they are often related to the infant.
  - ❑ The mother may think the infant is possessed by the devil, has special powers, or is destined for a terrible fate.
- While in a manic state, mothers need constant supervision when caring for their infants. Usually they are too preoccupied to provide child care.

Medical Management

- Postpartum psychosis is a psychiatric emergency, and the mother will probably need psychiatric hospitalization.
- Antipsychotics and mood stabilizers, such as lithium, are the treatments of choice.
  - ❑ Almost all psychotrophic medications are drugs for which the effects on breastfeeding newborns are unknown but still may be of concern.
  - ❑ All psychotrophic medications pass through breast milk; therefore the risks of using these medications must be weighed against the benefits associated with breastfeeding for the mother and infant.
  - ❑ If antidepressant medications are given to the breastfeeding woman, it is important to know that the amount of elapsed time between maternal dosing and infant feeding affects the amount of medication to which the breastfed infant is exposed; longer intervals will decrease exposure.
- Antidepressants should be used very cautiously even when depressive symptoms are present, because of the risk of precipitating rapid cycling.
- Bilaterally administered ECT is highly effective.
- Psychotherapy is indicated after the period of acute psychosis has passed.

SAFETY ALERT *Because women with PPD with psychotic features may harm their infants, extra caution is needed in assessment and intervention. The nurse needs to ask specifically if the mother has had thoughts about harming her baby.*

LOSS AND GRIEF

Many types of loss can be associated with pregnancy and birth.
- Miscarriage, premature labor and preterm birth, and cesarean birth involve a loss of the expected pregnancy and birth plans.
- Ectopic pregnancy, fetal death, and stillbirth are other types of loss, as is death of an infant who survives only a few hours or who dies after days, weeks, or months in an intensive care unit.
- Parents may grieve over the sex or appearance of their child or the birth of an infant who has a birth defect or chronic illness.
- Infertility may cause intense feelings of grief.
- The death of a baby in a multifetal gestation during pregnancy, labor, or birth or after birth requires parents to grieve and parent at the same time.

Grief Responses

- Grief or bereavement can be described as a cluster of painful responses experienced following a major loss or death.
- Parental grief responses occur in three overlapping phases: acute distress, intense grief, and reorganization.
  - Acute distress and shock are followed by intense grief that includes emotional, cognitive, behavioral, and physical responses.
  - Reorganization occurs months or years later.
- The duration of grief varies with the individual.
- Grief is a long-term process that can extend for months or years.
- Some aspects of grief never truly end.
- The grief of grandparents is often complicated by the emotional pain of witnessing and feeling the immense grief of their own child.
- The siblings of the expected infant also experience a profound loss.
- Physical symptoms of grief include fatigue, headaches, dizziness, backaches, and difficulty sleeping.
- Appetites may be depressed or voracious. Lack of sleep and inadequate nutrition and fluids can complicate other grief responses.

Management
Assessment

Key areas to address include the following:
- The nature of the parental attachment with the pregnancy or infant, the meaning of the pregnancy and infant to the parents, and the related losses they are experiencing.

- The circumstances surrounding the loss, the level of preparation for the loss, and the parents' level of understanding about the cause of the loss or death.
- The immediate response of the mother and father to the loss, whether their responses are complementary or problematic, and how their responses match with their past experiences, personalities, and behavioral and cultural backgrounds.
- The social support network of the parents and the extent to which it has been activated.
  - ❏ Some prefer to handle the tragedy alone for a time; others want assistance in calling other family members, friends, and clergy.

Interventions

- The parents need to be told honestly about the situation by their physician or others on the health care team.
- Caregivers must use the words "dead" and "died," rather than "lost" or "gone," to assist bereaved persons in accepting this reality.
- Parents need opportunities to tell their story about the events, experiences, and feelings surrounding the loss.
- Knowing the sex and naming the fetus or baby help actualize the loss.
  - ❏ Do not create the sense that the parents have to name the "baby," especially in the case of a miscarriage when the sex is not known.

> **NURSING ALERT**   *Cultural taboos and rules in some religious faiths prohibit naming an infant who has died. It is important to be sensitive to this possibility and not impose naming on parents.*

- It can be helpful for some parents to see the fetus or baby. A question such as, "Some parents have found it helpful to see their baby. Would you like time to consider this?" is useful. Mothers and fathers may differ in their desire; this should be an individual decision, not a joint one.
- Parents appreciate explanations and descriptions about what to expect when they see the baby. For example, babies may have red, peeling skin that resembles a bad sunburn, dark discoloration similar to bruises, molding of the head that makes the head look soft and swollen, or birth defects.

- If a baby has a congenital anomaly, the nurse can point out aspects of the baby that are normal.
- Provide the opportunity for parents to bathe and dress their baby, comb the hair, dress the baby in a special outfit, wrap the baby in a blanket, or place the baby in a crib.
- Parents need to be offered time alone with their baby. They also need to know when the nurse will return and how to call if they need anything.
- Provide privacy for the family (e.g., a private room with a rocking chair for the parents to sit in when holding their baby).
- Mark the door to the room with a special card to remind staff that this family has experienced a perinatal loss.
- Provide grandparents the same opportunities to hold, rock, swaddle, and love their grandchild so that their grief is started in a healthy way.

Decisions to Be Made

- An autopsy may be useful in determining the cause of death.
- Organ donation may help give some meaning to the loss. The most common donation is the cornea, which can occur if the baby was born alive at 36 weeks of gestation or later.
- Spiritual rituals may be helpful and important to parents. Support from clergy is an option that should be offered to all parents.
- Parents should be given information about the choices for the final disposition of their baby, regardless of gestational age.

Helping Bereaved Parents Acknowledge and Express Their Feelings

- Validate the experience and feelings of the parents by encouraging them to tell their stories and listening with care.
- Acknowledge the loss with a simple but sincere comment, such as, "I'm sorry about the baby."
- Ask the father about his views of what happened and his feelings of loss.
- Do not give advice or use clichés in offering support to the bereaved individuals (Box 6-4).
- When a bereaved person expresses feelings of anger, it can be helpful to identify the feeling by simply saying, "You sound angry" or "You look angry."

BOX 6-4

What to Say and What Not to Say to Bereaved Parents

WHAT TO SAY
- "I'm sad for you."
- "How are you doing with all of this?"
- "This must be hard for you."
- "What can I do for you?"
- "I'm sorry."
- "I'm here, and I want to listen."

WHAT NOT TO SAY
- "God had a purpose for her."
- "Be thankful you have another child."
- "The living must go on."
- "I know how you feel."
- "It's God's will."
- "You have to keep on going for her sake."
- "You're young; you can have others."
- "We'll see you back here next year, and you'll be happier."
- "Now you have an angel in heaven."
- "This happened for the best."
- "Better for this to happen now, before you knew the baby."
- "There was something wrong with the baby anyway."

Used with permission of Bereavement Services. Copyright Lutheran Hospital–La Crosse, Inc., a Gundersen Lutheran Affiliate, La Crosse, WI.

- Help parents to understand their grief responses and to feel they are not alone in these painful responses.
- Reassure them of the normality of their responses and prepare them for the length of their grief.
- Give books and pamphlets about grief to parents to take home.
- Help parents understand that they may respond and grieve in very different ways. Discourage dependence on drugs and alcohol.

Meeting Physical Needs of the Postpartum Bereaved Mother

- The mother should be given the opportunity to decide if she wants to remain on the maternity unit or be moved to another hospital unit after she hears the advantages and disadvantages of each choice.

- Mothers need ideas about how to cope with problems with sleep, such as decreasing food or fluids that contain caffeine, limiting alcohol and nicotine consumption, exercising regularly, using strategies for rest, taking a warm bath or drinking warm milk before bedtime, doing relaxation exercises, listening to restful music, or getting a massage.

Creating Memories for Parents to Take Home

- Parents may want tangible mementos of their baby to allow them to actualize the loss.
- Special memory books, cards, and information about grief and mourning are available for purchase by parents or hospitals or clinics through national perinatal bereavement organizations.
- The nurse can provide information about the baby's weight, length, and head circumference to the family.
- Footprints and handprints can be taken and placed with the other information on a special card or in a memory or baby book.
- Parents often appreciate articles that were in contact with or used in caring for the baby, such as the tape measure used to measure the baby, baby lotions, combs, clothing, hats, blankets, crib cards, and identification bands, or a lock of hair.
  - ❑ Parents must be asked for permission before cutting a lock of hair, which can be removed from the nape of the neck where it is not noticeable.
- Photographs should be taken whenever there is an identifiable baby and when it is culturally acceptable to the family.

Providing Sensitive Care at and After Discharge

- Leaving the hospital without a baby in her arms is a very empty and painful experience for a woman.
- Mothers should not be discharged at a time when other mothers with live babies are leaving.
- Giving the mother a special flower to carry in her arms can be a thoughtful gesture.
- Parents can be referred to a perinatal or parental grief support group.

The Newborn

CARE MANAGEMENT: FROM BIRTH THROUGH THE FIRST 2 HOURS

- Care begins immediately after birth and focuses on assessing and stabilizing the newborn's condition. As part of Standard Precautions, gloves are worn when handling the newborn until blood and amniotic fluid are removed by bathing.
- The nurse verifies that respirations have been established, dries the infant, and assesses temperature.
- Identical identification bracelets are placed on the infant and the mother. In some settings the father or partner also wears an identification bracelet. Information on the bracelet includes name, sex, date and time of birth, and identification number. Infants are footprinted by using a form that includes the mother's fingerprints, name, and date and time of birth. These identification procedures must be performed before the mother and infant are separated after birth.
- The infant can be placed on the mother's chest or abdomen to allow skin-to-skin contact, wrapped in a warm blanket and placed in the mother's arms, given to the partner to hold, or kept partially undressed under a radiant warmer. The infant can be admitted to a nursery or remain with the parents throughout the hospital stay.
- The initial examination of the newborn can occur while the nurse is drying and wrapping the infant, or observations can be made while the infant is lying on the mother's chest or abdomen or in her arms immediately after birth. Interference in the initial parent-infant acquaintance process should be minimized.

Apgar Score

- The nurse usually assigns the Apgar score at 1 and 5 minutes after birth. The Apgar score permits a rapid assessment of the newborn's transition to extrauterine life based on five signs

TABLE 7-1

Apgar Score

Sign	SCORE		
	0	**1**	**2**
Heart rate	Absent	Slow (<100 beats/min)	>100 beats/min
Respiratory effort	Absent	Slow, weak cry	Good cry
Muscle tone	Flaccid	Some flexion of extremities	Well flexed
Reflex irritability	No response	Grimace	Cry
Color	Blue, pale	Body pink, extremities blue	Completely pink

(Table 7-1). Scores of 0 to 3 indicate severe distress; scores of 4 to 6 indicate moderate difficulty; and scores of 7 to 10 indicate that the infant is having no difficulty adjusting to extrauterine life. If resuscitation is required, it should be initiated before the 1-minute Apgar score.

Initial Physical Assessment

■ If the infant is breathing effectively, is pink, and has no apparent life-threatening anomalies or risk factors requiring immediate attention (e.g., infant of a mother with diabetes), delay further examination until after the parents have had an opportunity to interact with the infant. Routine procedures and the admission process can be carried out in the mother's room or in a separate nursery.

■ The initial physical assessment includes a brief review of systems:

1. *External:* Note skin color, general activity, and position; assess nasal patency by covering one nostril at a time while observing respirations; assess skin for peeling or lack of subcutaneous fat (dysmaturity or postterm); note meconium staining of cord, skin, fingernails, or amniotic fluid (staining can indicate fetal release of meconium, often related to hypoxia; offensive odor can indicate intrauterine infection); note length of nails and creases on soles of feet.

2. *Chest:* Auscultate apical heart for rate and rhythm, heart tones, and presence of abnormal sounds; note character of respirations and presence of crackles or other adventitious sounds; note equality of breath sounds by auscultation.

3. *Abdomen:* Observe characteristics of abdomen (rounded, flat, concave) and absence of anomalies; auscultate bowel sounds; note number of vessels in cord.
4. *Neurologic:* Check muscle tone; assess Moro and suck reflexes; palpate anterior fontanel; note by palpation the presence and size of the fontanels and sutures.
5. *Genitourinary:* Note external sex characteristics and any abnormality of genitalia; check anal patency and presence of meconium; note passage of urine.
6. *Other observations:* Note gross structural malformations obvious at birth that require immediate medical attention.

■ A gestational age assessment is done within 2 hours of birth using forms readily available in nurseries.
■ An assessment of newborn reflexes (Table 7-2) and a more comprehensive physical assessment (Table 7-3) are completed within 24 hours of birth.

Stabilization

■ Generally the normal term infant born vaginally has little difficulty clearing the airway. Most secretions are moved by gravity and brought to the oropharynx by the cough reflex.
■ If the infant has excess mucus in the respiratory tract, the mouth and nasal passages can be suctioned with a bulb syringe.

Suctioning with a Bulb Syringe

■ Suction the mouth first to prevent the infant from inhaling pharyngeal secretions by gasping as the nares are touched.
  ❑ Compress the bulb, and insert into one side of the mouth.
  ❑ Avoid the center of the infant's mouth because this can stimulate the gag reflex.
  ❑ Suction the nasal passages one nostril at a time.
  ❑ Always keep the bulb syringe in the infant's crib.
  ❑ Demonstrate to the parents how to use the bulb syringe, and ask for a return demonstration.

Text continued on p. 312.

TABLE 7-2

Assessment of Newborn's Reflexes

Reflex	Eliciting the Reflex	Characteristic Response	Comments
Rooting and sucking	Touch infant's lip, cheek, or corner of mouth with nipple	Infant turns head toward stimulus, opens mouth, takes hold, and sucks	Response difficult if not impossible to elicit after infant has been fed; if response weak or absent, consider prematurity or neurologic defect
			Parental guidance: avoid trying to turn head toward breast or nipple, allow infant to root; response disappears after 3-4 mo* but can persist upto 1 yr
Swallowing	Feed infant; swallowing usually follows sucking and obtaining fluids	Swallowing usually coordinated with sucking and usually occurs without gagging, coughing, or vomiting	If response is weak or absent, may indicate prematurity or neurologic defect Sucking and swallowing often uncoordinated in preterm infant
Grasp:			
Palmar	Place finger in palm of hand	Infant's fingers curl around examiner's fingers	Palmar response lessens by 3-4 mo; parents enjoy this contact with infant; plantar response lessens by 8 mo
Plantar	Place finger at base of toes	Toes curl downward	
Extrusion	Touch or depress tip of tongue	Newborn forces tongue outward	Response disappears about fourth mo of life

Glabellar (Myerson)	Tap over forehead, bridge of nose, or maxilla of newborn whose eyes are open	Newborn blinks for first four or five taps	Continued blinking with repeated taps consistent with extrapyramidal disorder
Tonic neck or "fencing"	With infant falling asleep or sleeping, turn head quickly to one side	With infant facing left side, arm and leg on that side extend; opposite arm and leg flex (turn head to right, and extremities assume opposite postures)	Responses in leg are more consistent. Complete response disappears by 3-4 mo, incomplete response may be seen until third or fourth yr. After 6 wk, persistent response is sign of possible cerebral palsy

Classic pose in spontaneous tonic neck reflex. (Courtesy Marjorie Pyle, RNC, Lifecircle, Costa Mesa, CA.)

*All durations for persistence of reflexes are based on time elapsed after 40 wk of gestation; that is, if this newborn was born at 36 wk of gestation, add 1 mo to all time limits given.

Continued

TABLE 7-2

Assessment of Newborn's Reflexes—cont'd

Reflex	Eliciting the Reflex	Characteristic Response	Comments
Moro	Hold infant in semisitting position, allow head and trunk to fall backward to an angle of at least 30 degrees Place infant on flat surface, strike surface to startle infant	Symmetric abduction and extension of arms are seen; fingers fan out and form a C with thumb and forefinger; slight tremor may be noted; arms adducted in embracing motion and return to relaxed flexion and movement Legs may follow similar pattern of response Preterm infant does not complete "embrace"; instead, arms fall backward because of weakness	Response is present at birth; complete response may be seen until 8 wk; body jerk is seen only between 8 and 18 wk; response absent by 6 mo if neurologic maturation is not delayed; response may be incomplete if infant is deeply asleep; give parental guidance about normal response Asymmetric response may connote injury to brachial plexus, clavicle, or humerus Persistent response after 6 mo indicates possible brain damage

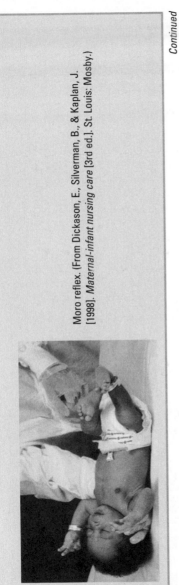

Moro reflex. (From Dickason, E., Silverman, B., & Kaplan, J. [1998]. *Maternal-infant nursing care* [3rd ed.]. St. Louis: Mosby.)

Continued

TABLE 7-2

Assessment of Newborn's Reflexes—cont'd

Reflex	Eliciting the Reflex	Characteristic Response	Comments
Stepping or "walking"	Hold infant vertically, allowing one foot to touch table surface	Infant will simulate walking, alternating flexion and extension of feet; term infants walk on soles of their feet, and preterm infants walk on their toes	Response normally present for 3-4 wk

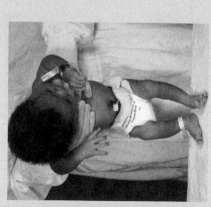

Stepping reflex. (From Dickason, E., Silverman, B., & Kaplan, J. [1998]. *Maternal-infant nursing care* [3rd ed.]. St. Louis: Mosby.)

Crawling	Place newborn on abdomen	Newborn makes crawling movements with arms and legs	Response should disappear about 6 wk of age
Deep tendon	Use finger instead of percussion hammer to elicit patellar, or knee-jerk, reflex; newborn must be relaxed	Reflex jerk present; even with newborn relaxed, nonselective overall reaction can occur	
Crossed extension	Infant should be supine; extend one leg, press knee downward, stimulate bottom of foot; observe opposite leg	Opposite leg flexes, adducts, and then extends as if attempting to push away stimulating agent	This reflex should be present during newborn period

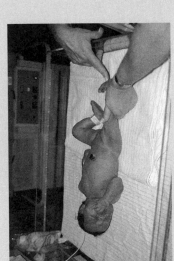

Crossed extension reflex. (Courtesy Marjorie Pyle, RNC, Lifecircle, Costa Mesa, CA.)

Continued

TABLE 7-2

Assessment of Newborn's Reflexes—cont'd

Reflex	Eliciting the Reflex	Characteristic Response	Comments
Babinski (plantar)	On sole of foot, beginning at heel, stroke upward along lateral aspect of sole, then move finger across ball of foot	All toes hyperextend, with dorsiflexion of big toe; recorded as a positive sign	Absence requires neurologic evaluation, should disappear after 1 yr of age

Babinski reflex. (From Hockenberry, M., & Wilson, D. [2011]. *Wong's nursing care of infants and children* [9th ed.]. St. Louis: Mosby.)

Pull-to-sit (traction)	Pull infant up by wrists from supine position with head in midline	Head will lag until infant is in upright position, then will be held in same plane with chest and shoulder momentarily before falling forward; infant will attempt to right head	Response depends on general muscle tone and maturity and condition of infant
Trunk incurvation (Galant)	Place infant prone on flat surface, run finger down back about 4-5 cm lateral to spine, first on one side and then down other	Trunk is flexed, and pelvis is swung toward stimulated side With transverse lesions of cord, no response below the level of the lesion is present	Response disappears by fourth wk Absence suggests general depression of nervous system Response can vary but should be obtainable in all infants, including preterm ones

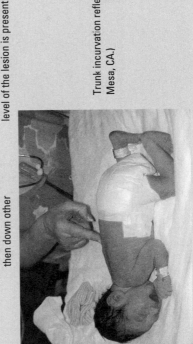

Trunk incurvation reflex. (Courtesy Marjorie Pyle, RNC, Lifecircle, Costa Mesa, CA.)

Continued

TABLE 7-2

Assessment of Newborn's Reflexes—cont'd

Reflex	Eliciting the Reflex	Characteristic Response	Comments
Magnet	Place infant in supine position, partially flex both lower extremities, and apply pressure to soles of feet	Both lower limbs should extend against examiner's pressure 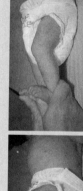 Magnet reflex. (Courtesy Michael S. Clement, MD, Mesa, AZ.)	Absence suggests damage to spinal cord or malformation Reflex can be weak or exaggerated after breech birth
Additional newborn responses: yawn, stretch, burp, hiccup, sneeze	Spontaneous behaviors	Can be slightly depressed temporarily because of maternal analgesia or anesthesia, fetal hypoxia, or infection	Parental guidance: most of these behaviors are pleasurable to parents Parents need to be assured that behaviors are normal Sneeze is usually response to lint, etc., in nose and not an indicator of a cold No treatment needed for hiccups; sucking may help

TABLE 7-3

Physical Assessment of Newborn

Area Assessed	Normal Findings	Deviations From Normal Range	Etiology
POSTURE Inspect newborn before disturbing	Arms, legs in moderate flexion; fists clenched Normal spontaneous movement bilaterally; asynchronous but equal extension in all extremities	Hypotonia Hypertonia Opisthotonos Frank breech: legs straighter and stiff Limitation of motion in any of extremities	Prematurity or hypoxia in utero, maternal medications Drug dependence, central nervous system (CNS) disorder CNS disturbance

Continued

TABLE 7-3

Physical Assessment of Newborn—cont'd

Area Assessed	Normal Findings	Deviations From Normal Range	Etiology
VITAL SIGNS			
Heart rate and pulses: Inspection Palpation Auscultation	Visible pulsations in left midclavicular line, fifth intercostal space	Tachycardia: persistent, >180 beats/min	Respiratory distress syndrome (RDS)
	Apical pulse, fourth intercostal space, 110-160 beats/min (listen for 1 full min); 80-100 beats/min (sleeping) to 180 beats/min (crying)	Bradycardia: persistent, <80 beats/min	Congenital heart block, maternal lupus
	Quality: first sound (closure of mitral and tricuspid valves) and second sound (closure of aortic and pulmonic valves) sharp and clear	Murmurs (if present, note other signs of cardiovascular dysfunction, such as tachypnea, tachycardia, pallor, cyanosis, absence of peripheral pulses, or poor perfusion)	Possibly functional
	Possible murmur	Arrhythmias: irregular rate (irregular heart rate not attributed to changes in activity or respiratory pattern should be further evaluated)	
		Sounds distant, poor quality, extra	Pneumomediastinum
		Heart on right side of chest	Dextrocardia, often accompanied by reversal of intestines

Peripheral pulses: femoral, brachial, popliteal, posterior tibial	Peripheral pulses equal and strong Femoral pulses equal and strong	Weak or absent peripheral pulses; unequal pulses Weak or absent femoral pulses	Decreased cardiac output, thrombus Hip dysplasia, coarctation of aorta if weak on left and strong on right, thrombophlebitis
Temperature: axillary method of choice	Axillary: 36.5°-37.2° C	Subnormal	Prematurity, infection, low environmental temperature, inadequate clothing, dehydration
		Increased	Infection, high environmental temperature, excessive clothing, proximity to heating unit or in direct sunshine, drug addiction, diarrhea and dehydration
	Temperature stabilized by 8-10 hr of age	Temperature not stabilized by 6-8 hr after birth	If mother received magnesium sulfate, maternal analgesics

Continued

TABLE 7-3

Physical Assessment of Newborn—cont'd

Area Assessed	Normal Findings	Deviations From Normal Range	Etiology
VITAL SIGNS—cont'd			
Check respiratory rate and effort when infant is at rest Count respirations for full min	30-60 breaths/min Shallow and irregular in rate, rhythm, and depth when infant is awake	Apneic episodes: >15 sec	Preterm infant: "periodic breathing," "rapid warming or cooling of infant
	Subnormal	Bradypnea: <25/min	Maternal narcosis from analgesics or anesthetics, birth trauma
	Breath sounds loud, clear	Tachypnea: >60/min	Narrowing of bronchi, RDS, congenital diaphragmatic hernia, transient tachypnea of the newborn
	Crackles may be heard after birth	Crackles, rhonchi, wheezes Expiratory grunt Distress evidenced by nasal flaring, retractions, chin tug, labored breathing	Fluid in lungs

Measure blood pressure (BP) using oscillometric monitor BP cuff; palpate Check electronic monitor BP cuff: BP cuff width affects readings, use appropriate size and palpate brachial, popliteal, or posterior tibial pulse (depending on measurement site)	80-90/40-50 (mm Hg)	Difference between upper and lower extremity pressures Hypotension Hypertension	Coarctation of aorta Sepsis, hypovolemia Coarctation of aorta, renal involvement, thrombus

Continued

TABLE 7-3

Physical Assessment of Newborn—cont'd

Area Assessed	Normal Findings	Deviations From Normal Range	Etiology
WEIGHT*			
Weigh at same time each day	2500-4000 g Acceptable weight loss: <10% Second baby weighs more than first	Weight <2500 g	Prematurity, small for gestational age, rubella syndrome
		Weight ≥4000 g	Large for gestational age, maternal diabetes, heredity—normal for these parents
	Birth weight regained within first 2 wk	Weight loss >10%-15%	Dehydration

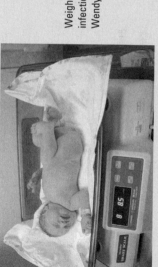

Weighing the infant. The scale is covered to protect against cross-infection. The nurse never leaves the infant alone on the scale. (Courtesy Wendy and Marwood Larson-Harris, Roanoke, VA.)

LENGTH

Length from top of head to heel

45-55 cm

<45 cm or >55 cm

Chromosomal abnormality, heredity—normal for these parents

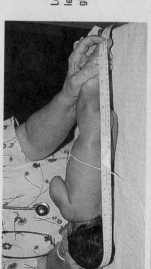

Length, crown to rump. To determine total length, include length of legs. If measurements are taken before the infant's initial bath, wear gloves. (Courtesy Marjorie Pyle, RNC, Lifecircle, Costa Mesa, CA.)

Continued

*NOTE: Weight, length, and head circumference all should be close to the same percentile for any newborn.

TABLE 7-3

Physical Assessment of Newborn—cont'd

Area Assessed	Normal Findings	Deviations From Normal Range	Etiology
HEAD CIRCUMFERENCE			
Occipito-frontal circumference	32-36.8 cm Circumference of head and chest approximately the same for first 1 or 2 days after birth	Small head, <32 cm: microcephaly Hydrocephaly: sutures widely separated, circumference ≥4 cm more than chest circumference Increased intracranial pressure	Prematurely, maternal rubella, toxoplasmosis, cytomegalic inclusion disease, fused cranial sutures (craniosynostosis) Maldevelopment, infection Hemorrhage, space-occupying lesion

Head circumference. (Courtesy Marjorie Pyle, RNC, Lifecircle, Costa Mesa, CA.)

CHEST CIRCUMFERENCE
Measure at nipple line

2-3 cm less than head circumference, averages between 30 and 33 cm

<30 cm

Prematurity

Chest circumference. (Courtesy Marjorie Pyle, RNC, Lifecircle, Costa Mesa, CA.)

Continued

TABLE 7-3

Physical Assessment of Newborn—cont'd

Area Assessed	Normal Findings	Deviations From Normal Range	Etiology
SKIN Color	Generally pink	Dark red	Prematurity, polycythemia
	Varying with ethnic origin	Gray	Hypotension, poor perfusion
	Acrocyanosis, especially if chilled	Pallor	Cardiovascular problem, CNS damage, blood dyscrasia, blood loss, twin-to-twin transfusion, nosocomial infection
	Mottling		
	Harlequin sign		
	Plethora		
	Telangiectasia ("stork bite" or capillary hemangioma)	Cyanosis	Hypothermia; infection; hypoglycemia; cardiopulmonary diseases; cardiac, neurologic, or respiratory malformations
	Erythema toxicum or neonatorum ("newborn rash")		
	Milia		
	Petechiae over presenting part	Petechiae over any other area	Clotting factor deficiency, infection

	Ecchymoses from forceps in vertex births or over buttocks, genitalia, and legs in breech births	Ecchymoses in any other area	Hemorrhagic disease, traumatic birth
Jaundice	None at birth Physiologic jaundice in up to 50% of term infants in first wk of life	Jaundice within first 24 hr	Increased hemolysis, Rh isoimmunization, ABO incompatibility
Birthmarks	Mongolian spots: Infants of African-American, Asian, and Native-American origin: 70%-85% Infants of Caucasian origin: 5%-13%	Hemangiomas Nevus flammeus: port-wine stain Nevus vasculosus: strawberry mark Cavernous hemangiomas	

Continued

TABLE 7-3

Physical Assessment of Newborn—cont'd

Area Assessed	Normal Findings	Deviations From Normal Range	Etiology
SKIN—cont'd			
Check condition	No skin edema	Edema on hands, feet; pitting over tibia	Overhydration
	Opacity: few large blood vessels visible indistinctly over abdomen	Texture thin, smooth, or of medium thickness; rash or superficial peeling visible	Prematurity, postmaturity
		Numerous vessels very visible over abdomen	Prematurity
		Texture thick, parchment-like; cracking, peeling	Postmaturity
		Skin tags, webbing	
		Papules, pustules, vesicles, ulcers, maceration	Impetigo, candidiasis, herpes, diaper rash
Gently pinch skin between thumb and forefinger over abdomen and inner thigh to check for turgor	After pinch released, skin returns to original state immediately	Dehydration: loss of weight best indicator	Prematurity, postmaturity, dehydration: fold of skin persisting after release of pinch
		Loose, wrinkled skin	

	Normal findings	Alterations and possible causes	
	Normal weight loss after birth: 7 to 10% of birth weight		
	Possibly puffy	Tense, tight, shiny skin	Edema, extreme cold, shock, infection
		Lack of subcutaneous fat, prominence of clavicle or ribs	Prematurity, malnutrition
Vernix caseosa: color and odor	Whitish, cheesy, odorless; usually more found in creases, folds	Absent or minimal	Postmaturity
		Excessive	Prematurity
		Green color	Possible in utero release of meconium or presence of bilirubin
Lanugo	Over shoulders, pinnae of ears, forehead	Odor	Possible intrauterine infection
		Absent	Postmaturity
		Excessive	Prematurity, especially if lanugo abundant and long and thick over back
HEAD Inspect palpate	Making up one fourth of body length	Cephalhematoma	Birth trauma
	Molding	Indentation	Fracture from trauma
	Caput succedaneum, possibly showing some ecchymosis	Severe molding	

Continued

TABLE 7-3

Physical Assessment of Newborn—cont'd

Area Assessed	Normal Findings	Deviations From Normal Range	Etiology
HEAD—cont'd			
Fontanels: open vs. closed	Anterior fontanel 5-cm diamond, increasing as molding resolves Posterior fontanel triangle, smaller than anterior	Full, bulging Large, flat, soft	Tumor, hemorrhage, infection Malnutrition, hydrocephaly, retarded bone age, hypothyroidism
Sutures	Palpable and unjoined sutures Possible overlap of sutures with molding	Depressed Widely spaced Premature closure	Dehydration Hydrocephaly Craniosynostosis
Hair	Silky, single strands lying flat; growth pattern toward face and neck, variation in amount	Fine, woolly Unusual swirls, patterns, or hairline or coarse, brittle	Prematurity Endocrine or genetic disorders

EYES

Eyeballs

Normal	Variations/Abnormal Findings	Cause
Both present and of equal size, both round, firm	Agenesis or absence of one or both eyeballs	Chromosomal disorders, such as Down, cri du chat syndromes
Eyes and space between eyes each one third the distance from outer-to-outer canthus	Epicanthal folds when present with other signs	
Epicanthal folds: normal racial characteristic		
Symmetric in size, shape	Small eyeball	Rubella syndrome
Blink reflex	Lens opacity or absence of red reflex	Congenital cataracts, possibly from rubella
No discharge	Discharge (purulent)	Infection
No tears	Chemical conjunctivitis	Eye medication (requires no treatment)
Subconjunctival hemorrhage	Lesions: coloboma (absence of part of iris)	
	Pink color of iris	Albinism
	Jaundiced sclera	Hyperbilirubinemia

Continued

TABLE 7-3

Physical Assessment of Newborn—cont'd

Area Assessed	Normal Findings	Deviations From Normal Range	Etiology
EYES—cont'd	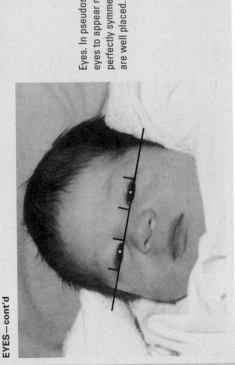	Eyes. In pseudostrabismus, inner epicanthal folds cause the eyes to appear misaligned; however, corneal light reflexes are perfectly symmetric. Eyes are symmetric in size and shape and are well placed.	

Characteristic	Normal Finding	Deviation	Potential Cause
Pupils	Present, equal in size, reactive to light	Pupils: unequal, constricted, dilated, fixed	Intracranial pressure, medications, tumors
Eyeball movement	Random, jerky, uneven, focus possible briefly, following to midline	Persistent strabismus	Increased intracranial pressure
	Transient strabismus or nystagmus until third or fourth month	Doll's eyes	Increased intracranial pressure
		Sunset	
Eyebrows	Distinct (not connected in midline)	Connection in midline	Cornelia de Lange syndrome
NOSE			
Shape	Midline		
Placement	Some mucus but no drainage	Copious drainage, with or without regular periods of cyanosis at rest and return of pink color with crying	Choanal atresia, congenital syphilis, chromosomal disorder
	Preferential nose breather	Malformed	Congenital syphilis
	Sneezing to clear nose		
Patency	Slight deformity (flat or deviated to one side) from passage through birth canal	Flaring of nares	Respiratory distress

Continued

TABLE 7-3

Physical Assessment of Newborn—cont'd

Area Assessed	Normal Findings	Deviations From Normal Range	Etiology
EARS Pinna	Correct placement: line drawn through inner and outer canthi of eyes reaching to top notch of ears (at junction with scalp)	Agenesis Low placement	Chromosomal disorder, mental retardation, kidney disorder
	Well-formed, firm cartilage	Lack of cartilage Preauricular tags Size: possibly overly prominent or protruding ears	Prematurity
Hearing	Responds to voice and other sounds State (e.g., alert, asleep) influences response	No response to sound	Deaf, rubella syndrome

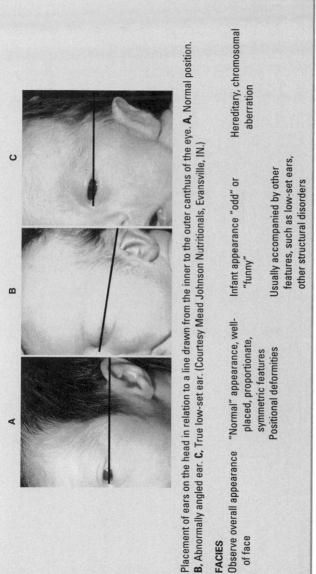

Placement of ears on the head in relation to a line drawn from the inner to the outer canthus of the eye. **A,** Normal position. **B,** Abnormally angled ear. **C,** True low-set ear. (Courtesy Mead Johnson Nutritionals, Evansville, IN.)

FACIES		
Observe overall appearance of face	"Normal" appearance, well-placed, proportionate, symmetric features	
	Positional deformities	Infant appearance "odd" or "funny"
		Usually accompanied by other features, such as low-set ears, other structural disorders
		Hereditary, chromosomal aberration

Continued

TABLE 7-3

Physical Assessment of Newborn—cont'd

Area Assessed	Normal Findings	Deviations From Normal Range	Etiology
MOUTH			
Lips	Symmetry of lip movement	Gross anomalies in placement, size, shape	Cleft lip and/or palate, gums
Buccal mucosa	Dry or moist Pink Transient circumoral cyanosis	Asymmetry in movement of lips Cyanosis, circumoral pallor	Cranial nerve VII paralysis Respiratory distress, hypothermia
Gums	Pink gums Inclusion cysts (Epstein pearls—Bohn nodules, whitish, hard nodules on gums or roof of mouth)	Teeth: predeciduous or deciduous	Hereditary
Tongue	Tongue not protruding, freely movable, symmetric in shape, movement Sucking pads inside cheeks	Macroglossia Short lingual frenulum Thrush: white plaques on cheeks or tongue that bleed if touched	Prematurity, chromosomal disorder *Candida albicans*
Palate (soft, hard): Arch	Soft and hard palates intact	Cleft, hard or soft palate	

Uvula	Uvula in midline Epstein pearls		
Chin	Distinct chin	Micrognathia	Pierre Robin sequence or other syndrome
Saliva	Mouth moist	Excessive saliva	Esophageal atresia, tracheoesophageal fistula
Reflexes: Rooting Sucking Extrusion	Reflexes present Reflex response dependent on state of wakefulness and hunger	Absent	Prematurity
NECK			
Sternocleidomastoid muscles	Short, thick, surrounded by skin folds; no webbing Head held in midline (sternocleidomastoid muscles equal), no masses Transient positional deformity Freedom of movement from side to side and flexion and extension, no movement of chin past shoulder	Webbing Restricted movement, holding of head at angle Absence of head control	Turner syndrome Torticollis (wryneck), opisthotonos Prematurity, Down syndrome
Thyroid gland	Thyroid not palpable	Masses Distended veins	Enlarged thyroid Cardiopulmonary disorder

Continued

TABLE 7-3

Physical Assessment of Newborn—cont'd

Area Assessed	Normal Findings	Deviations From Normal Range	Etiology
CHEST			
Thorax	Almost circular, barrel shaped	Bulging of chest, unequal movement	Pneumothorax, pneumomediastinum
	Tip of sternum possibly prominent	Malformation	Funnel chest—pectus excavatum
Respiratory movements	Symmetric chest movements, chest and abdominal movements synchronized during respirations	Retractions with or without respiratory distress, seesaw respirations	Prematurity, RDS
	Occasional retractions, especially when crying		
Clavicles	Clavicles intact	Fracture of clavicle; crepitus	Trauma

Ribs	Rib cage symmetric, intact; moves with respirations	Poor development of rib cage and musculature	Prematurity
Nipples	Prominent, well formed; symmetrically placed	Supernumerary, along nipple line Malpositioned or widely spaced	
Breast tissue	Breast nodule: approximately 3-10 mm in term infant Secretion of witch's milk	Lack of breast tissue Maternal hormones	Prematurity
ABDOMEN			
Umbilical cord	Two arteries, one vein Whitish gray Definite demarcation between cord and skin, no intestinal structures within cord Dry around base, drying Odorless Cord clamp in place for 24 hr Reducible umbilical hernia	One artery Meconium stained Bleeding or oozing around cord Redness or drainage around cord Herniation of abdominal contents into area of cord (e.g., omphalocele); defect covered with thin, friable membrane, possibly extensive	Renal anomalies Intrauterine distress Hemorrhagic disease Infection, possible persistence of urachus

Continued

302 Section 7

TABLE 7-3
Physical Assessment of Newborn—cont'd

Area Assessed	Normal Findings	Deviations From Normal Range	Etiology
ABDOMEN—cont'd			
	Rounded, prominent, dome shaped because abdominal musculature not fully developed	Gastroschisis: fissure of abdominal cavity	
	Some diastasis of abdominal musculature		
	Liver possibly palpable 1-2 cm below right costal margin		
	No other masses palpable		
	No distention	Distention at birth	Ruptured viscus, genitourinary masses or malformations: hydronephrosis, teratomas, abdominal tumors
		Mild	Overfeeding, high gastrointestinal tract obstruction

		Lower gastrointestinal tract obstruction, imperforate anus
	Marked	
		Overfeeding
	Intermittent or transient	Stenosis of bowel
	Partial intestinal obstruction	Obstruction
	Visible peristalsis	
	Malrotation of bowel or adhesions	
		Infection
	Sepsis	
Bowel sounds	Sounds present within minutes after birth in healthy term infants	
	Scaphoid, with bowel sounds in chest and respiratory distress	Diaphragmatic hernia
Stools	Meconium stool passing within 24-48 hr after birth	
	No stool	Imperforate anus
Color	Linea nigra possibly apparent	Hormone influence during pregnancy
Movement with respiration	Respirations primarily diaphragmatic, abdominal and chest movement synchronous	
	Decreased abdominal breathing	Intrathoracic disease, phrenic nerve palsy, diaphragmatic hernia
	"Seesaw"	Respiratory distress

Continued

TABLE 7-3

Physical Assessment of Newborn—cont'd

Area Assessed	Normal Findings	Deviations From Normal Range	Etiology
GENITALIA			
Female			
General appearance	Female genitalia	Ambiguous genitalia—enlarged clitoris with urinary meatus on tip, fused labia	Chromosomal disorder, maternal drug ingestion
Clitoris	Usually edematous	Virilized female; extremely large clitoris	Congenital adrenal hyperplasia, pregnancy hormones
Labia majora	Usually edematous, covering labia minora in term newborns		
	Increased pigmentation		
	Edema and ecchymosis after breech birth		
Labia minora	Possible protrusion over labia majora	Labia majora widely separated and labia minora prominent	Prematurity
Discharge	Smegma		

Vagina	Open orifice	Absence of vaginal orifice Fecal discharge	Fistula
	Some vernix caseosa between labia possible		
	Blood-tinged discharge from pseudomenstruation		Pregnancy hormones
	Mucoid discharge		
	Hymenal or vaginal tag		
Urinary meatus	Beneath clitoris, difficult to see (to watch for voiding)	Stenosed meatus	
Check urination	Voiding within 24 hr, amount adequate	No voiding	Absence of kidneys, obstruction
	Rust-stained urine†		Uric acid crystals
Male			
General appearance	Male genitalia	Increased size and pigmentation	Ambiguous genitalia Pregnancy hormones
Penis:			
Urinary meatus as slit	Meatus at tip of penis	Urinary meatus not on tip of glans penis	Hypospadias, epispadias Round meatal opening
Prepuce	Prepuce (foreskin) covering glans penis and not retractable	Prepuce removed if circumcised	
	Wide variation in size of genitalia		

†To determine whether rust color is caused by uric acid or blood, rinse diaper under running warm tap water; uric acid washes out, blood does not.

Continued

TABLE 7-3

Physical Assessment of Newborn—cont'd

Area Assessed	Normal Findings	Deviations From Normal Range	Etiology
GENITALIA—cont'd			
Scrotum:			
Covered with rugae (wrinkles)	Large, edematous, pendulous in term infant	Scrotal edema and ecchymosis if breech birth	Breech birth
		Scrotum smooth	Prematurity
Testes	Palpable on each side	Testes undescended	Prematurity, cryptorchidism
		Hydrocele, small, noncommunicating	Prematurity
		Bulge palpable in inguinal canal	Inguinal hernia
Check urination	Voiding within 24 hr, stream adequate, amount adequate	No voiding	Absence of kidneys, obstruction
	Rust-stained urine†		Uric acid crystals
Reflex: cremasteric	Testes retracted, especially when newborn is chilled		
EXTREMITIES			
Degree of flexion	Assuming of position maintained in utero	Limited motion	Malformations
Range of motion	Transient (positional) deformities	Poor muscle tone	Prematurity, maternal medications, CNS anomalies
Symmetry of motion		Positive scarf sign	

Muscle tone	Attitude of general flexion, Full range of motion, spontaneous movements, Slight tremors sometimes apparent, Contours and movement symmetric	Asymmetry of movement	Fracture or crepitus, brachial nerve trauma, malformations
Arms and hands: Intactness, Appropriate placement	Longer than legs in newborn period	Asymmetry of contour, Amelia or phocomelia, Palmar creases, Simian line with short, incurved little fingers	Malformations, fracture, Teratogens, Down syndrome
Color	Some acrocyanosis, especially when chilled		
Fingers	Five on each hand, Fist often clenched with thumb under fingers	Webbing of fingers: syndactyly, Polydactyly, Absence or excess of fingers, Strong, rigid flexion; persistent fists in front of mouth constantly	Familial trait, CNS disorder
Joints	Full range of motion	Increased tonicity, clonus, symmetric contour	CNS disorder, prolonged tremors

Continued

TABLE 7-3

Physical Assessment of Newborn—cont'd

Area Assessed	Normal Findings	Deviations From Normal Range	Etiology
EXTREMITIES—cont'd			
Humerus	Intact	Fractured humerus	Trauma
Legs and feet	Appearance of bowing because lateral muscles more developed than medial muscles	Amelia (absence of limbs), phocomelia (shortened limbs)	Chromosomal deficiency, teratogenic effect
	Feet appearing to turn in but can be easily rotated externally, positional defects tending to correct while infant is crying	Temperature of one leg different from that of the other	Circulatory deficiency CNS disorder
	Acrocyanosis		
Number of toes	Five on each foot	Webbing: syndactyly	Chromosomal defect
		Absence or excess of digits	Chromosomal defect, familial trait
Femur	Intact femur	Femoral fracture	Difficult breech birth

Soles of feet	No click heard, femoral head not overriding acetabulum Major gluteal folds even Soles well lined (or wrinkled) over two thirds of foot in term infants Plantar fat pad giving flat-footed effect	Developmental dysplasia or dislocation Soles of feet: Few lines Covered with lines Congenital clubfoot	Prematurity Postmaturity
Joints	Full range of motion, symmetric contour	Hypermobility of joints Asymmetric movement	Down syndrome Trauma, CNS disorder
BACK Spine	Spine straight and easily flexed	Limitation of movement	Fusion or deformity of vertebrae
Shoulders	Infant able to raise and support head momentarily when prone Temporary minor positional deformities, correction with passive manipulation		

Continued

TABLE 7-3

Physical Assessment of Newborn—cont'd

Area Assessed	Normal Findings	Deviations From Normal Range	Etiology
BACK—cont'd			
Scapulae Iliac crests	Shoulders, scapulae, and iliac crests lining up in same plane		
Base of spine— pilonidal area		Spina bifida cystica	Meningocele, myelomeningocele
		Pigmented nevus with tuft of hair	Often associated with spina bifida occulta
ANUS			
Patency	One anus with good sphincter tone	Low obstruction: anal membrane	
	Passage of meconium within 24-48 hr after birth	High obstruction: anal or rectal atresia	
		Absence of anal opening	
Sphincter response (active "wink" reflex)	Good "wink" reflex of anal sphincter	Drainage of fecal material from vagina in female or urinary meatus in male	Rectal fistula

STOOLS

Patency | No stool | Obstruction

Frequency, color, consistency | Meconium followed by transitional and soft yellow stools | Frequent watery stools | Infection, phototherapy

Use of Nasopharyngeal Catheter with Mechanical Suction Apparatus

- Deeper suctioning may be needed to remove tenacious mucus from the newborn's nasopharynx or posterior oropharynx.
- If wall suction is used, adjust the pressure to less than 80 mm Hg. Proper tube insertion and suctioning for 5 seconds or less per tube insertion help prevent laryngospasm and oxygen depletion.
- Lubricate the catheter in sterile water, then insert either orally along the base of the tongue or up and back into the nares.
- After the catheter is properly placed, create suction by placing your thumb intermittently over the control as the catheter is carefully rotated and gently withdrawn.
- Repeat the procedure until the infant's cry sounds clear and air entry into the lungs is heard by stethoscope.

Relieving Airway Obstruction

- Repositioning the infant and suctioning the mouth and nose with the bulb syringe may eliminate the problem.
- Auscultate the infant's respiration and lung sounds with a stethoscope to determine whether there are crackles, rhonchi, or inspiratory stridor. Fine crackles may be auscultated for several hours after birth.
- If air movement is adequate, the bulb syringe may be sufficient to clear the mouth and nose. If the bulb syringe does not clear mucus interfering with respiratory effort, use mechanical suction.
- If the newborn has an obstruction that is not cleared with suctioning, investigate further to determine if there is a mechanical defect (e.g., tracheoesophageal fistula or choanal atresia) causing the obstruction (see pp. 372, 375; Emergency box).

Maintaining Body Temperature

- Cold stress increases the need for oxygen and can deplete glucose stores. The infant can react to exposure to cold by increasing the respiratory rate and becoming cyanotic.
- Ways to stabilize the newborn's body temperature include the following:
    - ❑ Place the infant directly on the mother's chest or abdomen, and cover with a warm blanket (skin-to-skin contact).

EMERGENCY

Relieving Airway Obstruction

Back blow and chest thrusts are used to clear an airway obstructed by a foreign body.

BACK BLOWS
- Position the infant prone over forearm with the head down and the infant's jaw firmly supported.
- Rest the supporting arm on the thigh.
- Deliver four back blows forcefully between the infant's shoulder blades with the heel of the free hand.

TURN INFANT
- Place the free hand on the infant's back to sandwich the baby between both hands; one hand supports the neck, jaw, and chest while the other supports the back.
- Turn the infant over, and place the head lower than the chest, supporting the head and neck.
- Alternative position: Place the infant face down on your lap with the head lower than the trunk; firmly support the head. Apply back blows, and then turn the infant as a unit.

CHEST THRUSTS
- Provide four downward chest thrusts on the lower third of the sternum.
- Remove foreign body if it is visible.

OPEN AIRWAY
- Open airway with the head tilt–chin lift maneuver, and attempt to ventilate.
- Repeat the sequence of back blows, turning, and chest thrusts.
- Continue these emergency procedures until signs of recovery occur:
  ❑ Palpable peripheral pulses return.
  ❑ The pupils become normal in size and are responsive to light.
  ❑ Mottling and cyanosis disappear.
- Record the time and duration of the procedure and the effects of this intervention.

❑ Dry and wrap the newborn in warmed blankets immediately after birth.
❑ Keep the head covered.
❑ Maintain the ambient temperature of the nursery at 22° to 26° C (72° to 78° F).

- ❑ If the infant does not remain with the mother during the first 1 to 2 hours after birth, place the thoroughly dried unclothed infant under a radiant warmer or in an isolette until the body temperature stabilizes.
- ■ Use the infant's skin temperature as the point of control in a warmer with a servo-controlled mechanism.
  - ❑ The control panel usually is maintained between 36° and 37° C.
  - ❑ Maintain this setting at the healthy newborn's skin temperature of around 36.5° to 37.2° C.
  - ❑ Tape a thermistor probe (automatic sensor) to the right upper quadrant of the abdomen immediately below the right intercostal margin (never over a bone).
  - ❑ A reflector adhesive patch can be used over the probe to provide adequate warming. This will ensure detection of minor changes resulting from external environmental factors or neonatal factors (peripheral vasoconstriction, vasodilation, or increased metabolism) before a dramatic change in core body temperature develops.
  - ❑ The servo-controller adjusts the warmer temperature to maintain the infant's skin temperature within the desired range.
  - ❑ Check the sensor periodically to make sure it is securely attached to the infant's skin.
  - ❑ Check the newborn's axillary temperature every hour (or more often as needed) until the temperature stabilizes.

Because the time needed to stabilize and maintain body temperature varies, each newborn should be allowed time to achieve thermal regulation as necessary, and care should be individualized.

Examinations and activities are performed with the newborn under a heat panel to avoid heat loss. The initial bath is postponed until the newborn's skin temperature is stable and can adjust to heat loss from a bath. The optimal timing of the bath for each newborn is unknown.

Causes of Hypothermia

- ■ Inadequate drying and wrapping immediately after birth
- ■ A cold birthing room
- ■ Birth in a car on the way to the hospital

Warming the hypothermic infant is accomplished with care. Rapid warming can cause apneic spells and acidosis in an infant. The warming process is monitored to progress slowly over 2 to 4 hours.

Therapeutic Interventions

Eye Prophylaxis

- Installation of an agent in the eyes of all neonates as prophylaxis against ophthalmia neonatorum is mandatory in the United States.
- In the United States, if parents object to this treatment, ask them to sign an informed refusal form and note their refusal in the infant's record.
- The agent used for prophylaxis varies according to hospital protocols but usually includes forms of erythromycin, tetracycline, or silver nitrate.
- To instill medication, the thumb and forefinger are used to open the eye; medication is placed in the lower conjunctiva from the inner to the outer canthus (Fig. 7-1).
- Eye prophylaxis can be delayed until 1 hour or so after birth (up to 2 hours in Canada) so that eye contact and parent-infant attachment and bonding are facilitated (see the Medication Guide: Eye Prophylaxis: Erythromycin Ophthalmic Ointment, 0.5%, and Tetracycline Ophthalmic Ointment, 1%, in Appendix B).

Vitamin K Administration

Administering vitamin K is routine in the newborn period in the United States. A single intramuscular dose of 0.5 to 1 mg of vitamin K is given soon after birth to prevent hemorrhagic disorders (Fig. 7-2).

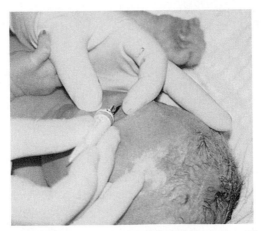

Fig. 7-1 Installation of medication into eye of newborn. (Courtesy Marjorie Pyle, RNC, Lifecircle, Costa Mesa, CA.)

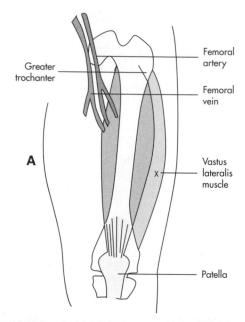

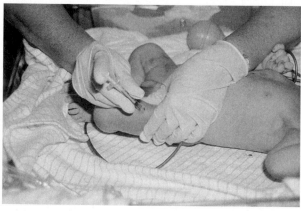

Fig. 7-2 Intramuscular injection. **A,** Acceptable intramuscular injection site for newborn infant. *X,* Injection site. **B,** Infant's leg stabilized for intramuscular injection. Nurse is wearing gloves to give injection. (**B,** Courtesy Marjorie Pyle, RNC, Lifecircle, Costa Mesa, CA.)

Administration can be delayed until after the first breastfeeding in the birthing room. By day 8, healthy newborns are able to produce their own vitamin K (see the Medication Guide: Vitamin K: Phytonadione [AquaMEPHYTON, Konakion] in Appendix B).

Umbilical Cord Care

Many hospitals have subscribed to the practice of "dry care," which consists of cleaning the periumbilical area with soap and water and wiping it dry.

- Others apply an antiseptic solution, such as erythromycin solution, triple dye, or alcohol.
- Recommendations for cord care by the Association of Women's Health, Obstetric and Neonatal Nurses (AWHONN) include cleaning the cord with sterile water or a neutral pH cleanser. Subsequent care entails cleaning with water.
- The stump and base of the cord should be assessed for edema, redness, purulent drainage, and odor with each diaper change.
- The cord clamp is removed when the cord is drying and no longer bleeding, typically in 24 to 48 hours.
- The average cord separation time is 10 to 14 days.

CARE MANAGEMENT: FROM 2 HOURS AFTER BIRTH UNTIL DISCHARGE

Gestational Age Assessment

- The simplified Assessment of Gestational Age is commonly used to assess gestational age of infants between 35 and 42 weeks. The total score correlates with a maturity rating of 26 to 44 weeks of gestation. The score is accurate to plus or minus 2 weeks and is accurate for infants of all races.
- The New Ballard Score, a revision of the original scale, can be used with newborns as young as 20 weeks of gestation. The scale overestimates gestational age by 2 to 4 days in infants younger than 37 weeks of gestation, especially at gestational ages of 32 to 37 weeks.

Classification of Newborns by Size, Gestational Age, and Mortality (Box 7-1)

- The infant's birth weight, length, and head circumference are plotted on standardized graphs that identify normal values for gestational age.
- Preterm birth and LBW commonly occur together (e.g., <32 weeks of gestation and birth weight <2500 g).

BOX 7-1

Classification of Infants According to Size, Gestational Age, and Mortality

CLASSIFICATION ACCORDING TO SIZE

- Low-birth-weight (LBW) infant: an infant whose birth weight is less than 2500 g, regardless of gestational age
- Very low-birth-weight (VLBW) infant: an infant whose birth weight is less than 1500 g
- Extremely low-birth-weight (ELBW) infant: an infant whose birth weight is less than 1000 g
- Appropriate for gestational age (AGA) infant: an infant whose birth weight falls between the 10th and 90th percentiles on intrauterine growth curves
- Small-for-date (SFD) or small for gestational age (SGA) infant: an infant whose rate of intrauterine growth was restricted and whose birth weight falls below the 10th percentile on intrauterine growth curves
- Large for gestational age (LGA) infant: an infant whose birth weight falls above the 90th percentile on intrauterine growth charts
- Intrauterine growth restriction (IUGR): found in infants whose intrauterine growth is restricted (sometimes used as a more descriptive term for the SGA infant)
  - ❏ Symmetric IUGR: growth restriction in which the weight, length, and head circumference are all affected
  - ❏ Asymmetric IUGR: growth restriction in which the head circumference remains within normal parameters while the birth weight falls below the 10th percentile

CLASSIFICATION ACCORDING TO GESTATIONAL AGE

- Premature (preterm): an infant born before completion of 37 weeks of gestation, regardless of birth weight
  - ❏ Late preterm: an infant born between 34 and 36 weeks of gestation, regardless of birth weight
- Full-term: an infant born between the beginning of 38 weeks and the completion of 42 weeks of gestation, regardless of birth weight
- Postterm (postdate): an infant born after completion of week 42 of gestation
- Postmature: an infant born after 42 weeks of gestation and showing effects of progressive placental insufficiency

BOX 7-1

Classification of Infants According to Size, Gestational Age, and Mortality—cont'd

CLASSIFICATION ACCORDING TO MORTALITY

- Live birth: birth in which the neonate manifests any heartbeat, breathes, or displays voluntary movement, regardless of gestational age
- Fetal death: death of the fetus after 20 weeks of gestation and before birth, with absence of any signs of life after birth
- Neonatal death: death that occurs in the first 27 days of life; early neonatal death occurs in the first week of life; late neonatal death occurs at 7 to 27 days
- Infant death: death of an infant younger than 1 year of age
- Infant mortality: numbers of deaths of infants younger than 1 year of age per 1000 live births
- Perinatal mortality: total number of fetal and early neonatal deaths per 1000 live births

NURSING ALERT *Late preterm infants are often the size and weight of term infants and are usually admitted to the healthy newborn nursery or mother/baby unit. Late preterm infants have risk factors resulting from their physiologic immaturity that require close attention. Compared with term infants, they have a greater tendency for respiratory distress, temperature instability, hypoglycemia, apnea, feeding difficulties, and jaundice and hyperbilirubinemia. Nurses must be continually vigilant for the development of these problems.*

COMMON PROBLEMS IN THE NEWBORN
Physical Injuries

Birth trauma is physical injury sustained by a newborn during labor and birth. Injury can occur because of factors such as uterine dysfunction or cephalopelvic disproportion, fetal macrosomia, multifetal gestation, abnormal or difficult presentation, and congenital anomalies. Intrapartum events include use of the scalp electrode or collection of fetal scalp blood, and obstetric birth techniques, such as forceps- or vacuum-assisted birth, external version, and cesarean birth. Most injuries are minor and resolve in the neonatal period without treatment; some types of trauma require intervention. A few are serious enough to be fatal. See Section 8 for a discussion of selected physical injuries.

Physiologic Jaundice

■ Every newborn is assessed for jaundice. To differentiate cutaneous jaundice from normal skin color, apply pressure with a finger over a bony area (e.g., nose, forehead, or sternum) for several seconds to empty all the capillaries in that spot. If jaundice is present the blanched area will appear yellow before the capillaries refill. The conjunctival sacs and buccal mucosa also are assessed, especially in darker-skinned infants. It is recommended to assess for jaundice in daylight because artificial lighting and reflection from nursery walls can distort the actual skin color.

■ Jaundice is noticeable first in the head, then progresses gradually toward the abdomen and extremities. If jaundice is suspected, evaluation of serum bilirubin level is needed.

❑ Noninvasive monitoring of bilirubin by cutaneous reflectance measurements (transcutaneous bilirubinometry [TcB]) allows for repetitive estimations of bilirubin levels.

❑ TcB monitors provide accurate measurements within 2 to 3 mg/dl in most neonatal populations at serum levels less than 15 mg/dl. After phototherapy has been initiated, TcB is no longer useful as a screening tool.

❑ Bilirubin levels are evaluated based on the newborn's age in hours. The American Academy of Pediatrics, Subcommittee on Hyperbilirubinemia recommends the use of a nomogram prior to hospital discharge to predict the risk of hyperbilirubinemia in infants at 35 weeks of gestation or greater.

❑ Risk factors that place infants in the high risk category include gestational age less than 38 weeks, breastfeeding, previous sibling with significant jaundice, and jaundice appearing before discharge.

❑ Healthy infants (35 weeks or greater) should receive follow-up care and assessment of bilirubin within 3 days of discharge if discharged at less than 24 hours.

Hypoglycemia

Hypoglycemia that warrants treatment is usually defined as blood glucose levels less than 40 mg/dl; some experts recommend treatment for levels less than 50 mg/dl.

- Signs of hypoglycemia can be transient or recurrent and include the following:
  - Jitteriness
  - Lethargy
  - Poor feeding
  - Hypotonia
  - Temperature instability
  - Respiratory distress
  - Apnea
  - Seizures

> **NURSING ALERT** *Hypoglycemia can be present without clinical manifestations.*

- Hypoglycemia in the low risk term infant is usually eliminated by feeding the infant. Occasionally the IV administration of glucose is required for newborns with persistently high insulin levels or those with depleted glycogen stores.

Hypocalcemia

- Hypocalcemia (serum calcium levels <7.8 to 8 mg/dl in term infants or <7 mg/dl in preterm infants) can occur in newborns of diabetic mothers, in newborns who had perinatal asphyxia or trauma, and in LBW and preterm infants. Early-onset hypocalcemia occurs within the first 24 to 48 hours after birth.
- Signs of hypocalcemia include the following:
  - Jitteriness
  - High-pitched cry
  - Irritability
  - Apnea
  - Intermittent cyanosis
  - Abdominal distention
  - Laryngospasm
- Some hypocalcemic infants are asymptomatic.
  - Early-onset hypocalcemia is usually self-limiting and resolves within 1 to 3 days. Treatment includes early feeding. In some cases (e.g., the medically unstable ELBW infant), IV elemental calcium and phosphorus are administered.

■ Jitteriness is a symptom of both hypoglycemia and hypocalcemia; therefore, hypocalcemia must be considered if the therapy for hypoglycemia proves ineffective. In some newborns jitteriness remains despite therapy and cannot be explained by hypoglycemia or hypocalcemia.

LABORATORY AND DIAGNOSTIC TESTS

Laboratory tests commonly performed in the newborn period include the following:
■ Blood glucose levels
■ Bilirubin levels
■ Complete blood count (CBC)
■ Newborn screening tests
■ Serum drug levels

Box 7-2 gives standard laboratory values for a term newborn.

Newborn Genetic Screening

■ Before hospital discharge, a heelstick blood sample is obtained to detect a variety of congenital conditions. All states in the United States screen for phenylketonuria (PKU) and hypothyroidism,

---

BOX 7-2

Standard Laboratory Values in a Term Newborn*

Hemoglobin	14.5-22.5 g/dl
Hematocrit	48%-69%
Glucose	40-60 mg/dl
Leukocytes (white blood cells)	9000-30,000/mm^3
Bilirubin, total serum	<2 mg/dl
Blood gases	
Arterial	pH 7.31-7.49
	Pco_2 26-41 mm Hg
	Po_2 60-70 mm Hg
Venous	pH 7.31-7.41
	Pco_2 40-50 mm Hg
	Po_2 40-50 mm Hg

*These values can change significantly in the first week of life.
Some data from Pagana, K., & Pagana, T. (2009). *Mosby's manual of diagnostic and laboratory tests* (4th ed.). St. Louis: Mosby.

but each state determines whether other tests, such as for galactosemia, cystic fibrosis, maple syrup urine disease, and sickle cell disease, are performed. In Canada, individual provinces determine which tests are performed.

- The screening test should be repeated at age 1 to 2 weeks if the initial specimen was obtained when the infant was younger than 24 hours.
- The advent of tandem mass spectrometry holds promise to increase the number of conditions (more than 50) that can be tested with the same minimal amount of blood. Information about which tests are required in a state can be obtained from state health departments and in provinces in Canada from www.savebabiescanada.org.

Newborn Hearing Screening

Universal newborn hearing screening is required by law in more than 30 states and is performed routinely in other states. Newborn hearing screening is completed before hospital discharge or before 1 month of age. Infants who do not pass are referred for repeated testing within the next 2 to 8 weeks. The practice of universal hearing screening reduces the age at which infants with hearing loss are identified and treated.

Collection of Specimens

Heelstick

- Warm the heel before the sample is taken; heat applied for 5 to 10 minutes helps dilate the vessels in the area. A cloth soaked with warm water and wrapped loosely around the foot provides effective warming. Disposable heel warmers are available from a variety of companies but should be used with caution to prevent burns.
- Wear gloves when collecting any specimen.
- Restrain the infant's foot with a free hand.
- Cleanse the area with alcohol.
- Identify an appropriate puncture site (Fig. 7-3).
- Make the puncture at the outer aspect of the heel, and do not penetrate deeper than 2.4 mm.
- A spring-loaded automatic puncture device causes less pain and requires fewer punctures than a manual lance blade.
- After the specimen has been collected, apply pressure with a dry gauze square; do not apply more alcohol because this will cause the site to continue to bleed.
- Cover the site with an adhesive bandage.
- Dispose of used equipment properly.

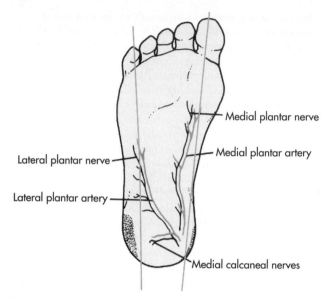

Fig. 7-3 Heelstick sites *(shaded areas)* on infant's foot for obtaining samples of capillary blood.

- Review the laboratory slip for correct identification.
- Check the specimen for accurate labeling and routing.

To reassure the infant and promote feelings of safety, the neonate should be cuddled and comforted when the procedure is complete and appropriate pain management measures taken to minimize the pain.

Venipuncture

- Venous blood samples can be drawn from antecubital, saphenous, superficial wrist, and rarely, scalp veins. If an IV site is used to obtain a blood specimen, it is important to consider the type of infusion fluid; contamination of the blood sample with the fluid can alter the results.
- Although regular venipuncture needles can be used, some practitioners prefer butterfly needles. A 25-gauge needle is adequate for blood sampling in neonates with minimal hemolysis occurring when the proper procedure is followed.
- A tourniquet is optional but can help increase blood flow with venipuncture.

- The mummy restraint commonly is used to help secure the infant.
- Crying, fear, and agitation affect blood gas values; therefore, every effort must be made to keep the infant quiet during the procedure.
- For blood gas studies, the blood sample tubes are packed in ice (to reduce blood cell metabolism) and are taken immediately to the laboratory for analysis.

The infant's tolerance of the procedure should be recorded. The infant should be cuddled and comforted when the procedure is completed.

NURSING ALERT *Pressure must be maintained over an arterial or femoral vein puncture with a dry gauze square for at least 3 to 5 minutes to prevent bleeding from the site. For 1 hour after any venipuncture, the nurse should observe the infant frequently for evidence of bleeding or hematoma formation at the puncture site.*

Obtaining a Urine Specimen

The urine sample should be fresh and analyzed within 1 hour of collection. A variety of urine collection bags are available, including clear plastic single-use bags with an adhesive material around the opening at the point of attachment.

- Remove the diaper, and place the infant in a supine position.
- Wash the genitalia, perineum, and surrounding skin, and dry thoroughly (the adhesive on the bag will not stick to moist, powdered, or oily skin surfaces).
- Remove the protective paper to expose the adhesive.
- In female infants, stretch the perineum to flatten skinfolds, and then press the adhesive area on the bag firmly onto the skin all around the urinary meatus and vagina. Start the application at the bridge of skin separating the rectum from the vagina and work upward.
- In male infants, tuck the penis and scrotum through the opening into the collection bag before removing the protective paper from the adhesive and pressing it firmly onto the perineum, making sure the entire adhesive is firmly attached to skin and the edges of the opening do not pucker. This helps ensure a leakproof seal and decreases the chance of contamination from stool.
- Cutting a slit in the diaper and pulling the bag through the slit helps prevent leaking.

- Replace the diaper, and check the bag frequently.
- When a sufficient amount of urine (this amount varies according to the test done) appears, remove the bag.
- Observe the infant's skin for signs of irritation while the bag is in place.
- Aspirate the specimen with a syringe, or drain the specimen directly from the bag. For some types of urine tests, urine can be aspirated directly from the diaper by means of a syringe without a needle. If the diaper has absorbent gel material that traps urine, a small gauze dressing or some cotton balls can be placed inside the diaper and the urine aspirated from them.

CARE MANAGEMENT

Hand hygiene between infant handlings is the single most important measure in the prevention of neonatal infection.

Therapeutic and Surgical Procedures
Intramuscular Injection

- It is routine to administer a single dose of 0.5 to 1 mg of vitamin K intramuscularly to an infant soon after birth.
- Hepatitis B (Hep B) vaccination is recommended for all infants (see the Medication Guide: Hepatitis B Vaccine [Recombivax; Engerix-B] in Appendix B). If the infant is born to an infected mother or to a mother who is a chronic carrier, hepatitis vaccine and hepatitis B immunoglobulin (HBIG) should be administered within 12 hours of birth (see the Medication Guide: Hepatitis B Immunoglobulin in Appendix B). The hepatitis vaccine is given in one site and the HBIG in another. For infants born to hepatitis B–negative women, the first dose of the vaccine can be given at birth or at 1 month of age.
- Obtain parental consent before administering these vaccines.

Therapy for Hyperbilirubinemia

The best therapy for hyperbilirubinemia is prevention. Because bilirubin is excreted in meconium, prevention can be facilitated by early feeding, which stimulates the passage of meconium. The goal of treatment of hyperbilirubinemia is to help reduce the newborn's serum levels of unconjugated bilirubin. The two principal ways of doing this are phototherapy and, rarely, exchange blood transfusion. Exchange transfusion is used to treat those infants whose levels of bilirubin are rising rapidly despite the use of intensive phototherapy.

Phototherapy

- During phototherapy the unclothed infant is placed beneath a bank of lights approximately 45 to 50 cm from the light source. The distance varies based on unit protocol and type of light used. The most effective therapy is achieved with a special blue light or a specially designed light-emitting diode (LED) light. The lamp energy should be monitored routinely during treatment with a photometer to ensure efficacy of therapy.
- Phototherapy is used until the infant's serum bilirubin level decreases to within an acceptable range. The decision to discontinue therapy is based on the observation of a definite downward trend in the bilirubin values.
- Several precautions must be taken while the infant is undergoing phototherapy:
  - Protect the infant's eyes with an opaque mask to prevent overexposure to the light (Fig. 7-4).
  - Cover the eyes completely with the eye shield, but do not occlude the nares.
  - Before applying the mask, gently close the infant's eyes to prevent excoriation of the corneas.
  - Remove the mask during infant feedings so that the eyes can be checked and the parents can have visual contact with the infant.
  - To promote optimal skin exposure during phototherapy, leave the diaper off, or make a "string bikini" from a disposable face mask to cover the infant's genital area.

> **SAFETY ALERT** *The metal strip must be removed from the face mask to prevent burning the infant. Lotions and ointments should not be used during phototherapy because they absorb heat, and this can cause burns.*

  - Monitor the infant's temperature.
  - Phototherapy lights increase insensible water loss, placing the infant at risk for fluid loss and dehydration; therefore, it is important that the infant is adequately hydrated.

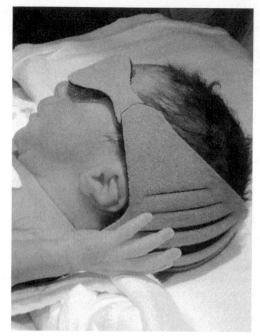

Fig. 7-4 Infant with eyes covered while receiving phototherapy. (Courtesy Cheryl Briggs, RNC, Annapolis, MD.)

❑ Hydration maintenance in the healthy newborn is accomplished with human milk or infant formula; glucose water and plain water do not promote excretion of bilirubin in the stools and perpetuate enterohepatic circulation, thus delaying bilirubin excretion.

❑ Urine output can be decreased or unaltered; the urine can have a brown or gold appearance.

❑ Monitor the number and consistency of stools. Bilirubin breakdown increases gastric motility, which results in the formation of loose stools that can cause skin excoriation and breakdown.

❑ Clean the infant's buttocks after each stool to help maintain skin integrity.

- ❑ A fine maculopapular rash can appear during phototherapy, but this is transient.
- ❑ Because visualization of the infant's skin color is difficult with blue light, implement appropriate cardiorespiratory monitoring based on the infant's overall condition.
- ❑ Record all aspects of the phototherapy treatment in the infant's record.
- ■ An alternative device for phototherapy that is safe and effective is a fiberoptic panel attached to an illuminator.
  - ❑ Use a combination of conventional lights and fiberoptic blankets when intensive therapy is warranted.
  - ❑ The fiberoptic blanket can be wrapped around the newborn's torso or placed flat in the bed, thus delivering continuous phototherapy.
  - ❑ Place a covering pad between the infant's skin and the fiberoptic device.
  - ❑ During treatment the newborn can remain in the mother's room in an open crib or in her arms.
  - ❑ Follow unit protocol for the use of eye patches.
  - ❑ The blanket can be used for home care.
- ■ Parent Education
  - ❑ Infants can leave the hospital as soon as 6 hours after birth.
  - ❑ Serum levels of bilirubin continue to rise until the fifth day of life.
  - ❑ Give written instructions to parents for assessing the infant's condition and the name of a contact person for reporting their findings and concerns.
  - ❑ Some agencies provide a home visit to evaluate the infant's condition and monitor the mother's health.
  - ❑ If it is necessary to measure serum bilirubin levels, a health care technician or nurse can draw the blood for the specimen or the parents can take the baby to a laboratory to have blood drawn.

Circumcision

- ■ Circumcision is the removal of the prepuce (foreskin) of the glans. The procedure is usually performed in the hospital before the infant's discharge. The circumcision of a Jewish male is commonly performed on the eighth day after birth and is done at home in a ceremony called a bris.

- Circumcision of newborn males is commonly performed in the United States. Parents usually decide to have their newborn circumcised for reasons of hygiene, religious conviction, tradition, culture, or social norms.
- Parents should be given unbiased information and the opportunity to discuss the benefits and risks of the procedure.
- Suggested medical benefits of circumcision for the infant include the following:
  - ❑ Decreased incidence of urinary tract infection
  - ❑ Decreased risk for sexually transmitted infections including HIV and human papillomavirus (HPV) infection
  - ❑ Decreased risk for penile cancer
- Risks and potential complications associated with circumcision include hemorrhage, infection, and penile injury (removal of excessive skin or damage to the meatus or glans).
- Procedure
  - ❑ The procedure itself takes only a few minutes.
  - ❑ Formula feedings are usually withheld up to 2 to 3 hours before the circumcision to prevent vomiting and aspiration.
  - ❑ Breastfed infants can nurse up until the procedure is done; this varies with unit protocol.
  - ❑ To prepare the infant for the circumcision, position him on a plastic restraint form, and cleanse the penis with soap and water or a preparatory solution, such as povidone-iodine (Fig. 7-5).
  - ❑ Drape the infant to provide warmth and a sterile field, and ready the sterile equipment for use.
  - ❑ After the procedure is completed, a small petrolatum gauze dressing or a generous amount of petrolatum is applied for 1 or 2 days to prevent the diaper from adhering to the site. If a PlastiBell is used for the circumcision, petrolatum need not be applied.
- Discomfort
  - ❑ Circumcision is painful, and the pain is characterized by both physiologic and behavioral changes in the infant. Analgesia or anesthesia should be used during the procedure.
  - ❑ Four types of anesthesia or analgesia are used in newborns who undergo circumcisions. These include (from most effective to less effective): ring block, dorsal penile nerve block (DPNB), topical anesthetic such as eutectic mixture of local anesthetic (EMLA) (prilocaine 2.5%-lidocaine 2.5%) or LMX4 (4% lidocaine), and concentrated sucrose given orally.

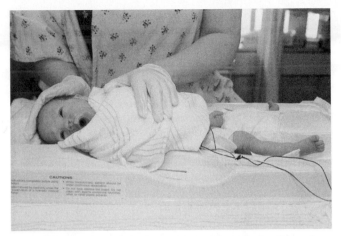

Fig. 7-5 Proper positioning of infant in Circumstraint. (Photo by Paul Vincent Kuntz, Texas Children's Hospital, Houston, TX.)

❑ A ring block is the injection of buffered lidocaine administered subcutaneously on each side of the penile shaft.

❑ A DPNB includes subcutaneous injections of buffered lidocaine at the 2 o'clock and 10 o'clock positions at the base of the penis. The circumcision should not be done for at least 5 minutes after these injections.

❑ A topical cream such as EMLA can be applied to the base of the penis at least 1 hour before the circumcision. The area where the prepuce attaches to the glans is well coated with 1 g of the cream and then covered with a transparent occlusive dressing or finger cot. Just before the procedure the cream is removed. Blanching or redness of the skin can occur.

❑ During the procedure, a concentrated oral sucrose solution can be given on a pacifier, or with a syringe or nipple.

❑ A combination of ring block or DPNB, topical anesthetic, nonnutritive sucking, oral acetaminophen, concentrated oral sucrose solution (2 ml of a 24% concentration given during the procedure on a pacifier, with a syringe or nipple), and swaddling has been shown to be the most effective at decreasing the pain associated with circumcision.

- After the circumcision the infant is comforted until he is quieted. If the parents were not present during the procedure, the infant is returned to them. The infant can be fussy for several hours, or he may be sleepy and difficult to awaken for feedings.
- Oral acetaminophen can be administered after the procedure every 4 hours (as ordered by the practitioner) for a maximum of five doses in 24 hours or a maximum of 75 mg/kg/day.

■ Care of the newly circumcised infant
  - Bleeding is the most common complication of circumcision.
  - Check the infant every 30 minutes for the first hour then hourly for the next 4 to 6 hours.
  - Monitor the urinary output; note and record the time and amount of the first voiding after the circumcision.
  - If bleeding occurs from the circumcision, apply gentle pressure to the site of bleeding with a folded sterile gauze square.
  - Absorbable gelatin sponge (Gelfoam) powder or sponge can be applied to stop bleeding.
  - If bleeding is not easily controlled, a blood vessel may require ligation. In this event one nurse notifies the primary health care provider and prepares the necessary equipment (circumcision tray and suture material) while another nurse maintains intermittent pressure until the primary health care provider arrives.

■ Parent education
  - If the parents take the baby home before the end of the 12-hour observation period, instruct them in postcircumcision care and when to notify the physician.
  - Before the infant is discharged, check to see that the parents have the physician's telephone number.
  - If the PlastiBell technique was used, instruct the parents to observe the position of the plastic ring on the glans; it should remain on the glans (not on the shaft of the penis) and should fall off within 5 to 7 days. Petrolatum is not usually needed when the PlastiBell is used.
  - Prepackaged commercial wipes for cleaning the diaper area should not be used because they contain alcohol, which delays healing and causes discomfort.
  - Wash the penis gently with water to remove urine and feces; apply fresh petrolatum to the glans with each diaper change.

❏ The glans becomes covered with a yellow exudate that can persist for several days. This is part of the normal healing process. Do not attempt to remove it.

NEONATAL PAIN
Assessment

Every newborn should have an initial pain assessment as well as a pain management plan. Pain can be assessed in behavioral, physiologic/autonomic, and metabolic categories.

Behavioral Responses

■ Vocalization or crying can range from a whimper to a distinctive, high-pitched, shrill cry.
■ Facial expressions of pain include grimacing, eye squeeze, brow contraction, deepened nasolabial furrows, a taut and quivering tongue, and an open mouth.
■ The infant will flex and adduct the upper body and lower limbs in an attempt to withdraw from the painful stimulus.
■ The preterm infant has a lower threshold for initiation of the flex response.
■ An infant who receives a muscle-paralyzing agent such as vecuronium will be unable to mount a behavioral or visible pain response.

Physiologic/Autonomic Response

■ Pain can result in significant changes in heart rate, blood pressure (increased or decreased), intracranial pressure, vagal tone, respiratory rate, and oxygen saturation.
■ Neonates respond to painful stimuli with release of epinephrine, norepinephrine, glucagon, corticosterone, cortisol, 11-deoxycorticosterone, lactate, pyruvate, and glucose.
■ In assessing pain, the health care provider needs to consider the following factors:
  ❏ Health of the neonate
  ❏ Type and duration of the painful stimulus
  ❏ Environmental factors
  ❏ Infant's state of alertness
  ❏ Severely compromised neonates may be unable to generate a pain response, although they are, in fact, experiencing pain

- CRIES is a pain assessment tool that can be used on infants between 32 weeks of gestation and 20 weeks after birth.
  - CRIES is an acronym for the physiologic and behavioral indicators of pain used in the tool: *c*rying, *r*equiring increased oxygen, *i*ncreased vital signs, *e*xpression, and *s*leeplessness. Each indicator is scored from 0 to 2. The total possible pain score, which represents the worst pain, is 10. A pain score greater than 4 should be considered significant.

Management of Neonatal Pain

Nonpharmacologic Management

- Containment, also known as swaddling, is effective in reducing excessive immature motor responses.
- Nonnutritive sucking on a pacifier, with or without sucrose, can be helpful in reducing pain with heel lance and venipuncture.
- Skin-to-skin contact with the mother during a painful procedure can help reduce pain.
- Breastfeeding helps to reduce pain during heel-lancing and blood collection.
- Combining these nonpharmacologic methods results in more effective pain reduction.
- Distraction with visual, oral, auditory, or tactile stimulation can be helpful in term neonates or older infants.

Pharmacologic Management

- Local anesthesia is used routinely during procedures such as chest tube insertion and circumcision.
- Topical anesthesia is used for circumcision, lumbar puncture, venipuncture, and heelsticks.
- Nonopioid analgesia (acetaminophen) is effective for mild to moderate pain from inflammatory conditions.
- Morphine and fentanyl by continuous or bolus intravenous infusion provide effective and safe pain control.
- Ketorolac (Toradol) is effective in managing postoperative pain.
- Postoperative neonatal pain should be managed with around-the-clock dosing or use of a continual drip. Dosing as needed (prn) is not effective in managing chronic or postoperative pain in infants.
- Epidural infusion, local and regional nerve blocks, and intradermal or topical anesthetics are also used to manage neonatal pain.
- Oral acetaminophen can be administered for painful procedures such as circumcision, venous puncture, and heelstick.

RECOMMENDED INFANT NUTRITION

The American Academy of Pediatrics recommends exclusive breast-feeding or human milk feeding for the first 6 months of life and that breastfeeding or human milk feeding continue as the sole source of milk for the next 6 months. See Section 5 for information on breast-feeding. Iron-fortified commercial infant formula should be fed to infants up to 1 year of age who are not receiving breast milk.

Bottle Feeding

- The first feeding of formula is given after the neonate's initial transition to extrauterine life.
- Feeding readiness cues include stability of vital signs, effective breathing patterns, presence of bowel sounds, an active sucking reflex, and signs described in Section 5 for breastfeeding babies.
- Infant formulas simulate the caloric content of human milk; standard formulas contain 20 kcal/oz.
- Typically a newborn will drink 15 to 30 ml of formula per feeding during the first 24 to 48 hours, with the intake gradually increasing during the first week of life. Most newborns are drinking 90 to 150 ml at a feeding by the end of the second week.
- Fill the bottle with 60 to 90 ml of formula. Discard the unused portion.
- Discard formula left at room temperature for more than 4 hours.
- Most newborn infants should be fed every 3 to 4 hours, even if that requires waking the baby for the feedings.
- An infant showing an adequate weight gain can be allowed to sleep at night and fed only on awakening.
- Most newborns need six to eight feedings in 24 hours.
- The infant's appetite usually increases at 7 to 10 days, 3 weeks, 6 weeks, 3 months, and 6 months. These appetite spurts correspond to growth spurts. The amount of formula per feeding should be increased by approximately 30 ml to meet the baby's needs.

Feeding Technique

- Babies should be held for all feedings. This provides an opportunity for parent-infant interaction.
- The bottle should be held so that fluid fills the nipple and none of the air in the bottle is allowed to enter the nipple.

- A bottle should never be propped with a pillow or other inanimate object and left with the infant. Such practices present a choking hazard.
- When the infant falls asleep, turns aside the head, or ceases to suck, it is usually an indication that enough formula has been consumed to satisfy the baby.
- Most babies swallow air when fed from a bottle and should be given a chance to burp several times during a feeding (Fig. 7-6).

Bottles and Nipples

- Most babies will feed well with any bottle and nipple. An angled bottle decreases the need for burping.
- Wash bottles and nipples in warm soapy water; use a bottle and nipple brush. They should be placed in boiling water for 5 minutes and allowed to air dry at least once prior to the first use and after each use unless they are cleaned in a dishwasher.
- Parents should avoid hard plastic bottles and containers containing bisphenol A (BPA).

Infant Formulas

- Commercial infant formulas are designed to resemble human milk as closely as possible, although none has ever duplicated it.
- Infants who are not breastfed or fed expressed breast milk should be given commercial formulas fortified with iron.
- The Women, Infants and Children (WIC) program provides iron-fortified commercial infant formula for low-income families.
- Cow's milk is the basis for most infant formulas, although soy-based and other specialized formulas are available for the infant who cannot tolerate cow's milk.

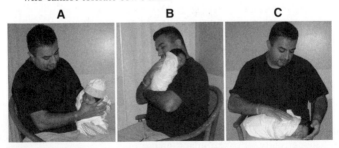

Fig. 7-6 Positions for burping an infant. **A,** Sitting. **B,** On the shoulder. **C,** Across the lap. (Courtesy Julie Perry Nelson, Loveland, CO.)

- Commercial formulas are available in three forms: powder, concentrate, and ready-to-feed. All are equivalent in terms of nutritional content, but they vary considerably in cost:
  - ❑ Powdered formula is the least expensive type. It is easily mixed by using one scoop for every 60 ml of water.
  - ❑ Concentrated formula is more expensive than powder. It is diluted with equal parts of water and can be stored in the refrigerator for 48 hours after opening.
  - ❑ Ready-to-feed formula is the most expensive but easiest to use. The desired amount is poured into the bottle. The opened can is safely refrigerated for 48 hours. This type of formula can be purchased in individual disposable bottles for the most convenient feeding.

Special Formulas

- Infants can have an allergic reaction to cow's-milk formula.
- Infants with cow's-milk allergy may better tolerate a soy-milk formula, although some can be allergic to soy protein.
- Other special formulas are available for infants with a variety of disorders, such as protein allergy, malabsorption syndromes, and inborn errors of metabolism.
- Formulas for preterm infants contain higher calorie concentration (22 to 24 cal/oz) and higher concentrations of some nutrients, such as protein, vitamin A, folic acid, and zinc.

Formula Preparation

Commercial infant formula includes directions for preparation and use with pictures and symbols for the benefit of people who cannot read. Some manufacturers translate the directions into languages such as Spanish, French, Vietnamese, Chinese, and Arabic, to prevent misunderstanding and errors in formula preparation.

NURSING ALERT   *It is important to impress on families that the proportions must not be altered—neither diluted to expand the amount of formula nor concentrated to provide more calories.*

- Sterilization of formula rarely is recommended for those families with access to a safe public water supply.
- It is usually safe to mix infant formula with cold tap water that has been boiled for 1 to 2 minutes and allowed to cool. Bottled water that is labeled as "sterile" is safe for mixing formula.

However, non-sterile bottled water should be boiled for 1 to 2 minutes and cooled.

■ When water from a private well is used, the family should contact the health department to have a chemical and bacteriologic analysis of the water. The presence of nitrates, excess fluoride, or bacteria can be harmful to the infant.

Vitamin and Mineral Supplementation

■ Commercial iron-fortified formula has all the nutrients the infant needs for the first 6 months of life. After 6 months the only mineral supplementation required is fluoride if the local water supply is not fluoridated.

■ Formula-fed infants who consume less than 32 ounces per day of vitamin-D–fortified milk should receive 400 International Units of vitamin D each day.

ANTICIPATORY GUIDANCE REGARDING THE NEWBORN

■ Anticipatory guidance helps prepare new parents for what to expect as their newborn grows and develops (see English-Spanish translations in Appendix C. See Figure 7-7 for a checklist for self-assessment of learning needs of new mothers.

■ Call the pediatric health care provider immediately if jaundice increases or if the infant exhibits any of the following signs of illness:

❑ Fever: temperature more than 38° C (100.4° F) axillary (under arm); also a continual increase in temperature

❑ Hypothermia: axillary temperature less than 36.5° C (97.7° F)

❑ Poor feeding or little interest in food: refusal of two feedings in a row

❑ Vomiting: frequent vomiting (over a 6-hour period) or more than one episode of forceful vomiting

❑ Diarrhea: two consecutive green, watery stools (NOTE: Stools of breastfed infants are normally yellow and looser than stools of formula-fed infants. Diarrhea leaves a water ring around the stool, whereas breast milk stools do not.)

❑ Decreased bowel movements: fewer than three soiled diapers per day after the third or fourth day of life

❑ Decreased urination: no wet diapers for 18 to 24 hours or fewer than six to eight wet diapers per day after 3 to 4 days

- Breathing difficulties: labored breathing (nasal flaring, retractions, cyanosis) or absence of breathing for more than 15 seconds (NOTE: A newborn's breathing is normally irregular and between 40 and 60 breaths/min. Count the breaths for a full minute.)
- Cyanosis whether or not accompanying a feeding
- Lethargy: sleepiness, difficulty waking, or periods of sleep longer than 6 hours (most newborns sleep for short periods, usually from 1 to 4 hours and wake to be fed)
- Inconsolable crying (attempts to quiet not effective) or continuous high-pitched cry
- Bleeding or purulent drainage from umbilical cord or circumcision
- Drainage developing in the eyes
■ Classes to teach infant CPR should be available (Emergency: Cardiopulmonary Resuscitation (CPR) for Infants.

EMERGENCY

Cardiopulmonary Resuscitation (CPR) for Infants

Perform hand hygiene before and after touching infant and equipment. Wear gloves if possible.

CHECK FOR RESPONSE
■ Observe color; tap or gently shake shoulders.
■ If infant is unresponsive and not breathing or only gasping, yell for help.

CHECK FOR BREATHING
■ If infant is unresponsive and not breathing, or only gasping, begin CPR.

START CHEST COMPRESSIONS
If infant is unresponsive and not breathing, give 30 chest compressions. Compress the sternum with 2 fingers placed just below the nipple line. Compress at least 1/3 the depth of the chest, about 4 cm. After each compression, allow complete recoil of the chest.

OPEN THE AIRWAY AND GIVE VENTILATIONS
■ Open the airway with the head tilt-chin lift method.
■ Place one hand on the infant's forehead, and tilt the head back.
■ Place the fingers of other hand under the bone of the lower jaw at the chin.

Continued

EMERGENCY—cont'd

- Use a mouth-to-mouth-and-nose technique.
- Take a breath.
- Place mouth over the infant's nose and mouth to create a seal.
- NOTE: When available, use a mask with a one-way valve.
- Give two breaths (1 second/breath), pausing to inhale between breaths.
- NOTE: Gently puff the volume of air in your cheeks into infant. Do not force air. The infant's chest should rise slightly with each puff; keep fingers on the chest wall to sense air entry.
- Continue the cycle of 30 compressions and 2 breaths for approximately 2 minutes before leaving to activate the emergency response system and obtain an automated external defibrillator (AED) if one is available.
- Return to the infant and use the AED (if available).
- Resume CPR starting with 30 chest compressions.
- Continue the cycle of 30 compressions and 2 breaths until emergency response rescuers arrive or the infant starts breathing spontaneously.

RECORD ACTIONS
- Record the time and duration of the procedure and the effects of intervention.

Source: Berg, J.D., Schexnayder, S.M., Chameides, L., Terry, M., Donoghue, A., Hickey, R.W., et al. (2010). Part 13: Pediatric basic life support: 2010 American Heart Association Guidelines for Cardiopulmonary Resuscitation and Emergency Cardiovascular Care. *Circulation, 122* (18 suppl 3), S862-S875.

Directions: Circle those items about which you would like information.

BABY CARE

Crying	■ Crying can indicate hunger, pain from not burping or gas, need for diaper change, or a too warm or too cold environment.
Hiccups and sneezing	■ Hiccups and sneezing are normal.
Bath: sponge/tub	■ Bathe as needed; daily bathing is not necessary. Keep creases and bottom clean and dry.
Soaps	■ Use mild soap (Dove, Neutrogena, baby care products).
Nail care	■ Use an emery board or baby scissors
Cord care	■ Keep clean and dry. Fold diaper below cord. Cord falls off in 1 to 2 weeks. There can be a few drops of blood when the cord falls off.
Skin care/diaper rash	■ Air dry, and use zinc oxide. Call for advice if no improvement in 2 days.
Diaper change	■ Wash girls front to back.
Genitalia (female)	■ White or pink discharge and cheesy material in the vagina are normal.
Circumcision care	■ Remove petrolatum (Vaseline) gauze 4 hours after the circumcision. ■ Apply petrolatum (Vaseline) to penis for 24 hours. ■ Glans becomes covered with a yellow exudate in 24 hours; this is normal; do not attempt to remove it.
Uncircumcised penis	■ It is not necessary to retract the foreskin (it will not retract until about 3 years of age).
Elimination	■ Bowel elimination should include meconium the first 1 to 2 days and change gradually to yellow, soft, and seedy. The infant urinates six to eight times daily after the first 3 to 4 days.
Axillary temperature	■ Normal axillary temperature is 36.5°-37.2° C. (97.7°-99° F). Call physician if higher than 37.7° C (99.8° F).
Clothing	■ Clothing should be flame retardant. Dress the infant comfortably; do not overdress.
Positioning	■ Position the infant on the back, not the abdomen for sleep. Use tummy time while awake.
Bulb syringe, choking	■ Keep syringe within reach; use to clear nose and mouth.

Fig. 7-7 Self-assessment checklist.

Continued

BABY CARE—cont'd

Handwashing	■ Viruses and bacteria are easily transmitted through hands. Wash frequently; wash after changing diaper and before feeding.
Environment	■ The environment should be smoke free, with a working smoke detector.
Car seat	■ A car seat is mandatory. Follow manufacturer's instructions for installation and use.
Breastfeeding Latch	■ Infant should take enough breast tissue into the mouth so that sucking causes mother no pain; she feels a strong tugging ensation as the baby sucks.
Position	■ Football (under the arm) hold, modified cradle (across the lap), cradling, and lying down (see Fig. 5-1).
Frequency	■ At least 8 to 12 times in 24 hours or about every 2 to 3 hours; a demand feeding schedule can be followed after the infant regains birth weight.
Length of feeding	■ Average feeding is 30 to 45 minutes or 15 to 20 minutes at each breast.
Care of breasts/ nipples	■ For sore nipples, check latch, vary feeding positions, rub breast milk into nipple, air dry, and try shorter, more frequent feedings; can apply purified lanolin or hydrogel pads, and breast shells. Use no soap on nipples (has drying effect).
	■ For breast engorgement, feed frequently, apply ice packs between feedings for 15 minutes, and stand in warm shower just before feeding; hand express or use breast pump to soften breast enough for baby to latch; can apply cabbage leaves for 15 minutes between feedings.
Milk expression/ storage	■ Can begin pumping after milk supply is established, although may need to pump if engorgement occurs.
	■ Freshly expressed breast milk can be stored safely at room temperature for up to 6 hours, in a refrigerator for 7 days, and in a freezer for 6 to 12 months.
Formula Feeding Feeding readiness cues	■ Hand-to-mouth or hand-to-hand movements
	■ Sucking and rooting motions
	■ Mouthing
	■ Don't wait for baby to cry.

Fig. 7-7 cont'd Self-assessment checklist.

BABY CARE—cont'd	
Feeding technique	■ Hold for all feedings. ■ Do not prop bottle. ■ Hold bottle so fluid fills nipple. ■ Burp infant several times during feeding. ■ Wash bottle and nipple in warm soapy water. ■ Do not use hard plastic bottles that contain bisphenol A (BPA).
Amount of feeding	■ 90 to 150 ml/feeding by end of second week
Frequency of feedings	■ Every 3 to 4 hours; 6 to 8 feeding in 24 hours; if adequate weight gain, allow to sleep at night
Appetite spurts/ growth spurts	■ At 7 to 10 days, 3 weeks, 6 weeks, 3 months, 6 months
Infant Quieting Techniques	

Provide security	■ Place baby skin-to skin on mother's or partner's chest
	■ Hold baby securely.
	■ Place in bassinet rather than crib.
	■ Swaddle snugly in a receiving blanket.
	■ Extra sucking
	  ❑ At breast
	  ❑ Pacifier
	  ❑ Thumb or finger

Rhythmic noise	■ Recording of heartbeat ■ Portable bassinet near dishwasher or washing machine
Movement	■ Rock in rocking chair or cradle ■ Change position; hold on shoulder; carry ■ Ride in car, stroller, carriage, or infant carrier ■ Place baby on stomach across lap, rock, pat on back
Close contact	■ Skin-to-skin contact with mother or partner, cover with warm blanket ■ Hold baby close to your face; talk to the baby.
Infant Safety	
Never	■ Never leave the baby alone on a bed, couch, or table. ■ Never put the baby on a cushion, pillow, beanbag, or waterbed to sleep. ■ Never leave the baby alone when bathing him or her ■ Never tie anything around the baby's neck. ■ Never shake the baby. ■ Never expose the baby to tobacco smoke. ■ Never heat the baby's bottle in the microwave.
Always	■ Always place infant on back to sleep.

Fig. 7-7 cont'd Self-assessment checklist.

Selected Newborn Complications

BIRTH TRAUMA

Birth trauma (injury) is physical injury sustained by a neonate during labor and birth. In theory, some birth injuries are avoidable. Fetal ultrasonography for antepartum diagnosis and elective cesarean birth can aid in preventing significant birth injury. The prompt reporting of signs that indicate deviations from normal permits early initiation of appropriate therapy.

Soft-Tissue Injuries

See Table 8-1 for a description of soft-tissue injuries, their causes, and treatment.

Skeletal Injuries

- Two types of *skull fractures* in the newborn are linear fractures and depressed fractures.
  - If an artery is torn as a result of the fracture, increased intracranial pressure (ICP) will follow. Unless a blood vessel is involved, linear fractures, which account for 70% of all fractures for this age-group, heal without special treatment.
  - Depressed fractures (or ping-pong ball indentations) can resolve without treatment or can be elevated by using a hand breast pump or vacuum extractor.
- The *clavicle* is the bone most often fractured during birth. Generally the break is in the middle third of the bone.
  - Risk factors in clavicular fracture are dystocia, particularly shoulder impaction, vacuum-assisted birth, and birth weight greater than 4000 g. Limitation of motion of the arm, crepitus over the bone, and the absence of the Moro reflex on the affected side are diagnostic.
  - Except for use of gentle rather than vigorous handling, no accepted treatment for fractured clavicle in the newborn exists, and the prognosis is good. The figure-eight bandage should not be used for the newborn.

TABLE 8-1

Soft-Tissue Injuries

Soft-Tissue Injury	Cause	Treatment
Subconjunctival and retinal hemorrhages	Rupture of capillaries caused by increased pressure during birth	Hemorrhages clear within 5 days after birth and present no further problems. Parents need explanation and reassurance.
Erythema, ecchymoses, petechiae, abrasions, lacerations, or edema of buttocks and extremities	Application of forceps or the vacuum cup Bruises on face from face presentation Bruising and swelling on buttocks or genitalia from breech presentation Ecchymoses and petechiae on head from tight nuchal cord Petechiae can extend over the upper trunk and face	Lesions are benign if they disappear within 2 or 3 days of birth and no new lesions appear. Ecchymoses and petechiae can be signs of a more serious disorder, such as thrombocytopenia.
Bruised caput or a linear mark across both sides of the face in the shape of the forceps blades	Application of vacuum cup or forceps	Keep areas clean to minimize the risk of infection.
Lacerations on the face, scalp, buttocks, and thighs	Accidental cuts with scalpel during a cesarean birth	Keep clean. Liquid skin adhesive or butterfly adhesive strips can hold together the edges of more serious lacerations. Rarely are sutures needed.

- The *humerus* and *femur* can be fractured during a difficult birth. Fractures in newborns generally heal rapidly. Immobilization is accomplished with slings, splints, swaddling, and other immobilization devices.

Management

- Support the parents in handling these infants because they often are fearful of hurting them.
- Encourage parents to practice handling, changing diapers, and feeding the injured neonate under the guidance of nursery personnel.
- Develop a plan for follow-up therapy.

Peripheral Nervous System Injuries

- *Erb-Duchenne palsy* or brachial plexus injury (brachial paralysis) of the upper portion of the arm results from a stretching or pulling of the head away from the shoulder during a difficult birth.
  - ❏ The arm hangs limp alongside the body. The shoulder and arm are adducted and internally rotated. The elbow is extended, and the forearm is pronated, with the wrist and fingers flexed; a grasp reflex can be present because finger and wrist movement remains normal.
  - ❏ Treatment is by intermittent immobilization across the upper abdomen, proper positioning, and range of motion (ROM) exercises starting about the tenth day to prevent additional injury to the brachial plexus. Immobilization can be accomplished with a brace or splint or by pinning the infant's sleeve to his or her shirt.
- Damage to the lower plexus, *Klumpke palsy,* is less common and results from severe stretching of the upper extremity while the trunk is relatively less mobile.
  - ❏ The wrist and hand are flaccid, the grasp reflex is absent, deep tendon reflexes are present, and dependent edema and cyanosis can be apparent (in the affected hand).
  - ❏ Treatment consists of placing the hand in a neutral position, padding the fist, and gently exercising the wrist and fingers.
- In a third and more severe form of brachial palsy, the entire arm is paralyzed and hangs limp and motionless at the side.
- The Moro reflex is absent on the affected side for all forms of brachial palsy.

- Parents are taught to position and immobilize the arm or wrist or both. They can gently massage and manipulate the muscles to prevent contractures while the arm is healing. If edema or hemorrhage is responsible for the paralysis, the prognosis is good, and recovery can be expected in a few weeks.

- Dress the infant beginning with the affected arm, and undress beginning with the unaffected arm to prevent unnecessary manipulation and stress on the paralyzed muscles.

- Teach parents to use the "football" (under the arm or clutch) position when holding the infant and to avoid picking the child up from under the axillae or by pulling on the arms.

- Full recovery is expected in 88% to 92% of infants. Complete recovery from stretched nerves usually takes 3 to 6 months.

- Facial paralysis (palsy) generally is caused by pressure on the facial nerve during birth. Risk factors include a prolonged second stage of labor and forceps-assisted birth. The face on the affected side is flattened and unresponsive to the grimace that accompanies crying or stimulation, the eye remains open on the affected side, and the forehead will not wrinkle. The infant's face appears distorted, especially when crying. Often the condition is transitory, resolving within hours or days of birth. Permanent paralysis is rare.

  ❏ Treatment involves assistance with feeding, prevention of damage to the cornea of the open eye with the application of artificial tears or taping the eye closed, and supportive care of the parents.

Central Nervous System Injuries

All types of intracranial hemorrhage (ICH) occur in newborns. ICH as a result of birth trauma is more likely to occur in the full-term, large infant. Risk factors for ICH include primiparity, advanced maternal age, vacuum- or forceps-assisted birth, precipitous or prolonged second stage of labor, and increased fetal size.

Subdural Hematoma

A subdural hematoma (hemorrhage) is most often produced by the stretching and tearing of the large veins in the tentorium of the cerebellum, the dural membrane that separates the cerebrum from the cerebellum.

- The typical history includes a primiparous mother, with total labor and birth lasting less than 2 or 3 hours; a difficult birth involving high- or midforceps application; or a large for gestational age (LGA) infant.
- Subdural hematoma occurs infrequently because of improvements in obstetric care. It is especially serious because of its inaccessibility to aspiration by subdural tap.

Subarachnoid Hemorrhage

Subarachnoid hemorrhage, the most common type of ICH, occurs in term infants as a result of trauma and in preterm infants as a result of hypoxia. Small hemorrhages are the most common. Bleeding is of venous origin, and underlying contusion also can occur.

- The clinical presentation of hemorrhage in the term infant can vary considerably. In many infants, signs are absent, and hemorrhaging is diagnosed only because of abnormal findings on lumbar puncture, such as red blood cells (RBCs) in the cerebrospinal fluid.
- The initial clinical manifestations of neonatal subarachnoid hemorrhage can be the early onset of alternating central nervous system (CNS) depression and irritability, with refractory seizures.
- Occasionally the infant appears normal initially, then has seizures on the second or third day of life, followed by no apparent sequelae.

Management

- Nursing care of an infant with ICH is supportive and includes monitoring ventilatory and intravenous therapy, observing and managing seizures, and preventing increased ICP. Handle the infant minimally to promote rest and reduce stress.

NEONATAL INFECTIONS
Sepsis

Sepsis is the presence of microorganisms or their toxins in the blood or other tissues and continues to be one of the most significant causes of neonatal morbidity and mortality.

- Table 8-2 outlines risk factors for neonatal sepsis. Special precautions for preventing infection, as well as prompt recognition when it occurs, are necessary for optimum newborn

TABLE 8-2

Risk Factors for Neonatal Sepsis

Source	Risk Factors
Maternal	Low socioeconomic status
	Late or no prenatal care
	Poor nutrition
	Substance abuse
	Recently acquired sexually transmitted infection
	Untreated focal infection (urinary tract infection, vaginal, cervical)
	Systemic infection
	Fever
Intrapartum	Premature rupture of fetal membranes
	Maternal fever
	Chorioamnionitis
	Prolonged labor
	Premature labor
	Use of fetal scalp electrode
Neonatal	Multiple gestation
	Male infant
	Birth asphyxia
	Meconium aspiration
	Congenital anomalies of skin or mucous membranes
	Metabolic disorders (e.g., galactosemia)
	Absence of spleen
	Low birth weight
	Preterm birth
	Malnourishment
	Formula feeding
	Prolonged hospitalization
	Mechanical ventilation
	Umbilical artery catheterization or use of other vascular catheters

Source: Edwards, M. (2006). Postnatal bacterial infections. In R. Martin, A. Fanaroff, & M. Walsh (Eds.), *Fanaroff and Martin's neonatal-perinatal medicine: Diseases of the fetus and infant* (8th ed.). Philadelphia: Mosby.

TABLE 8-3

Signs of Sepsis

System	Signs
Respiratory	Apnea, bradycardia
	Tachypnea
	Grunting, nasal flaring
	Retractions
	Decreased oxygen saturation
	Acidosis
Cardiovascular	Decreased cardiac output
	Tachycardia
	Hypotension
	Decreased perfusion
Central nervous	Temperature instability
	Lethargy
	Hypotonia
	Irritability, seizures
Gastrointestinal	Feeding intolerance
	Abdominal distention
	Vomiting, diarrhea
Integumentary	Jaundice
	Pallor
	Petechiae
Metabolic	Hypoglycemia
	Hyperglycemia
	Metabolic acidosis
Hematologic	Thrombocytopenia
	Neutropenia

Source: Edwards, M. (2006). Postnatal bacterial infections. In R. Martin, A. Fanaroff, & M. Walsh (Eds.), *Fanaroff and Martin's neonatal-perinatal medicine: Diseases of the fetus and infant* (8th ed.). Philadelphia: Mosby.

care. Neonatal infections can be health care–associated or acquired in utero or during birth or resuscitation. Table 8-3 outlines the clinical signs associated with neonatal sepsis.

Early-Onset or Congenital Sepsis

Early-onset or congenital sepsis usually manifests within 24 to 72 hours after birth, progresses more rapidly than later-onset infection, and has a mortality rate ranging between 3% and 50%.

- Early-onset infection is usually caused by microorganisms from the normal flora of the maternal vaginal tract, including group B streptococcus, *Haemophilus influenzae, Listeria monocytogenes, Escherichia coli,* and *Streptococcus pneumoniae.*
- Early-onset sepsis is associated with preterm labor, premature rupture of membranes, maternal fever during labor, and chorioamnionitis.

Late-Onset Infection

Late-onset sepsis occurs at 7 to 30 days of age and can include maternally derived infection or health care–associated infection.

- The organisms responsible include staphylococci, *Klebsiella,* enterococci, *E. coli, Pseudomonas,* and *Candida.* Additional infections of concern include methicillin-resistant *Staphylococcus aureus* (MRSA), vancomycin-resistant enterococci, and multidrug-resistant gram-negative pathogens.
- Bacterial invasion can occur through sites such as the umbilical stump; the skin; mucous membranes of the eye, nose, pharynx, and ear; and internal systems such as the respiratory, nervous, urinary, and gastrointestinal (GI) systems.

Septicemia

Septicemia refers to a generalized infection in the bloodstream.

Other Infections

- Pneumonia, the most common form of neonatal infection, is one of the leading causes of perinatal death, and is caused by many of the same organisms that cause sepsis.
- Bacterial meningitis affects 1 in 2500 live-born infants.
- Gastroenteritis is sporadic, depending on epidemic outbreaks.
- Local infections such as conjunctivitis and omphalitis occur frequently.

Management

- Maternal antepartum infection is treated with a number of antiviral medications to decrease viral replication and fetal transmission of disease; neonates can be treated with antiviral medications such as acyclovir and ganciclovir.
- Treatment with antibiotics is initiated after blood cultures are obtained in neonates; in high risk infants with significant illness, antiviral or antibiotic treatment can begin once cultures are

obtained. Once the pathogen is identified, antibiotic, antiviral, or antifungal therapy may be modified.

Viral Infections

Viral infections can cause intrauterine infection, congenital malformations, and acute neonatal disease. These pathogens also can cause chronic infection. It is important to recognize and treat the acute infection to prevent health care–associated infections in other infants and to anticipate effects on the infant's subsequent growth and development.

Fungal Infections

Fungal infections are of greatest concern in the immunocompromised or premature infant. Occasionally fungal infections such as thrush are found in otherwise healthy term infants.

Candidiasis

Candida albicans can cause disease in any organ system. It is a yeastlike fungus that can be acquired from a maternal vaginal infection during birth, by person-to-person transmission, or from contaminated hands, bottles, nipples, or other articles. It usually is a benign disorder in the neonate, often confined to the oral and diaper regions

- Candidal diaper dermatitis appears on the perianal area, inguinal folds, and lower portion of the abdomen. The affected area is intensely erythematous, with a sharply demarcated, scalloped edge, frequently with numerous satellite lesions that extend beyond the larger lesion. The source of the infection is through the gastrointestinal tract.
  - ❏ Treatment is with applications of an antifungal ointment, such as nystatin (Mycostatin) or miconazole 2% (Monistat), with each diaper change. The infant also can be given an oral antifungal preparation to eliminate any gastrointestinal source of infection.
- Oral candidiasis (thrush, or mycotic stomatitis) is characterized by the appearance of white plaques on the oral mucosa, gums, and tongue. The white patches are easily differentiated from milk curds; the patches cannot be removed and tend to bleed when touched. In most cases, the infant does not seem to be in discomfort from the infection. A few infants seem to have some difficulty swallowing.
  - ❏ Topical application of 1 ml nystatin over the surfaces of the oral cavity four times a day, or every 6 hours, is usually sufficient to prevent spread of the disease or prolongation of

its course. To prevent relapse, therapy should be continued for at least 2 days after the lesions disappear. Gentian violet solution can be used in long-term cases of oral thrush (gentian violet permanently stains clothing or other material).

■ Infants who are breastfed can acquire thrush from the mother; in the event that the mother is colonized, treatment for mother and infant is recommended. There is no need to stop breastfeeding even if the mother is receiving systemic antifungal medications.

■ Scrupulous cleanliness (by nursing personnel, parents, and others) must be maintained. Good hand hygiene is imperative.

Transplacental Infections

The occurrence of certain maternal infections during early pregnancy is known to be associated with various congenital malformations and disorders. The most common and best understood infections are traditionally represented by the acronym TORCH.

T	Toxoplasmosis
O	Other: gonorrhea, hepatitis B, syphilis, varicella-zoster virus, parvovirus B19, and human immunodeficiency virus (HIV)
R	Rubella
C	Cytomegalovirus
H	Herpes simplex virus (HSV)

Additional organisms known to cause congenital infection include enteroviruses and parvovirus, leading some clinicians to suggest the need for a new, more comprehensive acronym.

Toxoplasmosis

Toxoplasmosis is a multisystem disease caused by the protozoan *Toxoplasma gondii* commonly found in cats, dogs, pigs, sheep, and cattle, with cats being the most common host. In the United States risk factors for acquisition of toxoplasmosis include exposure to contaminated soil and consumption of raw or undercooked meats or seafood (oysters, clams, or mussels). The transplacental transmission rate increases as pregnancy progresses: 15% in the first trimester, 30% in the second trimester, and 60% in the third trimester.

■ Severe toxoplasmosis is associated with preterm birth, growth restriction, microcephaly or hydrocephaly, microphthalmos, chorioretinitis, CNS calcification, thrombocytopenia, jaundice, and fever. Petechiae or a maculopapular rash can also be evident.

> **NURSING ALERT**   *To differentiate hemorrhagic areas from skin rashes and discolorations, try to blanch the skin with two fingers. Petechiae and ecchymoses do not blanch because extravasated blood remains within the tissues, whereas skin rashes and discolorations do blanch.*

■ Maternal treatment with spiramycin can prevent fetal infection. The affected infant can be treated with pyrimethamine, as well as oral sulfadiazine, but folic acid supplementation is required to prevent anemia.

Gonorrhea

Gonorrhea is caused by *Neisseria gonorrhoeae*. The incidence of gonococcal infection in pregnant women ranges from 2.5% to 7.3%.

■ After rupture of membranes, ascending infection can result in orogastric contamination of the fetus. The organism can also invade mucosal surfaces, such as the conjunctiva (ophthalmia neonatorum), rectal mucosa, and pharynx. Neonatal gonococcal arthritis, septicemia, meningitis, vaginitis, and scalp abscesses can also develop.

■ Eye prophylaxis (e.g., with 0.5% erythromycin ointment) is administered within the first hour after birth to prevent ophthalmia neonatorum. Eye prophylaxis alone does not prevent systemic infection; therefore, infants with a gonococcal eye infection should receive one dose of ceftriaxone. Infants with systemic gonococcal infection require hospitalization and 7 days of IV antibiotic therapy. Rarely, infants die of overwhelming infection in the early neonatal period.

Syphilis

Syphilis is caused by the spirochete *Treponema pallidum*. If syphilis during pregnancy is untreated, 40% to 50% of neonates born to these women will have symptomatic congenital syphilis. If maternal infection is treated adequately before the eighteenth week, neonates seldom demonstrate signs of the disease. Treatment failure can occur, particularly when treatment is given in the third trimester; therefore, infants born to women treated within 4 weeks of birth should be evaluated for congenital syphilis.

■ Early congenital syphilis can result in prematurity, hydrops fetalis, and failure to thrive. Hepatosplenomegaly and jaundice are common. Hematologic findings include anemia, leukocytosis, and thrombocytopenia. Characteristic bony lesions occur in the long bones, the cranium, and the spine and include osteochondritis, osteomyelitis, and periostitis. Other findings include snuffles, mucocutaneous lesions, edema, and a copper-colored maculopapular dermal rash on the palms, the soles, and in the perioral, perinasal, and the diaper region (Fig. 8-1). The maculopapular lesions can become vesicular and confluent and extend over the trunk and extremities. Poor feeding, slight hyperthermia, and snuffles can be nonspecific signs.

- If the mother was adequately treated before giving birth and serologic testing of the infant does not show syphilis, generally the infant is not treated with antibiotics. The infant is checked for antibody titer (received from the mother through the placenta) every 2 weeks for 3 months, at which time the test result should be negative. Some physicians recommend antibiotic therapy for asymptomatic or inconclusive cases.

- Treatment should be carried out in the following situations: when the diagnosis of congenital syphilis is confirmed or suspected, when maternal treatment status is unknown, when the mother is treated within 4 weeks of giving birth or does not respond to treatment, when medications other than penicillin are used to treat the mother, and when inadequate neonatal follow-up is anticipated.

Varicella Zoster

The varicella-zoster virus, responsible for chickenpox and shingles, is a member of the herpes family. Approximately 90% of women in their childbearing years are immune; therefore, the risk of infection in pregnancy is low.

- When transmission to the fetus occurs in the early part of pregnancy (relatively infrequently, about 2%), the effects on the fetus include

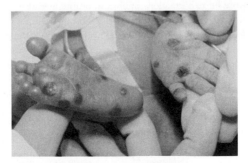

Fig. 8-1 Neonatal syphilis lesions on hands and feet. (Courtesy Mahesh Kotwal, MD, Phoenix, AZ.)

limb atrophy, neurologic abnormalities (hydrocephalus or microcephaly), and eye abnormalities. When maternal infection occurs in the last 3 weeks of pregnancy, 25% of infants born to these mothers will develop clinical varicella. The severity of the infant's illness increases greatly if maternal infection occurred within 5 days before or 2 days after birth. The mortality in severe illness is 30%.

- Infants born to mothers who develop chickenpox between 5 days before birth and 48 hours after birth should be given varicella-zoster immune globulin (VZIG) at birth because of the risk of severe disease. Acyclovir can be used to treat infants with generalized involvement and pneumonia.

- Term infants exposed to chickenpox after birth have a mild or no infection if they are born to immune mothers. In those born to nonimmune mothers, chickenpox can develop but the course is not usually severe. Experts are divided as to whether this group of infants should receive VZIG. Infants younger than 28 weeks are at risk regardless of their mother's status and probably benefit from VZIG if exposed to chickenpox.

Hepatitis B Virus

Transmission of hepatitis B virus (HBV) occurs transplacentally, serum to serum, and by contact with contaminated urine, feces, saliva, semen, or vaginal secretions during birth. The transmission rate of HBV to the newborn is high when the mother is seropositive for both hepatitis B surface antigen (HBsAg) and hepatitis B e antigen (HBeAg). Diagnosis is made by viral culture of amniotic fluid as well as the presence of HBsAg and immunoglobulin M (IgM) in the cord blood or newborn's serum.

- There is no association between infection during pregnancy and an increase in malformations, stillbirths, or intrauterine growth restriction (IUGR); however, there is a significant risk for preterm birth. Infants can be symptom free at birth or show evidence of acute hepatitis with changes in liver function. The mortality for full-blown hepatitis is 75%. Infants who become carriers are at high risk for chronic hepatitis, cirrhosis of the liver, or liver cancer even years later.

- Infants whose mothers have antibodies for HBsAg or who have developed hepatitis during pregnancy or the postpartum period should be treated with hepatitis B immunoglobulin (HBIG), 0.5 ml intramuscularly, as soon as possible after birth or within the first 12 hours of life. Hepatitis B vaccine should also be given concurrently but at a different site.

- The second dose of vaccine is given at 1 month and the third dose at 6 months of age. After the infant has been cleansed thoroughly and has received the vaccine, breastfeeding can be initiated.
- Vaccination for infants not exposed to maternal HBV is recommended before discharge from the hospital; breastfeeding for these infants can begin before the vaccine is given.

Human Immunodeficiency Virus (Type 1)

Transmission of HIV from the mother to the infant can occur transplacentally at various gestational ages. The majority of cases of pediatric acquired immunodeficiency syndrome (AIDS) (90% or more) result from maternal-to-fetal transmission.

- With antepartum, intrapartum, and neonatal zidovudine (ZDV) treatment the incidence of neonatal HIV infection is decreased to 5% to 8%, and compliance with highly active antiretroviral therapy (HAART) is said to further reduce newborn infection rates to 1% to 2%.
- Postpartum transmission can occur, with an additional risk of 14% attributed to breast milk contact. Diagnosis of HIV infection in the neonate is complicated by the presence of maternal immunoglobulin G (IgG) antibodies, which cross the placenta after 32 weeks of gestation.
- The most accurate test for newborns and infants younger than 18 months is the HIV-1 DNA polymerase chain reaction (PCR) assay, which is performed on neonatal blood, not cord blood.
- Typically the HIV-infected neonate is asymptomatic at birth. Early-onset illness (i.e., virus detected within 48 hours of birth) is attributed to prenatal infection and occurs in 10% to 15% of infected infants. These infants develop opportunistic infections (*Candida* and *Pneumocystis jiroveci* pneumonia) and rapid progression of immunodeficiency, which progresses to death in the first 1 to 2 years of life. The presenting signs and symptoms of HIV infection vary from severe immunodeficiency to nonspecific findings such as growth failure, parotitis, and recurrent or persistent upper respiratory tract infections.
- Universal counseling and screening of pregnant women are recommended in the United States and Canada.
- Standard Precautions are used to protect the infant from further exposure to maternal blood and body fluids.

- In the United States, breastfeeding by the HIV-positive mother is contraindicated. However, in developing countries, the risks versus benefits in relation to number of infant deaths attributed to poor sanitary conditions and availability of an appropriate food supply for infants are considered. The World Health Organization recommends that HIV-positive mothers who are taking antiretroviral medications should breastfeed for at least 12 months.

- Children who are HIV positive can be treated with a combination of three antiretroviral drugs: two nucleoside reverse transcriptase inhibitors, such as zidovudine and stavudine, plus either a protease inhibitor such as nelfinavir, lopinavir, or saquinavir, or a nonnucleoside reverse transcriptase such as nevirapine.

- If the infant is diagnosed with HIV infection, the family should be counseled about conventional and investigational treatment options, the care of the mother herself, the family's care of the infant, and future pregnancies. The risk for transmission among members of the same household is minimal. Social services are required in these cases.

Rubella Infection

Since rubella vaccination was begun in 1969, cases of congenital rubella infection have been reduced by 99%. Vaccination failures, lack of compliance, and the migration of nonimmunized persons result in periodic outbreaks of rubella, also known as German, or 3-day, measles. The risk of a congenitally infected infant varies with the gestational age of the fetus when maternal infection occurs. Abnormalities are most severe if the mother contracts the virus during the first trimester and rare if the disease occurs after that time.

- More than two thirds of infected infants have no symptoms obvious at birth, but sequelae can develop years later.

- Hearing loss, the most common result, appears to be progressive after birth.

- Congenital rubella syndrome includes cataracts or glaucoma, hearing loss, and cardiac defects (pulmonary artery stenosis, patent ductus arteriosus, or coarctation of the aorta).

- Multiple other abnormalities can be present including IUGR, microphthalmia, hypotonia, hepatosplenomegaly, thrombocytopenic purpura, dermatoglyphic abnormalities, bony radiolucencies, microcephaly, and brain wave abnormalities.

- Severe infection can result in fetal death.
- The rubella virus has been cultured in infants for up to 18 months after their birth. These infants are a serious source of infection to susceptible individuals, particularly women in the childbearing years. Extended pediatric isolation is mandatory until the noncontagious stage of rubella has been reached. The infant should be isolated until pharyngeal mucus and the urine are free of virus.

Cytomegalovirus Infection

Cytomegalovirus (CMV) infection during pregnancy can result in congenital or neonatal cytomegalic inclusion disease (CMID). It is the most common cause of congenital viral infections in the United States. Most (90%) affected infants are asymptomatic at birth; however, hearing loss and learning disabilities have been reported in 10% to 15% of previously asymptomatic infants.

- The neonate with full-blown CMV has IUGR, microcephaly, rash, jaundice, and hepatosplenomegaly. Anemia, thrombocytopenia, and hyperbilirubinemia are common. Intracranial, periventricular calcification often is noted on radiography. Inclusion bodies ("owl's eye" figures) in cells sedimented from freshly voided urine or in liver biopsy specimens are typical.
- The virus can be isolated from urine or saliva of the newborn. CMV can be transmitted through breast milk while the mother has acute CMV infection. In preterm infants, postnatal acquisition of CMV can result in pneumonia, hepatitis, thrombocytopenia, and long-term neurologic sequelae.
- Treatment of the infected newborn with ganciclovir is effective in decreasing neurologic sequelae, in particular sensorineural hearing loss.

Herpes Simplex Virus

HSV infections among newborns are being diagnosed more frequently and are estimated to occur in as many as 1 in 3000 to 1 in 20,000 births. HSV type 2 is the most common cause of illness in neonates (75%). The neonate can acquire the virus by any of four modes of transmission: (1) transplacental infection, (2) ascending infection by way of the birth canal, (3) direct contamination during passage through an infected birth canal, and (4) direct transmission from infected personnel or family.

- Congenital infection is rare and is characterized by in utero destruction of normally formed organs. Affected infants are growth restricted. They have severe psychomotor delays, intracranial calcifications, microcephaly, hypertonicity, and seizures as well as eye involvement, including microphthalmos, cataracts, chorioretinitis, blindness, and retinal dysplasia. Some infants have patent ductus arteriosus, limb anomalies, recurrent skin vesicles, and a short life expectancy. Most infants are infected directly during passage through the birth canal.

- Standard Precautions should be observed when caregivers have contact with these infants.

- Nursery personnel with cold sores should practice strict hand hygiene and wear a mask, but no evidence indicates they should be removed from the nursery unless they have a herpetic whitlow (primary HSV infection of the terminal segment of a finger).

- The neonate's eyes, oral cavity, and skin are inspected carefully for lesions. Cultures are obtained from the mouth, eyes, and any lesions.

- Circumcision, if performed, is delayed until the infant is ready to be discharged.

- The infant can be discharged with the mother if his or her cultures are negative for the virus.

- As long as no suspicious lesions are on the mother's breasts, breastfeeding is encouraged.

- For the infant at risk, prophylactic topical eye ointment (vidarabine) is administered for 5 days to prevent keratoconjunctivitis.

- Blood, urine, and cerebrospinal fluid (CSF) specimens should be cultured when indicated clinically.

- Therapy includes general supportive measures, as well as treatment with acyclovir or vidarabine. Ophthalmic ointment should be administered simultaneously.

Bacterial Infections

Group B Streptococci

The most common cause of neonatal sepsis and meningitis in the United States is group B streptococci (GBS).

- Early-onset GBS infection in the neonate occurs in the first 7 days of life but most commonly manifests in the first 24 hours following birth.

- Risk factors for the development of early-onset GBS include low birth weight, preterm birth, rupture of membranes of more than 18 hours, maternal fever, previous GBS infant, maternal GBS bacteriuria, and multiple gestation.
- Early-onset disease is usually the result of vertical transmission from the birth canal and causes a respiratory illness that mimics the symptoms of severe respiratory distress. The infant can rapidly develop septic shock, which has a significant mortality rate.
- The practice of giving prophylactic antibiotics to women in labor who are GBS positive has significantly reduced the incidence and severity of early-onset GBS infection in the newborn.
- The neonate is treated with penicillin and an aminoglycoside.

Escherichia coli

E. coli is the second most common cause of neonatal sepsis and meningitis in the United States. It is found in the GI tract soon after birth and makes up the bulk of human fecal flora.

- In addition to chorioamnionitis in the mother, *E. coli* can cause a variety of neonatal infections including omphalitis, diarrheal illness, pneumonia, peritonitis, urinary tract infections, and meningitis.
- Increasing use of ampicillin in labor as prophylaxis against GBS infection can result in more virulent *E. coli* infection resulting from ampicillin-resistant organisms.
- Risk factors for the development of *E. coli* infections in the newborn include maternal infection, low birth weight, prolonged rupture of membranes, and septic or traumatic birth.
- Clinical signs of *E. coli* sepsis are relatively nonspecific and include fever, temperature instability, apnea, cyanosis, jaundice, hepatomegaly, lethargy or irritability, vomiting, abdominal distention, and diarrhea.

Listeriosis

Listeria monocytogenes is a bacterium capable of producing significant intrapartum illness.

- Two forms of neonatal listeriosis are recognized: early onset and late onset.
- Early-onset infections usually present at birth with meconium-stained amniotic fluid, respiratory distress, cyanosis, apnea, and evidence of pneumonia.
- Listeriosis also can manifest as meningitis in a late-onset infection.

Chlamydia Infection

Chlamydia trachomatis is an intracellular bacterium that causes neonatal conjunctivitis and pneumonia.

- Conjunctivitis, with minimal discharge, develops 5 to 14 days after birth. Inclusion conjunctivitis is usually self-limiting, but if untreated, chronic follicular conjunctivitis (trachoma) with conjunctival scarring and corneal microgranulations can develop.
- Chlamydial pneumonia has a gradual onset, between 4 and 11 weeks of age, beginning with rhinorrhea and progressing to tachypnea and coughing. Signs can be quite subtle and often are not recognized.
- Ophthalmic silver nitrate is not effective against *C. trachomatis*; but erythromycin or tetracycline ointment may prevent ophthalmic infection; therefore, infants at risk should be treated with systemic antibiotics such as oral erythromycin syrup. Erythromycin administration in infants younger than 6 weeks has been associated with an increased risk of infantile hypertrophic pyloric stenosis (IHPS); therefore, parents should be educated regarding the symptoms of the condition (feeding intolerance, projectile vomiting, and abdominal distention).

SUBSTANCE ABUSE

Maternal habits hazardous to the fetus and neonate include recreational and prescription drug abuse, tobacco use, and alcohol abuse. Drug dependence in the neonate is physiologic, not psychologic.

- The adverse effects of exposure of the fetus to drugs vary. They include transient behavioral changes, such as fetal breathing movements, and irreversible effects, such as fetal death, IUGR, structural malformations, or mental retardation.
- Critical determinants of the effect of the drug on the fetus include the specific drug, the dosage, the route of administration, the genotype of the mother or fetus, and the timing of the drug exposure. Determining the specific effects of individual drugs on the fetus is made difficult by the common practice of polydrug use, errors or omissions in reporting drug use, and variations in the strength, purity, and types of additives found in street drugs.

Table 8-4 summarizes the effects of commonly abused substances on the neonate.

TABLE 8-4

Neonatal Effects of Commonly Abused Substances

Substance	Neonatal Effects	Nursing Considerations
Alcohol	*Fetal alcohol syndrome (FAS)*: craniofacial anomalies including short eyelid opening, flat midface, flat upper lip groove, thin upper lip; microcephaly; hyperactivity; developmental delays; attention deficits *Alcohol-related birth defects (ARBDs)*: milder forms of FAS, cardiac anomalies, failure to thrive	Alcohol enters breast milk.
Cocaine	Prematurity; small for gestational age; placental or cerebral infarctions, hyperactivity; difficult to console; hypersensitivity to noise and external stimuli, reduction in verbal reasoning.	Cocaine enters breast milk. Caution mothers about this hazard to their infants.
Heroin	Low birth weight, small for gestational age, neonatal abstinence syndrome (see Table 8-5)	Sudden infant death syndrome (SIDS) risk is increased. Usually the following drugs are given singly or in combination: phenobarbital, diluted tincture of opium (paregoric), or morphine. Use of naloxone (Narcan) is contraindicated in these infants because it can exacerbate narcotic abstinence syndrome and cause seizures.

Continued

TABLE 8-4

Neonatal Effects of Commonly Abused Substances—cont'd

Substance	Neonatal Effects	Nursing Considerations
Marijuana	Possible neonatal tremors; low birth weight; growth restriction	Secondhand smoke is a hazard if mother continues to use.
Amphetamines	Small for gestational age; prematurity; poor weight gain; lethargy	Monitor for heart rate abnormalities; encourage oral intake.
Tobacco	Prematurity; low birth weight; increased risk for SIDS; increased risk for bronchitis, pneumonia, developmental delays	Secondhand smoke is a hazard. Counsel parents about effects.

Management

- Use a multidisciplinary approach that includes home health or community resource personnel (e.g., regulatory agencies such as child protective services). Involve the parents in the care.
- Review the mother's prenatal record. Note any history of drug abuse and detoxification.
- Observe infant for signs of drug withdrawal.
- Assess infant for neonatal abstinence syndrome (NAS) (Table 8-5; Fig. 8-2).
- Correct fluid and electrolyte in balance and provide nutrition, infection control, and respiratory care.
- Swaddling, holding, reducing environmental stimuli (dim lights and decreased noise level), and feeding can help to ease withdrawal.
- Protect hyperactive infants from skin abrasions on the knees, toes, and cheeks that are caused by rubbing on bed linens while awake and in a prone position.
- Pharmacologic treatment to decrease withdrawal side effects includes neonatal tincture of opium (paregoric) and phenobarbital which can be used to control symptoms.

TABLE 8-5

Signs of Neonatal Abstinence Syndrome

System	Signs
Respiratory	Irregular respirations, tachypnea, apnea, nasal flaring, chest retractions, intermittent cyanosis, rhinorrhea, nasal congestion
Neurologic	Irritability, tremors, shrill cry, incessant crying, hyperactivity, disturbed sleep pattern, seizures, hypertonicity, increased deep tendon reflexes, exaggerated Moro reflex
Autonomic dysfunction	Frequent yawning, frequent sneezing, tearing, excessive generalized sweating, mottling of skin, fever
Gastrointestinal	Abnormal feeding pattern, uncoordinated and ineffectual sucking and swallowing reflexes, incessant hunger, frantic sucking, refusal to feed, vomiting, regurgitation, diarrhea

Source: Fike, D. (2007). Substance-exposed newborn. In C. Kenner, & J. Lott (Eds.), Comprehensive neonatal care: An interdisciplinary approach (4th ed.). St. Louis: Saunders.

- Breastfeeding is encouraged as long as the mother is not actively using drugs.
- Parents should be involved in their child's care and opportunities for parent-child attachment encouraged.
- Refer the infants to early intervention programs, including child health care, parental drug treatment, individualized developmental care, and parenting education.

HEMOLYTIC DISORDERS

Hemolytic Disease of the Newborn

Hemolytic diseases occur when the blood groups of the mother and newborn differ; the most common of these are ABO and Rh factor incompatibilities. Hemolytic disorders occur when maternal antibodies are present naturally or form in response to an antigen from the fetal blood crossing the placenta and entering the maternal circulation. The maternal antibodies of the IgG class cross the placenta, causing hemolysis of the fetal RBCs, resulting in hyperbilirubinemia and jaundice.

NEONATAL ABSTINENCE SCORING SYSTEM

SYSTEM	SIGNS AND SYMPTOMS	SCORE	AM					PM					COMMENTS
													Daily Weight:
CENTRAL NERVOUS SYSTEM DISTURBANCES	Excessive High Pitched (Or Other) Cry	2											
	Continuous High Pitched (Or Other) Cry	3											
	Sleeps <1 Hour After Feeding	3											
	Sleeps <2 Hours After Feeding	2											
	Sleeps <3 Hours After Feeding	1											
	Hyperactive Moro Reflex	2											
	Markedly Hyperactive Moro Reflex	3											
	Mild Tremors Disturbed	1											
	Moderate-Severe Tremors Disturbed	2											
	Mild Tremors Undisturbed	3											
	Moderate-Severe Tremors Undisturbed	4											
	Increased Muscle Tone	2											
	Excoriation (Specific Area)	1											
	Myoclonic Jerks	3											
	Generalized Convulsions	5											

		Score	
METABOLIC/VASOMOTOR/RESPIRATORY DISTURBANCES	Sweating	1	
	Fever <101° (99-100.8° F./37.2-38.2° C.)	1	
	Fever >101° (38.4° C. and Higher)	2	
	Frequent Yawning (>3 or 4 Times/Interval)	1	
	Mottling	1	
	Nasal Stuffiness	1	
	Sneezing (>3 or 4 Times/Interval)	1	
	Nasal Flaring	2	
	Respiratory Rate >60/min	1	
	Respiratory Rate >60/min with Retractions	2	
GASTROINTESTINAL DISTURBANCES	Excessive Sucking	1	
	Poor Feeding	2	
	Regurgitation	2	
	Projectile Vomiting	3	
	Loose Stools	2	
	Watery Stools	3	
	TOTAL SCORE		
	INITIALS OF SCORER		

Fig. 8-2 Neonatal abstinence scoring (NAS) system, developed by L. Finnegan. (From Nelson, N. [1980]. *Current therapy in neonatal-perinatal medicine* [2nd ed.]. St. Louis: Mosby.)

Rh Incompatibility

Rh incompatibility, or isoimmunization, occurs when an Rh-negative mother has an Rh-positive fetus who inherits the dominant Rh-positive gene from the father. The Rh blood group consists of several antigens, with D being the most significant because it causes the most antibody production in a person who is Rh negative.

- Maternal sensitization (antibody formation) can occur during pregnancy, birth, miscarriage or induced abortion, amniocentesis, external cephalic version, or trauma. Usually women become sensitized in their first pregnancy with an Rh-positive fetus but do not produce enough antibodies to cause lysis (destruction) of fetal blood cells.

- Severe Rh incompatibility results in marked fetal hemolytic anemia because the fetal erythrocytes are destroyed by maternal Rh-positive antibodies. Although the placenta usually clears the bilirubin resulting from the RBC breakdown, in extreme cases fetal bilirubin levels increase. The fetus compensates for the anemia by producing large numbers of immature erythrocytes to replace those hemolyzed, thus the name for this condition: erythroblastosis fetalis.

- In hydrops fetalis, the most severe form of this disease, the fetus has marked anemia, cardiac decompensation, cardiomegaly, and hepatosplenomegaly. Intrauterine or early neonatal death can occur as a result of hydrops fetalis, although intrauterine transfusions and early birth of the fetus can avert this.

- Intrauterine transfusion involves the infusion of Rh-negative, type O blood into the umbilical vein. The frequency of intrauterine transfusions can vary according to institution and fetal status, but it can be as often as every 2 weeks until the fetus reaches pulmonary maturity at approximately 37 to 38 weeks of gestation.

ABO Incompatibility

ABO incompatibility is more common than Rh incompatibility but causes less severe problems in the affected infant. It occurs if the fetal blood type is A, B, or AB and the maternal type is O. It occurs rarely in infants with type B blood born to mothers with type A blood. The incompatibility arises because naturally occurring anti-A and anti-B antibodies are transferred across the placenta to the fetus.

- Unlike the situation that pertains to Rh incompatibility, first-born infants can be affected because mothers with type O blood already have anti-A and anti-B antibodies in their blood.

Such a newborn can have a weakly positive direct Coombs' test (also referred to as a direct antiglobulin test [DAT]). The cord bilirubin level usually is less than 4 mg/dl, and any resulting hyperbilirubinemia usually can be treated with phototherapy.

Glucose-6-Phosphate Dehydrogenase Deficiency

Glucose-6-phosphate dehydrogenase (G6PD) deficiency can cause an exaggerated jaundice in a newborn within 24 to 48 hours of birth. G6PD red cells hemolyze at a greater rate than healthy red cells, thus overwhelming the immature neonatal liver's ability to conjugate the indirect bilirubin.

- Because it is a sex-linked disease, male offspring are more often affected. Treatment is the same as for any newborn with rapidly rising serum bilirubin levels.
- Other metabolic and inherited conditions that increase hemolysis and can cause jaundice in the infant include galactosemia, Crigler-Najjar disease, and hypothyroidism.

Management
Coombs' Test

- At birth the neonate's cord blood is sent to the laboratory to determine the infant's blood type and Rh status. A direct Coombs' test is performed on this cord blood to determine whether there are maternal antibodies in the fetal blood. If antibodies are present, the titer, which indicates the degree of maternal sensitization, is measured. If the titer is 1:64, an exchange transfusion is indicated.
- In addition, the prevention of or prompt therapy for perinatal asphyxia, acidosis, cold stress, sepsis, and hypoglycemia decreases the newborn's risk for severe hemolytic disease and susceptibility to kernicterus.
- Early feeding is initiated to stimulate stooling and facilitate the removal of bilirubin.

Exchange Transfusion

Exchange transfusions are needed infrequently because of the decreased incidence of severe hemolytic disease in newborns resulting from isoimmunization.

- In an exchange transfusion, 5 to 20 ml of the infant's blood is removed at a time and replaced with an equal amount of warmed donor blood. The total amount of blood exchanged is approximately 170 ml/kg of body weight, or approximately 87% of the infant's total blood volume. If the infant has Rh incompatibility, type O Rh-negative blood is used for transfusion. After the procedure, phototherapy is continued and the bilirubin level is monitored every 4 hours.
- Preservatives in donor blood lower the infant's serum calcium and magnesium levels; therefore, calcium gluconate is often given during the exchange transfusion.
- The neonate is monitored closely for signs of a blood transfusion reaction as well as hypotension, temperature instability, cardiorespiratory compromise, and hypoglycemia.
- Potential complications of exchange transfusion include transfusion reaction, infection, metabolic instability, and complications related to placement of the umbilical catheter.

CONGENITAL ANOMALIES

- Congenital anomalies (structural defects) occur in approximately 2% of all live births.
- Major congenital defects are the leading cause of death in infants younger than 1 year of age in the United States and account for 20% of neonatal deaths.
- The most common congenital anomalies that cause serious problems in the neonate are congenital heart disease, neural tube defects (NTDs), cleft lip or palate, clubfoot, and developmental dysplasia of the hip.

Cardiovascular System Anomalies

Congenital heart defects (CHDs) are anatomic abnormalities of the heart that are present at birth, although they may not be diagnosed immediately. Ventricular septal defect is the most common type of heart defect with increased pulmonary blood flow (acyanotic lesion) and tetralogy of Fallot is the most common type of heart defect with decreased pulmonary blood flow (cyanotic lesion). After prematurity, CHDs are the next major cause of death in the first year of life.

- The etiology of CHD is multifactorial. Maternal factors associated with a higher incidence of CHD include maternal rubella and cytomegalovirus, alcohol intake, diabetes mellitus, systemic lupus erythematosus, phenylketonuria (PKU), poor nutrition, radiation exposure, ingestion of folic acid antagonists, progesterone, estrogen, lithium, warfarin, isotretinoin, or anticonvulsant medications, maternal age greater than 40 years.

- Chromosomal abnormalities are highly associated with CHDs. Half of the children with trisomy 21, or Down syndrome, have a cardiac defect. Most children who have trisomy 18 or trisomy 13 have a cardiac anomaly.
- Increasingly, CHDs are diagnosed prenatally with ultrasound.
- Severe CHDs are often evident immediately after birth, especially those defects that cause central cyanosis despite 100% oxygen administration. Infants with these anomalies are transferred directly to an intensive care nursery or pediatric intensive care unit.
- The affected newborn's activity level varies from restlessness to lethargy, and possibly unresponsiveness, except to pain. Persistent bradycardia, a resting heart rate of less than 80 beats/min, or tachycardia, a rate exceeding 160 beats/min, can be noted. The cardiac rhythm can be abnormal, and various murmurs can be heard. Signs of congestive heart failure and decreased tissue perfusion can also become evident.
- Respiratory rate should be assessed when the newborn is in a resting state. Abnormal findings can include tachypnea, which is a rate of 60 breaths/min or more; retractions with nasal flaring; grunting occurring with or without exertion; and dyspnea, which can worsen with crying and activity. Signs that are indicative of congestive heart failure include feeding difficulties and increasing respiratory distress, especially tachypnea such that the baby has to stop feeding to breathe.

Care Management

Administer oxygen as ordered. Give cardiotonic medications to increase cardiac output, medications (e.g., prostaglandin) to prevent closure of the ductus arteriosus, and diuretic agents as needed to rid the body of accumulated fluid. Decrease the workload of the heart by maintaining a thermoneutral environment and feeding by gavage if necessary. Diagnostic tests, such as echocardiography and cardiac catheterization, are performed to obtain specific information about the defect and the need for surgical intervention.

Central Nervous System Anomalies

Most congenital anomalies of the CNS result from defects in the closure of the neural tube during fetal development (Table 8-6). Maternal folic acid deficit has a direct bearing on failure of the neural tube to close; therefore, folic acid supplementation is recommended for women of childbearing age.

Respiratory System Anomalies

Respiratory distress at birth or shortly thereafter can be the result of lung immaturity or anomalous development. Congenital laryngeal web and bilateral choanal atresia are readily apparent at birth. Respiratory distress caused by congenital diaphragmatic hernia and tracheoesophageal fistula can appear immediately or be delayed, depending on the severity of the defect.

Laryngeal Web and Choanal Atresia

A laryngeal web results from the incomplete separation of the two sides of the larynx and is most often between the vocal cords. Choanal atresia is the most common congenital anomaly of the nose; it is a bony or membranous septum located between the nose and the pharynx. Inability to pass a suction catheter through the nose into the pharynx or cyanosis without obvious respiratory distress usually leads to its detection. Nearly half of the infants with choanal atresia have other anomalies.

Congenital Diaphragmatic Hernia

Congenital diaphragmatic hernia (CDH) results from a defect in the formation of the diaphragm, allowing the abdominal organs to be displaced into the thoracic cavity. This can cause severe respiratory distress and represent a neonatal emergency.

Management

Infants with either a laryngeal web or choanal atresia require emergency surgery. The condition of the infant with CDH is stabilized until surgical repair can be done. These infants are cared for in neonatal intensive care units (NICUs) or pediatric intensive care units.

TABLE 8-6

Central Nervous System Anomalies

Anomaly	Definition	Treatment and Nursing Considerations
Encephalocele	Herniation of the brain and meninges through a skull defect	Surgical repair and shunting to relieve hydrocephalus. Infant can have cognitive deficit.
Anencephaly	Absence of both cerebral hemispheres and of the overlying skull	Incompatible with life; infant can be stillborn or die within a few days of birth. Comfort measures are provided until the infant dies of temperature instability and respiratory failure.
Spina bifida occulta	Posterior portion of the laminae fails to close, but the spinal cord or meninges do not herniate or protrude through the defect	Usually asymptomatic and often is not diagnosed unless there are associated problems.
Spina bifida cystica	Includes meningocele and myelomeningocele	
Meningocele	External sac that contains meninges and CSF and that protrudes through a defect in the vertebral column	Visible at birth, most often in the lumbosacral area. Sac usually covered with a very fragile, thin membrane that can tear easily, allowing CSF to leak out and providing an entry for infectious agents into the CNS. Motor and sensory deficits below the lesion in myelomeningocele. Usually develops hydrocephalus. Scheduled cesarean birth to try to prevent rupture of the meningeal sac.

Continued

TABLE 8-6

Central Nervous System Anomalies—cont'd

Myelomeningo-cele	External sac that contains meninges and CSF and nerves and that protrudes through a defect in the vertebral column	Protect sac from injury, rupture, and resultant risk of CNS infection. Before surgical repair (within the first 24-48 hr), position in side-lying or prone position to prevent pressure on the sac. Skin around defect must be cleansed and dried carefully to prevent breakdown. Sac should be covered with a sterile, moist, nonadherent dressing and cared for using sterile technique. Provide support and information to parents.
Hydrocephalus	Ventricles of the brain enlarged as a result of an imbalance between production and absorption of CSF, often occurs in conjunction with myelomeningocele	Bulging anterior fontanel and head circumference that increases at an abnormal rate. Enlargement of the forehead with depressed eyes that are rotated downward, causing a "setting sun" sign, occurs as the condition worsens. Surgical shunting of excess CSF from the brain should be done soon after birth to prevent irreversible neurologic damage from increased ICP, as evidenced by palpably widening sutures and fontanels, distended scalp veins, lethargy, poor feeding, vomiting, irritability, opisthotonic positioning, and a high-pitched, shrill cry. Head circumference is measured and neurologic assessments are done frequently. A sheepskin or a special pressure-sensitive air mattress is placed under the infant; position is changed frequently to prevent skin breakdown on the enlarged head.
Microcephaly	Head circumference that measures more than three standard deviations below the mean for age and sex	Mental retardation is common. Infants require supportive nursing care and medical observation to determine the extent of the psychomotor retardation that almost always accompanies this abnormality. There is no treatment. Parents need support to learn to care for a child with a cognitive impairment.

CNS, Central nervous system; *CSF,* cerebrospinal fluid; *ICP,* intracranial pressure.

Gastrointestinal System Anomalies
Cleft Lip and Palate

Cleft lip or palate is a congenital midline fissure, or opening, in the lip or palate resulting from failure of the primary palate to fuse. Cleft lip with or without cleft palate is more common in males, and cleft palate alone is more common in females.

Management

Treatment of the infant with cleft lip is surgical; repair usually occurs between 6 and 12 weeks of age. Cleft palate repair is generally postponed until 12 to 18 months of age to take advantage of palatal changes that take place with normal growth.

Parents of infants with a cleft lip or palate need much support, particularly in the case of a cleft lip because this is both a cosmetic and a functional defect. These defects can interfere with normal parent-infant bonding in the neonatal period.

- Feeding is difficult because the cleft lip renders the newborn unable to maintain a seal around a nipple; with a cleft palate, the infant is unable to form a vacuum to maintain suction when feeding.
- The inability to suck and swallow allows milk to pool in the nasopharynx, which increases the likelihood of aspiration. Milk can come out through the cleft and out of the nares.
- Feeding problems are greater in infants with a cleft palate than in those with a cleft lip alone. Breastfeeding is successful in some infants.
- Special nipples, bottles, and appliances are available to aid in feeding.
- Parents of infants with these defects need a great deal of education and support as they learn to feed their baby.

Esophageal Atresia and Tracheoesophageal Fistula

Esophageal atresia (EA) and tracheoesophageal fistula (TEF) often occur together. In EA the esophagus ends in a blind pouch or narrows into a thin cord and fails to form a continuous passageway to the stomach. TEF is an abnormal connection between the esophagus and trachea.

- Infants with the life-threatening anomaly EA with TEF show significant respiratory difficulty immediately after birth. EA with or without TEF results in excessive oral secretions, drooling, and feeding intolerance. Typically when fed, the infant sucks and swallows, then coughs and gags as fluid returns through the nose and mouth. Respiratory distress can result from aspiration or from the acute gastric distention produced by the TEF. Choking, coughing, and cyanosis occur after even a small amount of fluid is taken by mouth.

- Nursing interventions are supportive until surgery is performed.
  - ❏ The infant with EA and TEF should have the head of the bed raised to 30 to 45 degrees to facilitate respiratory efforts and prevent reflux and aspiration of gastric contents. The baby with an isolated EA can be placed in the normal supine position.
  - ❏ An orogastric (Replogle) tube is placed in the proximal esophageal pouch and attached to low continuous suction to remove secretions and decrease the possibility of aspiration.
  - ❏ The infant requires close observation and intervention to maintain a patent airway.
- Other supportive measures include thermoregulation, maintaining fluid and electrolyte balance intravenously as well as acid-base balance, and preventing further complications as a result of an associated defect.
- Surgical correction, done in one stage if possible, consists of ligating the fistula and anastomosing the two segments of the esophagus.

Omphalocele and Gastroschisis

An omphalocele is a covered defect of the umbilical ring into which varying amounts of the abdominal organs can herniate. The sac can rupture during or after birth. Many of the infants born with an omphalocele are preterm and have other serious syndromes or anomalies involving the GI, cardiac, genitourinary, musculoskeletal, and nervous systems.

Gastroschisis is the herniation of the bowel through a defect in the abdominal wall to the right of the umbilical cord. No membrane covers the contents as occurs with an omphalocele. Unlike infants with omphalocele, these infants have less likelihood of associated anomalies. If associated anomalies are present, most are cardiac.

- The preoperative nursing care is similar for infants with either defect. Immediately after birth, the neonate's torso should be placed in an impermeable clear plastic bowel bag to decrease insensible water losses, maintain thermoregulation, and prevent contamination of the exposed viscera.
- The baby is placed in a side-lying position and the viscera supported with a blanket roll to prevent vascular compromise. Prior to surgery the exposed viscera is kept covered with sterile moistened saline gauze and plastic wrap.
- Gastric decompression with a Replogle tube connected to low intermittent wall suction is also necessary to prevent aspiration pneumonia and to allow as much bowel as possible to be placed into the abdomen during surgery.
- Antibiotics, fluid and electrolyte replacement, and thermoregulation are needed for physiologic support.
- Surgery is performed soon after birth. If complete closure is impossible because of the small size of the defect and the large amount of viscera to be replaced, a Silastic silo pouch (Dow Corning, Midland, MI) is created and sewn to the fascia of the abdominal defect. The defect is closed surgically after the reduction of the contents that have been exposed is completed, which usually takes 7 to 10 days.

Imperforate Anus

Imperforate anus includes a wide range of congenital disorders involving the anus and rectum and, in many cases, the genitourinary system. Occurring more often in male than in female infants, these congenital defects result from the failure of anorectal development in weeks 7 and 8 of gestational life. Such infants have no anal opening, and commonly there is also a fistula from the rectum to the perineum or genitourinary system.

- Extensive surgical repair is often required in stages for the more complex types of anorectal malformations. The preoperative nursing care is similar to that described for other GI obstructions.

Gastrointestinal Obstruction

Congenital intestinal obstruction can occur anywhere in the GI tract and takes one of the following forms: atresia, which is a complete obliteration of the passage; partial obstruction, in which the symptoms can vary in severity and sometimes not be detected in the neonatal period; or malrotation of the intestine, which leads to twisting of the intestine (volvulus) and obstruction.

- Esophageal atresia, discussed previously, is a type of GI obstruction.
- Duodenal atresia, midgut malrotation and volvulus, jejunoileal atresia, necrotizing enterocolitis, and meconium ileus are the most common causes of neonatal intestinal obstruction.
- Meconium ileus is an obstruction caused by impacted meconium; over 90% of infants who with meconium ileus have cystic fibrosis, a life-threatening chronic illness.
- Signs of neonatal intestinal obstruction occur early. It can be suspected in infants born to women who had polyhydramnios during pregnancy.
  - ❏ The neonate with an intestinal obstruction displays the following cardinal signs: bilious vomiting, abdominal distention, and failure to pass normal amounts of meconium in the first 24 hours.
  - ❏ High intestinal obstruction is characterized by vomiting, even if the infant is not being fed orally.
  - ❏ Distention usually indicates a low obstruction, with vomiting occurring later. Abdominal distention can elevate the diaphragm, which can cause respiratory difficulties.
- Nursing care is aimed at supporting the infant until surgical intervention can be carried out to eliminate the obstruction.
  - ❏ Oral feedings are withheld, an orogastric tube is placed to low intermittent wall suction, and intravenous therapy is initiated to provide needed fluid and electrolytes.
- Surgery consists of resecting the obstructed area of bowel and anastomosing the nonaffected bowel, or creating an ostomy and allowing the bowel to rest. In recent years the survival rate for these infants has risen to 90% to 95% as a result of improved medical and nursing management, as well as a better understanding of the total problem.

Musculoskeletal System Anomalies

The two most common musculoskeletal system anomalies in neonates are developmental dysplasia of the hip and congenital clubfoot. Both of these conditions must be detected and treated early for successful correction.

Developmental Dysplasia of the Hip

Developmental dysplasia of the hip (DDH) (formerly known as congenital hip dysplasia or congenital dislocation of the hip) describes disorders related to abnormal development of the hip that can occur at any time during fetal life, infancy, or childhood. DDH more properly reflects a variety of hip abnormalities in which there is a shallow acetabulum, subluxation, or dislocation. There are three degrees of DDH.

- *Acetabular dysplasia* (preluxation) is the mildest form of DDH, in which there is neither subluxation nor dislocation. The femoral head remains in the acetabulum.
- *Subluxation* is incomplete dislocation of the hip. The femoral head remains in contact with the acetabulum, but a stretched capsule and ligamentum teres cause the head of the femur to be partially displaced. Pressure on the cartilaginous roof inhibits ossification and produces a flattening of the socket.
- In *dislocation* the femoral head loses contact with the acetabulum and is displaced posteriorly and superiorly over the fibrocartilaginous rim. The ligamentum teres is elongated and taut.

DDH is often not detected at the initial examination after birth. In the newborn period dysplasia usually appears as hip joint laxity rather than as outright dislocation. Subluxation and the tendency to dislocate can be demonstrated by the Ortolani or Barlow tests. Other signs of DDH are shortening of the limb on the affected side (Galeazzi sign or Allis sign), asymmetric thigh and gluteal folds, and broadening of the perineum (in bilateral dislocation).

NURSING ALERT *The Ortolani and Barlow tests must be performed by an experienced clinician to prevent fracture or other damage to the hip.*

- Treatment is begun as soon as the condition is recognized. The treatment varies with the age of the child and the extent of the dysplasia. The goal of treatment is to obtain and maintain a safe, congruent position of the hip joint to promote normal hip joint development and ambulation.
- The hip joint is maintained by dynamic splinting in a safe position with the proximal femur centered in the acetabulum in an attitude

of flexion and abduction. Of the numerous devices available, the Pavlik harness is the most widely used, and with time, motion, and gravity, the hip works into a more abducted, reduced position. The harness is worn continuously until the hip is proved stable on clinical and radiographic examination, typically around 3 months. Follow-up care is necessary, as is psychosocial support for the family.

NURSING ALERT   *The former practice of double- or triple-diapering for DDH is not recommended because it promotes hip extension, thus impeding proper hip development.*

Clubfoot

The most frequently occurring type of clubfoot is the composite deformity talipes equinovarus (TEV), in which the foot appears C-shaped, pointing downward and inward; the ankle is inverted; and the Achilles tendon is shortened.

Unilateral clubfoot is more common than bilateral clubfoot and can occur as an isolated defect or in association with other disorders or syndromes, such as chromosomal aberrations, arthrogryposis (a generalized immobility of the joints), cerebral palsy, or spina bifida.

- The goal of treatment for clubfoot is to achieve a painless, plantigrade (able to walk on the sole of the foot with the heel on the ground), and stable foot.
- Serial casting is begun shortly after birth, before discharge from the nursery. Successive casts allow for gradual stretching of skin and tight structures on the medial side of the foot. Manipulation and casting are repeated frequently (every week) to accommodate the rapid growth of early infancy.
- Because these infants are often placed in a cast before discharge, the nurse must teach parents necessary care, including how to protect the cast and assess the toes for neurovascular compromise.

Polydactyly

Occasionally infants are born with extra digits on their hands or feet; this is known as polydactyly. In some instances, it is hereditary. If there is little or no bone involvement, the extra digit is tied with silk suture soon after birth. The digit falls off within a few days, leaving a small scar. When there is bone involvement, surgical repair is indicated.

Genitourinary System Anomalies
Hypospadias and Epispadias

Hypospadias constitutes a range of penile anomalies associated with an abnormally located urinary meatus. The meatus can open below the glans penis or anywhere along the ventral surface of the penis, the scrotum, or the perineum. It is classified according to the location of the meatus and the presence or absence of chordee, which is a ventral curvature of the penis.

- Mild cases of hypospadias are often repaired for cosmetic reasons and involve a single surgical procedure. In more severe cases several operations are required to reconstruct the urethral opening and correct the chordee, thereby straightening the penis.
- The goals are to improve the appearance of the genitalia and make it possible for the child to urinate in a standing position and have a sexually adequate organ. These infants are not circumcised because the foreskin can be needed during surgical repair. Repair is done early, between 6 and 12 months of age.

Epispadias results from failure of urethral canalization. About half of the affected infants are males who have a widened pubic symphysis and a broad spadelike penis with the urethral opening on the dorsal surface. In females there is a wide urethra and a bifid clitoris. Severity ranges from a mild anomaly to a severe one that is associated with exstrophy of the bladder. Surgical correction is necessary and affected males should not be circumcised.

Exstrophy of the Bladder

The most common bladder anomaly is *exstrophy*, which often occurs in conjunction with epispadias.

Epispadias results from the abnormal development of the bladder, abdominal wall, and pubic symphysis that causes the bladder, the urethra, and the ureteral orifices to be exposed. The bladder is visible in the suprapubic area as a red mass with numerous folds, with urine draining from it.

- Immediately after birth the exposed bladder should be covered with a sterile nonadherent dressing to protect its delicate surface until closure can be performed. It is recommended that reconstructive surgery be started in the neonatal period, such that the bladder is closed within 48 hours. Parents need much support as they deal with caring for an infant who has such an obvious defect.

Ambiguous Genitalia

Ambiguous genitalia are discovered during physical examination. Abnormal sexual differentiation can be a genetic aberration such as congenital adrenal hypoplasia, which can be life threatening because it involves deficiency of all adrenocortical hormones.

■ Therapeutic intervention, including counseling and surgery, should be started as soon as possible. An appropriate gender assignment should be based on age at presentation, potential for mature sexual function, potential fertility, and the long-term psychologic and intellectual effect on the child and family. Parents need much support as they learn to deal with this challenging situation.

GENETIC DIAGNOSIS AND NEWBORN SCREENING

Diagnostic procedures for the detection of genetic disorders are performed after birth at any time from the postnatal period through adulthood. Many tests exist for various disorders; only the most commonly used ones are discussed here.

■ Newborns are routinely screened for inborn errors of metabolism (IEMs), such as PKU, galactosemia, hemoglobinopathy (sickle cell disease, thalassemias), and hypothyroidism; these are the minimum mandatory newborn screening tests in most states in the United States.

■ Tandem mass spectrometry has the potential for identifying more than 50 IEMs in addition to the standard IEMs. With tandem mass spectrometry, earlier identification of IEMs can prevent further developmental delays and morbidities in affected children.

Phenylketonuria

PKU results from a deficiency of the enzyme phenylalanine dehydrogenase. The test for PKU is not reliable until the newborn has ingested an ample amount of the amino acid phenylalanine, a constituent of both human and cow's milk.

NURSING ALERT   *The nurse must document the initial ingestion of milk; the test must be performed at least 24 hours after that time.*

■ When infants are discharged early, a subsequent sample must be obtained before 2 weeks of age if the initial specimen is collected before the newborn is 24 hours old.

■ Infants with PKU should be fed a special formula that contains protein, but no phenylalanine. Breastfeeding is possible and often recommended, but must be combined with supplementary feedings of low phenylalanine or phenylalanine-free formula. Throughout childhood, adolescence, and generally for life, individuals with PKU must remain on a phenylalanine restricted diet. However, despite compliance with treatment, many affected children have some intellectual impairment.

Galactosemia

Galactosemia, caused by a deficiency of the enzyme galactose-1-phosphate uridyltransferase, results in the inability to convert galactose to glucose. Galactosemia can be detected by measuring the blood levels of galactose or testing for galactosuria in newborns suspected of having the disease who have ingested formula containing galactose.

■ Early symptoms are vomiting, weight loss, persistent jaundice, and CNS symptoms, including poor feeding, drowsiness, and seizures.

■ If the disorder is untreated, the galactose levels will continue to increase and the affected infant will show failure to thrive, mental retardation, cataracts, jaundice, hepatomegaly, and cirrhosis of the liver, with death possibly occurring in the first month of life.

■ Therapy consists of eliminating galactose from the diet. This condition precludes breastfeeding because lactose is present in breast milk.

Hypothyroidism

Congenital hypothyroidism results from a deficiency of thyroid hormones. Newborns are routinely screened for hypothyroidism by measuring thyroxine (T_4) in a drop of blood obtained from a heelstick at 2 to 5 days of age. At this time the normally expected increase in T_4 is lacking in newborns with hypothyroidism.

■ Treatment is thyroid hormone replacement. If the infant is untreated, symptoms usually appear after 6 weeks and include bradycardia; hypothermia; hypotension; hyporeflexia; abdominal distention; umbilical hernia; coarse, dry hair; thick, dry skin that feels cold; anemia; and widely patent cranial sutures. The most disabling problem, however, is delayed development of the nervous system, leading to severe developmental delay.

THE PRETERM INFANT

Classification of infants at risk according to birth weight, gestational age, and predominant pathophysiologic problems is presented in Box 7-1, pp. 318–319.

Preterm infants, those born before 37 weeks of gestation, are at risk because their organ systems are immature and they lack adequate physiologic reserves to function in an extrauterine environment.

Complications in Preterm Infants

Respiratory Distress Syndrome

Respiratory distress syndrome (RDS) is a lung disorder affecting preterm infants, although a small percentage of term or late preterm infants are affected. Perinatal asphyxia, hypovolemia, male infant, Caucasian race, maternal diabetes (types 1 and 2), second-born twin, familial predisposition, maternal hypotension, cesarean birth without labor, hydrops fetalis, and third-trimester bleeding place an infant at increased risk for RDS. RDS is caused by a lack of pulmonary surfactant that leads to progressive atelectasis, loss of functional residual capacity, and ventilation-perfusion imbalance with an uneven distribution of ventilation.

- These respiratory signs usually present immediately after birth or within 6 hours of birth:
  - ❑ Tachypnea
  - ❑ Grunting
  - ❑ Nasal flaring
  - ❑ Retractions
  - ❑ Cyanosis
  - ❑ Labored breathing
  - ❑ Hypercapnia
  - ❑ Respiratory or mixed acidosis
  - ❑ Hypotension and shock
- Physical examination reveals crackles, poor air exchange, pallor, the use of accessory muscles (retractions) and, occasionally, apnea.
- Radiographic findings include uniform reticulogranular appearance and air bronchograms.
- RDS is a self-limiting disease with respiratory symptoms abating after 72 hours. The treatment for RDS is supportive.
  - ❑ Adequate ventilation and oxygenation must be established and maintained.

TABLE 8-7

Normal Arterial Blood Gas Values for Neonates

Value	Range
pH	7.35-7.45
Arterial oxygen pressure (Pao_2)	60-80 mm Hg
Carbon dioxide pressure ($Paco_2$)	35-45 mm Hg
Bicarbonate (HCO_3)	18-26 mEq/L
Base excess	(-5) to (+5)
Oxygen saturation	92%-94%

Source: Wood, A., & Jones, D. (2011). Acid-base homeostasis and oxygenation. In S. Gardner, B. Carter, M. Enzman-Hines, & J. Hernandez (Eds.), *Merenstein & Gardner's handbook of neonatal intensive care* (7th ed.). St. Louis: Mosby.

- ❏ Exogenous surfactant can be administered at or shortly after birth.
- ❏ Positive-pressure ventilation, continuous positive airway pressure (CPAP), and oxygen therapy can be required during the respiratory illness.
- ❏ Prevention of complications (pulmonary interstitial emphysema, pneumothorax, pneumomediastinum, and pneumopericardium) associated with mechanical ventilation is critical.
- ❏ Acid-base balance is evaluated by monitoring arterial blood gas (ABG) values (Table 8-7).
- ❏ A neutral thermal environment (NTE) must be maintained.
- ❏ Fluid and nutrition must be maintained.

Complications Associated with Oxygen Therapy
Retinopathy of Prematurity

Retinopathy of prematurity (ROP) is a complex, multicausal disorder that affects the developing retinal vessels of preterm infants. The mechanism of injury is unclear, but it is associated with oxygen therapy. Once the retina is completely vascularized, the retinal vessels are not susceptible to ROP.

- ■ Oxygen tensions that are too high for the level of retinal maturity initially result in vasoconstriction. After oxygen therapy is discontinued, neovascularization occurs in the retina and vitreous, with capillary hemorrhages, fibrotic resolution, and possible retinal detachment. Cicatricial (scar) tissue formation and consequent visual impairment can be mild or severe.

- Changes are detected through ophthalmologic examinations.
- The key to management of ROP is prevention of preterm birth and early detection of the condition.
- Circumferential cryopexy, laser photocoagulation, vitamin E therapy, and decreased intensity of ambient light are used in the treatment of ROP, with varying results.
- Arrange for an examination by an ophthalmologist before discharge, and provide a schedule for repeat examinations for the parents' guidance.

Bronchopulmonary Dysplasia

Bronchopulmonary dysplasia (BPD) is a chronic pulmonary iatrogenic condition caused by barotrauma from pressure ventilation and oxygen toxicity. The etiology of BPD is multifactorial and includes pulmonary immaturity, surfactant deficiency, lung injury and stretch, barotrauma, inflammation caused by oxygen exposure, fluid overload, ligation of a patent ductus arteriosus (PDA), and a familial predisposition. With the advent of prenatal administration of maternal steroids when preterm birth is expected coupled with use of exogenous surfactant in the neonate, most BPD or chronic lung disease (CLD) has been eliminated.

- Clinical signs of BPD
  - Tachypnea
  - Retractions
  - Nasal flaring
  - Labored breathing
  - Exercise intolerance (to handling and feeding)
  - Tachycardia
- Auscultation of the lung fields in affected infants typically reveals crackles, decreased air movement, and occasionally expiratory wheezing.
- The treatment for BPD includes oxygen therapy, nutrition, fluid restriction, and medications (diuretics, corticosteroids, bronchodilators). However, the key to the management of BPD is preventing prematurity and RDS and using surfactant and other less toxic therapies. Use of high-frequency ventilation and nitric oxide has contributed to the decline of this condition.

- The prognosis for infants with BPD depends on the degree of pulmonary dysfunction. Most deaths occur within the first year of life as a result of cardiorespiratory failure, sepsis, or respiratory infection; in some infants, the deaths are sudden and unexplained.

Patent Ductus Arteriosus

When the fetal ductus arteriosus fails to close after birth, patent ductus arteriosus (PDA) occurs. Ductal closure usually occurs within hours or days in the term infant but can be delayed in preterm infants.

- Clinical manifestations
  - ❑ Systolic murmur
  - ❑ Active precordium
  - ❑ Bounding peripheral pulses
  - ❑ Tachycardia, tachypnea, crackles
  - ❑ Hepatomegaly
  - ❑ Cardiac enlargement and pulmonary edema are typically seen on radiographic studies of infants with a large shunting PDA
  - ❑ Hypercarbia and metabolic acidosis
- The PDA can be managed medically or surgically.
  - ❑ Medical management consists of ventilatory support, fluid restriction, and the administration of diuretics and indomethacin. Ventilatory support is adjusted based on ABG values. Fluid restriction is implemented to decrease cardiovascular volume overload in association with the diuretic therapy.
  - ❑ Surgical ligation is performed when a PDA is clinically significant and medical management has failed.
- Nursing care focuses on supportive care: an NTE, adequate oxygenation, meticulous fluid balance, and parental support.

Germinal Matrix Hemorrhage–Intraventricular Hemorrhage (GMH-IVH)

GMH-IVH is one of the most common types of brain injury that occurs in neonates and is among the most severe in both short- and long-term outcomes. The average incidence of GMH-IVH ranges from 5% to 11%. GMH-IVH events typically occur within the first hours or days of life.

- GMH-IVH is classified according to a grading system of I to III, with grade I being the least severe, and grade III, the most severe.

The long-term neurodevelopmental outcome is determined by the severity of the GMH-IVH.

- Nursing care focuses on recognition of factors that increase the risk of GMH-IVH and interventions to decrease the risk of bleeding, and supportive care to infants who have bleeding episodes.
  - ❑ Position the infant with the head in the midline.
  - ❑ Elevate the head of the bed slightly to prevent or minimize fluctuations in intracranial blood pressure (BP).
  - ❑ Maintain an NTE and oxygenation.
  - ❑ Avoid rapid infusions of fluids.
  - ❑ Monitor the BP closely for fluctuations.
  - ❑ Monitor infant closely for signs of pneumothorax because it often precedes GMH-IVH.

Necrotizing Enterocolitis

Necrotizing enterocolitis (NEC) is an acute inflammatory disease of the GI mucosa, commonly complicated by perforation. This often fatal disease occurs in about 2% to 5% of newborns in NICUs. Breast-feeding seems to lower the incidence of NEC, as does use of minimal enteral nutrition. The onset of NEC in the term infant usually occurs between 4 and 10 days after birth. In the preterm infant the onset can be delayed for up to 30 days.

- Signs of developing NEC are nonspecific
  - ❑ Decreased activity and hypotonia
  - ❑ Pallor or cyanosis
  - ❑ Recurrent apnea and bradycardia
  - ❑ Decreased oxygen saturation values
  - ❑ Respiratory distress
  - ❑ Metabolic acidosis
  - ❑ Oliguria
  - ❑ Hypotension
  - ❑ Decreased perfusion
  - ❑ Temperature instability
- GI signs include:
  - ❑ Abdominal distention
  - ❑ Increasing or bile-stained residual gastric aspirates
  - ❑ Vomiting (bile or blood)
  - ❑ Grossly bloody stools
  - ❑ Abdominal tenderness
  - ❑ Erythema of the abdominal wall

- Radiographic examination reveals bowel loop distention, pneumatosis intestinalis, pneumoperitoneum, portal air, or a combination of these findings
- Treatment of infants with NEC is supportive.
    - Discontinue oral or tube feedings to rest the GI tract.
    - Place an orogastric tube to low wall suction.
    - Begin parenteral therapy (often by total parenteral nutrition [TPN]).
    - NEC is an infectious disease; control of infection is imperative. Careful hand hygiene is essential.
    - Give systemic antibiotic therapy as ordered.
- Surgical resection is done if perforation or clinical deterioration occurs.
- Intestinal transplantation has been successful in some infants with NEC-associated short-gut syndrome.

THE LATE PRETERM INFANT

Late preterm infants are those born between 34 0/7 and 36 6/7 weeks of gestation. When compared with term infants, these infants are at increased risk for problems with thermoregulation, hypoglycemia, hyperbilirubinemia, sepsis, and respiratory function. Discharge before 48 hours after birth is not recommended for late preterm infants.

- In the postnatal unit, assess at least every 4 hours.
- Provide routine parent teaching.
    - Review signs and symptoms of respiratory distress.
    - Have parents attend an infant cardiopulmonary resuscitation (CPR) class or view a video on infant CPR.
    - Teach parents to take the infant's temperature.
    - Assist with feedings. Late preterm infants can have difficulty coordinating sucking, swallowing, and breathing.
    - Breastfeeding can be more problematic if the infant is sleepy and difficult to arouse for feedings.
    - Late preterm infants are prone to early fatigue during feedings and fall asleep before consuming adequate volumes of milk. They should be fed at least every 3 to 4 hours and according to feeding cues.
- Observe for jaundice; late preterm infants are more likely to have jaundice.

THE POSTMATURE INFANT

Postterm infants are those whose gestation is prolonged beyond 42 weeks, regardless of birth weight; the infant is called postmature. The cause of prolonged pregnancy is unknown; it can be associated with placental insufficiency.

- Characteristics of a postmature infant
  - ❑ Thin, emaciated appearance (dysmature)
  - ❑ Meconium-stained fingernails
  - ❑ Long hair and nails
  - ❑ Absence of vernix
  - ❑ Peeling skin
- Insufficient gas exchange in the postmature placenta also increases the likelihood of intrauterine hypoxia, which can result in the passage of meconium in utero, thereby increasing the risk for meconium aspiration syndrome (MAS).
- General supportive care is provided.

Meconium Aspiration Syndrome

Meconium staining of the amniotic fluid can indicate fetal distress, especially in a vertex presentation. It appears in 8% to 20% of all births. The presence of meconium in the amniotic fluid necessitates careful supervision of labor and close monitoring of fetal well-being.

- The neonatal resuscitation team is required at the birth of any infant with meconium-stained amniotic fluid.
- The mouth and nares of the infant born through meconium are not routinely suctioned on the perineum before the infant's first breath. However for infants with meconium staining who are not vigorous and are hypotonic, have a heart rate less than 100, and depressed respirations, endotracheal suctioning should be performed immediately. Vigorous infants need no special handling.
- If the infant is very depressed and the meconium is not removed from the airway at birth, it can migrate down to the terminal airways, causing mechanical obstruction leading to MAS.
- The fetus can aspirate meconium in utero, which can cause a chemical pneumonitis.
- These infants can develop persistent pulmonary hypertension of the newborn (PPHN), further complicating their management.
- One method of prevention of MAS is lavage with surfactant immediately after birth.

Persistent Pulmonary Hypertension of the Newborn

Persistent pulmonary hypertension of the newborn is a term applied to the combined findings of pulmonary hypertension, right-to-left shunting, and a structurally normal heart.

- PPHN can occur either as a single entity or as the main component of MAS, CDH, RDS, hyperviscosity syndrome, or neonatal pneumonia or sepsis.
- PPHN is also called persistent fetal circulation (PFC) because the syndrome includes reversion to fetal pathways for blood flow.
- The infant with PPHN is typically born at term or postterm, and has tachycardia and cyanosis. Management depends on the underlying cause of the PPHN. The use of inhaled nitric oxide (INO), extracorporeal membrane oxygenation (ECMO), and high-frequency ventilation has improved the chances of survival of these infants.
- Exogenous surfactant can be used.

OTHER PROBLEMS RELATED TO GESTATION
Small for Gestational Age Infants and Intrauterine Growth Restriction

Infants who are small for gestational age (SGA) (i.e., weight is below the 10th percentile expected at term) or infants who have intrauterine growth restriction (IUGR) (i.e., rate of growth does not meet expected growth pattern) are considered high risk.

- Common problems that affect SGA infants and those with IUGR are as follows:
  - Perinatal asphyxia
  - Meconium aspiration
  - Hypoglycemia
  - Polycythemia
  - Temperature instability

Perinatal Asphyxia

Commonly, IUGR infants have been exposed to chronic hypoxia for varying periods before labor and birth. The chronically hypoxic infant is severely compromised even by a normal labor and has difficulty compensating after birth. The alert, wide-eyed appearance of the new-born is attributed to prolonged fetal hypoxia.

Hypoglycemia

All stressed infants are at risk for the development of hypoglycemia. Such stress can include perinatal asphyxia and IUGR.

- Hypoglycemia occurring within the first 3 days of life in the term infant is defined as a blood glucose level of less than 40 mg/dl; that occurring in the preterm infant within the same time frame is defined as a blood glucose level of less than 25 mg/dl.
- Symptoms of hypoglycemia include:
  - ❑ Poor feeding, hypothermia, and diaphoresis
  - ❑ CNS symptoms such as tremors and jitteriness, weak cry, lethargy, floppy posture, convulsions, or coma.
- Diagnosis is confirmed by blood glucose determinations performed by the laboratory or by unit visual methods with reagent strips such as Chemstrip-BG or Dextrostix. To prevent or treat hypoglycemia, breastfeeding or bottle feeding should be instituted; if levels remain low despite feeding, IV dextrose is warranted.

Large for Gestational Age Infants

The LGA infant is defined as an infant weighing 4000 g or more at birth. An infant is also considered LGA when the weight is above the 90th percentile on growth charts or two standard deviations above the mean weight for gestational age.

- Birth trauma, especially associated with breech or shoulder presentation, is a serious hazard for the oversized neonate. Asphyxia, CNS injury, or both can occur.
- All large fetuses are monitored during a trial of labor, and preparation is made for a cesarean birth if fetal distress or poor progress of labor occurs.
- LGA newborns can be preterm, term, or postterm; they can be the infants of mothers who are diabetic (or prediabetic); and they can be postmature. Each of these problems has special concerns. Regardless of any coexisting potential problems, the oversized infant is at risk just by virtue of its size.
- Assess the LGA infant for hypoglycemia and trauma resulting from vaginal or cesarean birth.

- Monitor the blood glucose levels of LGA infants and correct hypoglycemia.
- Identify and treat birth injuries.

Infants of Mothers with Diabetes

All infants born to mothers with diabetes are at some risk for complications. Compared with nondiabetic pregnancies, mothers with diabetes have an increased risk of stillbirth, congenital anomalies including NTDs, microcephaly, caudal regression syndrome, and congenital heart disease. Problems seen in infants of mothers with diabetes include macrosomia, birth trauma, perinatal asphyxia, RDS, hypoglycemia, hypocalcemia, hypomagnesemia, cardiomyopathy, hyperbilirubinemia, and polycythemia.

- Congenital anomalies occur in up 10% of infants born to mothers with diabetes. The most frequently occurring anomalies involve the cardiac, renal, musculoskeletal, and central nervous systems.
- Common congenital heart lesions include coarctation of the aorta, transposition of the great vessels, and atrial or ventricular septal defects.
- Common renal problems include renal agenesis and obstruction of the urinary tract.
- Common CNS anomalies include anencephaly, encephalocele, myelomeningocele, and hydrocephalus.
- The musculoskeletal system can be affected by caudal regression syndrome (i.e., sacral agenesis, with weakness or deformities of the lower extremities, malformation and fixation of the hip joints, and shortening or deformity of the femurs).
- GI atresia can occur.

Macrosomia

Despite improvements in the control of maternal blood sugar levels, the incidence of macrosomia is 50% in the infants of mothers with gestational diabetes and 40% in mothers with pregestational type 1 diabetes.

- At birth the typical macrosomic infant has a round, cherubic ("tomato" or cushingoid) face, a chubby body, and a plethoric or flushed complexion.
- The infant has enlarged internal organs (i.e., hepatosplenomegaly, splanchnomegaly, cardiomegaly) and increased body fat, especially around the shoulders.

- The placenta and umbilical cord are larger than average.
- Because insulin does not cross the blood-brain barrier, the brain is the only organ that is not enlarged. Infants of mothers with diabetes can be LGA but physiologically immature.
- The macrosomic infant is at risk for hypoglycemia, hypocalcemia, hyperviscosity, and hyperbilirubinemia.
- The excessive shoulder size in these infants often leads to dystocia, because the head can be smaller in proportion to the shoulders than in a nonmacrosomic infant.
- Macrosomic infants born vaginally or by cesarean birth after a trial of labor can incur birth trauma such as clavicle fracture or Erb-Duchenne palsy.
- Assess infant for hypoglycemia, hypocalcemia, hyperviscosity, hyperbilirubinemia, congenital anomalies, and birth trauma. Treat any symptoms identified; record and report to the primary health care provider any anomalies noted or signs of birth trauma.

Laboratory Values for Pregnant and Nonpregnant Women

Values	Nonpregnant	Pregnant
HEMATOLOGIC		
Complete Blood Count (CBC)		
Hemoglobin (g/dl)	12-16*	>11*
Hematocrit, PCV (%)	37-47	>33*
Red blood cell (RBC) volume (per ml)	1400	1650
Plasma volume (per ml)	2400	40%-60% increase
RBC count (million per mm³)	4.2-5.4	5-6.25
White blood cells (total per mm³)	5000-10,000	5000-15,000
Neutrophils (%)	55-70	60-85
Lymphocytes (%)	20-40	15-40
Erythrocyte sedimentation rate (mm/hr)	20	Elevated in second and third trimesters
Mean corpuscular hemoglobin concentration (MCHC) (g/dl packed RBCs)	32-36	No change
Mean corpuscular hemoglobin (MCH) (pg)	27-31	No change
Mean corpuscular volume (MCV), per mm³	80-95	No change
Blood Coagulation and Fibrinolytic Activity†		
Factor VII	65-140	Increases in pregnancy, returns to normal in early puerperium
Factor VIII	55-145	Increases during pregnancy and immediately after birth

Continued

Values	Nonpregnant	Pregnant
Factor IX	60-140	Same as factor VII
Factor X	45-155	Same as factor VII
Factor XI	65-135	Decreases in pregnancy
Factor XII	50-150	Same as factor VII
Prothrombin time (PT) (sec)	11-12.5	Slight decrease in pregnancy
Partial thromboplastin time (PTT) (sec)	60-70	Slight decrease in pregnancy and decrease during second and third stage of labor (indicates clotting at placental site)
Bleeding time (min)	1-9 (Ivy)	No appreciable change
Coagulation time (min)	6-10 (Lee/White)	No appreciable change
Platelets (mm^3)	150,000-400,000	No significant change until 3-5 days after birth and then a rapid increase (may predispose woman to thrombosis) and gradual return to normal
Fibrinolytic activity	Normal	Decreases in pregnancy and then abruptly returns to normal (protection against thromboembolism)
Fibrinogen (mg/dl)	200-400	Increased levels late in pregnancy
Mineral and Vitamin Concentrations		
Vitamin B$_{12}$, folic acid, ascorbic acid	Normal	Moderate decrease
Serum Proteins		
Total (g/dl)	6.4-8.3	5.5-7.5
Albumin (g/dl)	3.5-5	Slight increase
Globulin, total (g/dl)	2.3-3.4	3-4

Values	Nonpregnant	Pregnant
Blood Glucose		
Fasting (mg/dl)	70-105	Decreases
2-hr postprandial (mg/dl)	<140	<140 after a 100-g carbohydrate meal is considered normal
Acid-Base Values in Arterial Blood		
P_{O_2} (mm Hg)	80-100	104-108 (increased)
P_{CO_2} (mm Hg)	35-45	27-32 (decreased)
Sodium bicarbonate (HCO_3) (mEq/L)	21-28	18-31 (decreased)
Blood pH	7.35-7.45	7.40-7.45 (slightly increased, more alkaline)
HEPATIC		
Bilirubin, total (mg/dl)	≤1	Unchanged
Serum cholesterol (mg/dl)	120-200	Increases from 16-32 wk of pregnancy; remains at this level until after birth
Serum alkaline phosphatase, units/L	30-120	Increases from wk 12 of pregnancy to 6 wk after birth
Serum albumin (g/dl)	3.5-5	Slight increase
RENAL		
Bladder capacity (ml)	1300	1500
Renal plasma flow (RPF) (ml/min)	490-700	Increases by 25%-30%
Glomerular filtration rate (GFR) (ml/min)	88-128	Increases by 30%-50%
Nonprotein nitrogen (NPN) (mg/dl)	25-40	Decreases
Blood urea nitrogen (BUN) (mg/dl)	10-20	Decreases
Serum creatinine (mg/dl)	0.5-1.1	Decreases
Serum uric acid (mg/dl)	2.7-7.3	Decreases but returns to prepregnancy level by end of pregnancy

Continued

Values	Nonpregnant	Pregnant
Urine glucose	Negative	Present in 20% of pregnant women
Intravenous pyelogram (IVP)	Normal	Slight to moderate hydroureter and hydronephrosis; right kidney larger than left kidney

*At sea level. Permanent residents of higher altitudes (e.g., Denver) require higher levels of hemoglobin.

†Pregnancy represents a hypercoagulable state.

ng, Nanogram; *PCV*, packed cell volume; *pg*, picogram.

Sources: Blackburn, S. (2007). *Maternal, fetal, & neonatal physiology: A clinical perspective* (3rd ed.). St. Louis: Saunders; Gordon, M. (2007). Maternal physiology. In S. Gabbe, J. Niebyl, & J. Simpson (Eds.), *Obstetrics: Normal and problem pregnancies* (5th ed.). Philadelphia: Churchill Livingstone; Pagana, K., & Pagana, T. (2009). *Mosby's diagnostic and laboratory test reference* (9th ed.). St. Louis: Mosby.

Medication Guides

MEDICATIONS

PREGNANCY

Antenatal Glucocorticoid Therapy with Betamethasone or Dexamethasone

Action

- Stimulates fetal lung maturation by promoting release of enzymes that induce production or release of lung surfactant. NOTE: The FDA has not approved these medications for this use (i.e., this is an unlabeled use for obstetrics).

Indication

- To prevent or reduce the severity of neonatal respiratory distress syndrome by accelerating lung maturity in fetuses between 24 and 34 weeks of gestation.

Dosage and Route

- Betamethasone: 12 mg IM for two doses 24 hours apart
- Dexamethasone: 6 mg IM for four doses 12 hours apart

Adverse Effects

- Pulmonary edema (if given with beta-adrenergic medications)
- May worsen maternal condition (diabetes, hypertension)

Nursing Considerations

- Give deep IM in ventral gluteal or vastus lateralis muscle.
- Teach signs of pulmonary edema.
- Assess blood glucose levels and lung sounds.

Text continued on p. 411.

Pharmacologic Control of Hypertension in Pregnancy

Action	Target Tissue	EFFECTS		Nursing Actions
		Maternal Effects	Fetal Effects	
HYDRALAZINE (APRESOLINE, NEOPRESOL)				
Arteriolar vasodilator	Peripheral arterioles: to decrease muscle tone, decrease peripheral resistance; hypothalamus and medullary vasomotor center for minor decrease in sympathetic tone	Headache, flushing, palpitations, tachycardia, some decrease in uteroplacental blood flow, increase in heart rate and cardiac output, increase in oxygen consumption, nausea and vomiting	Tachycardia; late decelerations and bradycardia if maternal diastolic pressure <90 mm Hg	Assess for effects of medication; alert mother (family) to expected effects of medication; assess blood pressure frequently because precipitous drop can lead to shock and perhaps placental abruption; if giving multiple doses, wait at least 20 min after the first dose is given to administer an additional dose to allow time to assess the effects of the initial dose; assess urinary output; maintain bed rest in a lateral position with side rails up; use with caution in presence of maternal tachycardia.

Continued

Pharmacologic Control of Hypertension in Pregnancy—cont'd

Action	Target Tissue	EFFECTS		
		Maternal Effects	Fetal Effects	Nursing Actions
LABETALOL HYDROCHLORIDE (NORMODYNE, TRANDATE)				
Combined alpha- and beta-blocking agent causing vasodilation without significant change in cardiac output	Peripheral arterioles (see hydralazine)	Minimal: flushing, tremulousness, orthostatic hypotension; minimal change in pulse rate	Minimal, if any	See hydralazine; less likely to cause excessive hypotension and tachycardia; less rebound hypertension than hydralazine.
METHYLDOPA (ALDOMET)				
Maintenance therapy if needed: 250-500 mg orally every 8 hr (α_2-receptor agonist)	Postganglionic nerve endings: interferes with chemical neurotransmission to reduce peripheral vascular resistance; causes CNS sedation	Sleepiness, postural hypotension, constipation; rare: drug-induced fever in 1% of women and positive Coombs test result in 20% of women	After 4 mo maternal therapy, positive Coombs test result in infant	See hydralazine.

NIFEDIPINE (ADALAT, PROCARDIA)

Calcium channel blocker	Arterioles: to reduce systemic vascular resistance by relaxation of arterial smooth muscle	Headache, flushing; possible potentiation of effects on CNS if administered concurrently with magnesium sulfate; may interfere with labor	Minimal	See hydralazine; use caution if patient is also receiving magnesium sulfate.

CNS, Central nervous system.

Tocolytic Therapy for Preterm Labor

Medication and Action	Dosage and Route†	Adverse Effects	Nursing Considerations
MAGNESIUM SULFATE			
• CNS depressant; relaxes smooth muscles including uterus	• IV fluid should contain 40 g in 1000 ml, piggyback to primary infusion, and administer using controller pump • Loading dose: 4-6 g over 20-30 min • Maintenance dose: 1-4 g/hr • Use for stabilization only • Discontinue within 24-48 hr at the maintenance dose or if intolerable adverse effects occur	Maternal: • Hot flushes, sweating, burning at the IV insertion site, nausea and vomiting, dry mouth, drowsiness, blurred vision, diplopia, headache, ileus, generalized muscle weakness, lethargy, dizziness • Hypocalcemia • Shortness of breath • Transient hypotension • Some reactions may subside when loading dose is completed Intolerable: • Respiratory rate fewer than 12 breaths/min • Pulmonary edema • Absent DTRs • Chest pain • Severe hypotension • Altered level of consciousness • Extreme muscle weakness	• Assess woman and fetus to obtain baseline before beginning therapy and then before and after each increment; follow frequency of agency protocol • Monitor serum magnesium levels with higher doses; therapeutic range is between 4 and 7.5 mEq/L or 5-8 mg/dl • Discontinue infusion and notify physician if intolerable adverse effects occur • Ensure that calcium gluconate 1 g (10 ml of 10% solution) or calcium chloride (normal dose is 500 mg IV infused over 30 min) is available for emergency administration to reverse magnesium sulfate toxicity

- Urine output less than 25-30 ml/hr or less than 100 ml/4 hr
- Serum magnesium level of 10 mEq/L (9 mg/dl) or greater

Fetal (uncommon):
- Decreased breathing movement
- Reduced FHR variability
- Nonreactive NST

- Should not be given to women with myasthenia gravis
- Total IV intake should be limited to 125 ml/hr

BETA-ADRENERGIC AGONIST (BETA-MIMETIC)

Terbutaline (Brethine)

- Relaxes smooth muscles, inhibiting uterine activity and causing bronchodilation

- Subcutaneous injection of 0.25 mg every 4 hr
- Treatment should last no longer than 24 hr
- Discontinue use if intolerable adverse effects occur

Maternal: (most are mild and of limited duration)
- Tachycardia, chest discomfort, palpitations, arrhythmias
- Tremors, dizziness, nervousness
- Headache
- Nasal congestion
- Nausea and vomiting
- Hypokalemia
- Hyperglycemia
- Hypotension

- Should not be used in women with a history of cardiac disease, pregestational or gestational diabetes, severe gestational hypertension, severe preeclampsia or eclampsia, migraine headaches, or hyperthyroidism, or with significant hemorrhage
- Myocardial infarction leading to death has been reported after use

Continued

Tocolytic Therapy for Preterm Labor—cont'd

Medication and Action	Dosage and Route†	Adverse Effects	Nursing Considerations
BETA-ADRENERGIC AGONIST (BETA-MIMETIC), cont'd			
		Intolerable: • Tachycardia greater than 130 beats/min • BP less than 90/60 • Chest pain • Cardiac arrhythmias • Myocardial infarction • Pulmonary edema Fetal: • Tachycardia • Hyperinsulinemia • Hyperglycemia	• Validate that woman is in PTL and is >20 and <35 wk of gestation • Assess woman and fetus according to agency protocol, being alert for adverse effects • Assess maternal glucose and potassium levels before treatment is initiated and periodically during treatment. Significant hyperglycemia (greater than 180 mg/dl) and hypokalemia (less than 2.5 mEq/L) may occur • Notify physician if the woman exhibits the following: • Maternal heart rate greater than 130 beats/min; arrhythmias, chest pain

- BP less than 90/60 mm Hg
- Signs of pulmonary edema (e.g., dyspnea, crackles, decreased Sao_2)
- FHR greater than 180 beats/min
- Hyperglycemia occurs more frequently in women who are being treated simultaneously with corticosteroids
- Ensure that propranolol (Inderal) is available to reverse adverse effects related to cardiovascular function

Continued

Tocolytic Therapy for Preterm Labor—cont'd

Medication and Action	Dosage and Route[†]	Adverse Effects	Nursing Considerations
CALCIUM CHANNEL BLOCKERS			
Nifedipine (Adalat, Procardia)			
• Relaxes smooth muscles including the uterus by blocking calcium entry	• Initial dose: 10-20 mg, orally, every 3 to 6 hr until contractions are rare, followed by long-acting formulations of 30 or 60 mg every 8-12 hr for 48 hr while corticosteroids are being given (however, the ideal dose has not been established)	Maternal (most effects are mild) • Hypotension • Headache • Flushing • Dizziness, • Nausea Fetal: • Hypotension (questionable)	• Avoid concurrent use with magnesium sulfate because skeletal muscle blockade can result • Should not be given simultaneously with or immediately after terbutaline because of effects on heart rate and blood pressure • Assess woman and fetus according to agency protocol, being alert for adverse effects • Do not use sublingual route of administration

PROSTAGLANDIN SYNTHETASE INHIBITORS (NSAIDs)

Indomethacin (Indocin)

- Relaxes uterine smooth muscle by inhibiting prostaglandins

- Loading dose: 50 mg orally, then 25-50 mg orally every 6 hr for 48 hr

Maternal (common):
- Nausea and vomiting
- Heartburn

Less common, but more serious:
- GI bleeding
- Prolonged bleeding time
- Thrombocytopenia
- Asthma in aspirin-sensitive patients

Fetal:
- Constriction of ductus arteriosus
- Oligohydramnios, caused by reduced fetal urine production
- Neonatal pulmonary hypertension

- The long-acting formulations decrease the incidence of adverse effects
- Used when other methods fail only if gestational age is <32 wk
- Administer for 48 hr or less
- Do not use in women with renal or hepatic disease, active peptic ulcer disease, poorly controlled hypertension, asthma, or coagulation disorders
- Can mask maternal fever
- Assess woman and fetus according to agency policy, being alert for adverse effects

Continued

Tocolytic Therapy for Preterm Labor—cont'd

Medication and Action	Dosage and Route[†]	Adverse Effects	Nursing Considerations
PROSTAGLANDIN SYNTHETASE INHIBITORS (NSAIDs), cont'd			
Indomethacin (Indocin), cont'd			• Determine amniotic fluid volume and function of fetal ductus arteriosus before initiating therapy and within 48 hr of discontinuing therapy; assessment is critical if therapy continues for more than 48 hr • Administer with food to decrease GI distress • Monitor for signs of postpartum hemorrhage

Note: There are variations in recommended administration protocols; always consult agency protocol, which should be evidence based.

BP, Blood pressure; *CNS*, central nervous system; *DTRs*, deep tendon reflexes; *FHR*, fetal heart rate; *GI*, gastrointestinal; *NSAIDs*, nonsteroidal antiinflammatory drugs; *NST*, nonstress test; *PTL*, preterm labor; *SaO₂*, arterial oxygen saturation; *SOB*, shortness of breath.

Sources: Gilbert, E. (2011). *Manual of high risk pregnancy and delivery* (5th ed.). St. Louis: Mosby; Iams, J., & Romero, R. (2007). Preterm birth. In S. Gabbe, J. Niebyl, & J. Simpson (Eds.), *Obstetrics: Normal and problem pregnancies* (5th ed.). Philadelphia: Churchill Livingstone; Iams, J., Romero, R., & Creasy, R. (2009). Preterm labor and birth. In R. Creasy, R. Resnik, J. Iams, C. Lockwood, & T. Moore (Eds.), *Creasy and Resnik's maternal-fetal medicine: Principles and practice* (6th ed.). Philadelphia: Saunders.

LABOR
Opioid Agonist Analgesics
(Fentanyl Citrate [Sublimaze]
Sufentanil Citrate [Sufenta])

Action

Opioid agonist analgesics that stimulate both mu and kappa opioid receptors to decrease the transmission of pain impulses, rapid action with short duration (0.5-1 hr IV; 1-2 hr epidural); sufentanil citrate has a more potent analgesic action than fentanyl citrate with less passage across the placenta to the fetus.

Indication

Because of their short duration of action when given intravenously, they are most commonly administered epidurally or intrathecally, alone or in combination with a local anesthetic agent, to relieve moderate to severe labor pain and postoperative pain after cesarean birth.

Dosage and Route

- *Fentanyl citrate:* 25 to 50 mcg IV; 1 to 2 mcg with 0.125% bupivacaine at rate of 8 to 10 ml/hr epidurally
- *Sufentanil citrate:* 10 to 15 mcg with 0.125% bupivacaine at rate of 10 ml/hr epidurally

Adverse Effects

Dizziness, drowsiness, allergic reactions, rash, pruritus, maternal and fetal or neonatal respiratory depression, nausea and vomiting, urinary retention

Nursing Considerations

Assess for respiratory depression; naloxone should be available as an antidote.

Opioid Agonist–Antagonist Analgesics (Butorphanol Tartrate [Stadol] Nalbuphine Hydrochloride [Nubain])

Action

Mixed agonist-antagonist analgesics that stimulate kappa opioid receptors and block or weakly stimulate mu opioid receptors, resulting in good analgesia but with less respiratory depression and nausea and vomiting when compared with opioid agonist analgesics

Indications

Moderate to severe labor pain and postoperative pain after cesarean birth

Dosage and Route

- *Butorphanol tartrate:* 1 mg (range 0.5-2 mg) IV every 3 to 4 hours as needed; 2 mg (range 1-4 mg) IM every 3 to 4 hours as needed
- *Nalbuphine hydrochloride:* 5 to 10 mg IV every 3 to 4 hours as needed; 10 to 20 mg IM every 3 to 4 hours as needed

Adverse Effects

Confusion, sedation, hallucinations, "floating" feeling, drowsiness, headache, dizziness, nervousness, sweating; maternal palpitations and tachycardia or bradycardia; transient nonpathologic sinusoidal-like fetal heart rate rhythm; respiratory depression; nausea and vomiting; difficulty with urination (retention, urgency)

Nursing Considerations

May precipitate withdrawal symptoms in opioid-dependent women and their newborns. Assess maternal vital signs, degree of pain, FHR, and uterine activity before and after administration; observe for maternal respiratory depression, notifying primary health care provider if maternal respirations are ≤12 breaths/min; encourage voiding every 2 hours and palpate for bladder distention; if birth occurs within 1 to 4 hours of dose administration, observe newborn for respiratory depression; implement safety measures as appropriate, including use of side rails and assistance with ambulation; continue use of nonpharmacologic pain relief measures.

Oxytocin (Pitocin)

Action

- Oxytocin is a hormone produced in the posterior pituitary gland that stimulates uterine contractions and aids in milk let-down. Pitocin is a synthetic form of this hormone.

Indications

- Oxytocin is used primarily for labor induction and augmentation.

Dosage and Route

- The IV solution containing oxytocin should be mixed in a standard concentration. Concentrations often used are 10 units in 1000 ml of fluid, 20 units in 1000 ml of fluid, or 30 units in 500 ml of fluid.
- Oxytocin is administered intravenously through a secondary line connected to the main line at the proximal port (connection closest to the intravenous insertion site). Oxytocin is always administered by pump.
- Begin oxytocin administration at 1 milliunit/minute. Increase the rate by 1 to 2 milliunits/min, no more frequently than every 30 to 60 minutes, based on the response of the maternal-fetal unit and the progress of labor.
- The goal of oxytocin administration is to produce acceptable uterine contractions as evidenced by:
  - ❑ Consistent achievement of 200 to 220 MVUs *or*
  - ❑ A consistent pattern of 1 contraction every 2 to 3 minutes, lasting 80 to 90 seconds, and strong to palpation

Adverse Effects

- Possible maternal adverse effects include uterine tachysystole, placental abruption, uterine rupture, unnecessary cesarean birth caused by abnormal (nonreassuring) FHR and patterns, postpartum hemorrhage, and infection.
- Possible fetal adverse effects include hypoxemia and acidosis, eventually resulting in abnormal (nonreassuring) FHR and patterns.

Nursing Considerations

- Patient and partner teaching and support
  - ❏ Reasons for use of oxytocin (e.g., to start or improve labor)
  - ❏ Effects to expect concerning the nature of contractions: the intensity of the contraction increases more rapidly, holds the peak longer, and ends more quickly; contractions will come regularly and more often
  - ❏ Monitoring to anticipate
  - ❏ Continue to keep woman and her partner informed regarding progress.
- Remember that women vary greatly in their response to oxytocin; some require only very small amounts to produce adequate contractions, whereas others need larger doses.
- Assessment
  - ❏ Fetal status using electronic fetal monitoring; evaluate tracing every 15 minutes and with every change in dose during the first stage of labor and every 5 minutes during the active pushing phase of the second stage of labor.
  - ❏ Monitor the contraction pattern and uterine resting tone every 15 minutes and with every change in dose during the first stage of labor and every 5 minutes during the second stage of labor.
  - ❏ Monitor blood pressure, pulse, and respirations every 30 to 60 minutes and with every change in dose.
  - ❏ Assess intake and output; limit IV intake to 1000 ml in 8 hours; urine output should be 120 ml or more every 4 hours.
  - ❏ Perform vaginal examination as indicated.
  - ❏ Monitor for side effects, including nausea, vomiting, headache, hypotension.
  - ❏ Observe emotional responses of woman and her partner.
- Use a standard definition for uterine tachysystole that does not include an abnormal (nonreassuring) FHR and pattern or the woman's perception of pain.
- The rate of oxytocin infusion should be continually titrated to the lowest dose that achieves acceptable labor progress. Usually the oxytocin dose can be decreased or discontinued after rupture of membranes and in the active phase of first stage labor.
- Documentation
  - ❏ The time the oxytocin infusion is begun, and each time the infusion is increased, decreased, or discontinued
  - ❏ Assessment data as described previously

❑ Interventions for uterine tachysystole and abnormal (nonreassuring) FHR and patterns and the response to the interventions
❑ Notification of the primary health care provider and that person's response

Prostaglandin E₁ (PGE₁): Misoprostol (Cytotec)
Action

■ PGE₁ ripens the cervix, making it softer and causing it to begin to dilate and efface; stimulates uterine contractions.

Indications

■ PGE₁ is used for preinduction cervical ripening (ripen cervix before oxytocin induction of labor when the Bishop score is 4 or less) and to induce labor or abortion (abortifacient agent); it has not yet been approved by the FDA for cervical ripening or labor induction.
■ Should not be used if the woman has a history of previous cesarean birth or other major uterine surgery.

Dosage and Route

■ Misoprostol is available either as a 100- or a 200-mcg tablet. Therefore, tablets must be broken to prepare the correct dose. This preparation should take place in the pharmacy to ensure accurate doses.
■ Recommended initial dose is 25 mcg. Insert intravaginally into the posterior vaginal fornix using the tips of index and middle fingers without the use of a lubricant. Repeat every 3 to 6 hours up to 6 doses in a 24-hour period or until an effective contraction pattern is established (three or more uterine contractions in 10 minutes), the cervix ripens (Bishop score of 8 or greater), or significant adverse reactions occur.

Adverse Effects

■ Higher doses (e.g., 50 mcg every 6 hours) are more likely to result in adverse reactions such as nausea and vomiting, diarrhea, fever, uterine tachysystole with or without an abnormal (nonreassuring) FHR and pattern, or fetal passage of meconium. The risk for adverse reactions is reduced with lower dosages and longer intervals between doses.

Nursing Considerations

- Explain the procedure to the woman and her family. Ensure that an informed consent has been obtained as per agency policy.
- Assess the maternal-fetal unit before each insertion and during treatment following agency protocol for frequency. Assess maternal vital signs and health status, FHR and pattern, and status of pregnancy, including indications for cervical ripening or induction of labor, signs of labor or impending labor, and the Bishop score. Recognize that an abnormal (nonreassuring) FHR and pattern; maternal fever, infection, vaginal bleeding, or hypersensitivity; and regular, progressive uterine contractions contraindicate the use of misoprostol.
- Use caution if the woman has a history of asthma, glaucoma, or renal, hepatic, or cardiovascular disorders.
- Have the woman void prior to insertion.
- Assist the woman to maintain a supine position with a lateral tilt or a side-lying position for 30 to 40 minutes after insertion.
- Prepare to swab the vagina to remove unabsorbed medication using a saline-soaked gauze wrapped around fingers or to administer terbutaline 0.25 mg subcutaneously if significant adverse reactions occur.
- Initiate oxytocin for induction of labor no sooner than 4 hours after last dose of misoprostol was administered, following agency protocol, if ripening has occurred and labor has not begun.
- Document all assessment findings and administration procedures.

Prostaglandin E_2 (PGE$_2$): Dinoprostone (Cervidil Insert; Prepidil Gel)

Action

- PGE_2 ripens the cervix, making it softer and causing it to begin to dilate and efface; stimulates uterine contractions. Dinoprostone is the only FDA-approved medication for cervical ripening or labor induction.

Indications

- PGE_2 is used for preinduction cervical ripening (ripen cervix before oxytocin induction of labor when the Bishop score is 4 or less) and for inducement of labor or abortion (abortifacient agent). It is not recommended for use if the woman has a history of previous cesarean birth or other major uterine surgery.

Dosage and Route
Cervidil Insert

- Dosage is 10 mg of dinoprostone designed to be gradually released (approximately 0.3 mg/hr) over 12 hours. Insert is placed transvaginally into the posterior fornix of the vagina. The insert is removed after 12 hours or at the onset of active labor or earlier if tachysystole or abnormal (nonreassuring) FHR and patterns occur.

Prepidil Gel

- Dosage is 0.5 mg of dinoprostone in a 2.5-ml syringe. Gel is administered through a catheter attached to the syringe into the cervical canal just below the internal cervical os. Dose may be repeated every 6 hours as needed for cervical ripening up to a maximum cumulative dose of 1.5 mg (3 doses) in a 24-hour period.

Adverse Effects

- Potential adverse effects include headache, nausea and vomiting, diarrhea, fever, hypotension, uterine tachysystole with or without an abnormal (nonreassuring) FHR and pattern, or fetal passage of meconium.

Nursing Considerations

- Explain the procedure to the woman and her family. Ensure that an informed consent has been obtained as per agency policy.
- Assess the maternal-fetal unit before each insertion and during treatment following agency protocol for frequency. Assess maternal vital signs and health status, FHR and pattern, and status of pregnancy, including indications for cervical ripening or induction of labor, signs of labor or impending labor, and the Bishop score. Recognize that an abnormal (nonreassuring) FHR and pattern; maternal fever, infection, vaginal bleeding, or hypersensitivity; and regular, progressive uterine contractions contraindicate the use of dinoprostone.
- Use caution if the woman has a history of asthma, glaucoma, or renal, hepatic, or cardiovascular disorders.

- Bring the gel to room temperature just before administration. Do not force the warming process by using a warm-water bath or other source of external heat such as microwave because heat may cause inactivation.
- Keep the insert frozen until just before insertion. No warming is needed.
- Have the woman void before insertion.
- Assist the woman to maintain a supine position with a lateral tilt or a side-lying position for at least 30 minutes after insertion of the gel or for 2 hours after placement of the insert.
- Allow the woman to ambulate after the recommended period of bed rest and observation.
- Prepare to pull the string to remove the insert and to administer terbutaline 0.25 mg subcutaneously if significant adverse effects occur. There is no effective way to remove the gel from the vagina if uterine tachysystole or abnormal (nonreassuring) FHR and patterns occur.
- Delay the initiation of oxytocin for induction of labor for 6 to 12 hours after the last instillation of the gel or for 30 to 60 minutes after removal of the insert, or follow agency protocol for induction if ripening has occurred but labor has not begun.
- Document all assessment findings and administration procedures.

POSTPARTUM
Medications Used to Manage Postpartum Hemorrhage

Drug	Action	Side Effects	Contraindications	Dosage and Route	Nursing Considerations
Oxytocin (Pitocin)	Contraction of uterus; decreases bleeding	Infrequent: water intoxication, nausea and vomiting	None for postpartum hemorrhage	10-40 units/L diluted in lactated Ringer's solution or normal saline at 125-200 milliunits/min IV or 10-20 units IM	Continue to monitor vaginal bleeding and uterine tone
Methylergonovine (Methergine)*	Contraction of uterus	Hypertension, nausea, vomiting, headache	Hypertension, cardiac disease	0.2 mg IM every 2-4 hr up to five doses; may also be given intrauterine or orally	Check blood pressure before giving and do not give if >140/90 mm Hg; continue monitoring vaginal bleeding and uterine tone
15-Methylprostaglandin $F_{2\alpha}$ (Prostin/15m; Carboprost Hemabate)	Contraction of uterus	Headache, nausea and vomiting, fever, tachycardia, hypertension, diarrhea	Avoid with asthma or hypertension, fever	0.25 mg IM or intrauterine every 15-90 min, up to eight doses	Continue monitoring vaginal bleeding and uterine tone

Continued

Medications Used to Manage Postpartum Hemorrhage—cont'd

Drug	Action	Side Effects	Contraindications	Dosage and Route	Nursing Considerations
Dinoprostone (Prostin E$_2$)	Contraction of uterus	Headache, nausea and vomiting, fever, chills, diarrhea	Avoid with asthma hypotension	20 mg vaginal or rectal suppository every 2 hr	Continue to monitor vaginal bleeding and uterine tone
Misoprostol (Cytotec)	Contraction of uterus	Headache, nausea and vomiting, diarrhea	History of allergy to prostaglandins	800 to 1000 mcg rectally once	Continue to monitor vaginal bleeding and uterine tone

*Information about methylergonovine may also be used to describe ergonovine (Ergotrate).

Rh Immunoglobulin, RhoGAM, Gamulin Rh, HypRho-D, Rhophylac

Action

- Suppression of immune response in nonsensitized women with Rh-negative blood who receive Rh-positive blood cells because of fetomaternal hemorrhage, transfusion, or accident

Indications

- Routine antepartum prevention at 28 to 30 wk of gestation in women with Rh-negative blood; suppresses antibody formation after birth, miscarriage or pregnancy termination, abdominal trauma, ectopic pregnancy, amniocentesis, version, or chorionic villus sampling

Dosage and Route

- Standard dose is one vial (300 mcg) IM in deltoid or gluteal muscle; microdose is one vial (50 mcg) IM in deltoid muscle; Rhophylac can be given IM or IV (available in prefilled syringes)

Adverse Effects

- Myalgia, lethargy, localized tenderness and stiffness at injection site, mild and transient fever, malaise, headache
- Rarely nausea, vomiting, hypotension, tachycardia, possible allergic response

Nursing Considerations

- Give standard dose to mother at 28 wk of gestation as prophylaxis or after an incident or exposure risk that occurs after 28 wk of gestation (e.g., amniocentesis, second-trimester miscarriage or abortion, after version) and within 72 hr after birth if baby is Rh positive.
- Give microdose for first-trimester miscarriage or abortion, ectopic pregnancy, chorionic villus sampling.
- Verify that the woman is Rh negative and has not been sensitized, that Coombs' test is negative, and that baby is Rh positive. Provide explanation to the woman about procedure, including the purpose, possible side effects, and effect on future pregnancies. Have the woman sign a consent form if required by agency. Verify correct dosage and confirm lot number and woman's identity before giving

injection (verify with another registered nurse or other procedure per agency policy); document administration per agency policy. Observe woman for allergic response for at least 20 min after administration.

■ The medication is made from human plasma (a consideration if woman is a Jehovah's Witness). The risk of transmitting infectious agents, including viruses, cannot be completely eliminated.

NEWBORN

Eye Prophylaxis: Erythromycin Ophthalmic Ointment, 0.5%, and Tetracycline Ophthalmic Ointment, 1%

Action

■ These antibiotic ointments are both bacteriostatic and bactericidal. They provide prophylaxis against *Neisseria gonorrhoeae* and *Chlamydia trachomatis.*

Indication

■ These medications are applied to prevent ophthalmia neonatorum in newborns of mothers who are infected with gonorrhea, conjunctivitis, or chlamydia.

Neonatal Dosage

■ Apply a 1- to 2-cm ribbon of ointment to the lower conjunctival sac of each eye; also may be used in drop form.

Adverse Reactions

■ May cause chemical conjunctivitis that lasts 24 to 48 hr; vision may be blurred temporarily.

Nursing Considerations

■ Administer within 1 to 2 hr of birth. Wear gloves. Cleanse eyes if necessary before administration. Open eyes by putting a thumb and finger at the corner of each lid and gently pressing on the periorbital ridges. Squeeze the tube, and spread the ointment from the inner canthus of the eye to the outer canthus. Do not touch the tube to the eye. After 1 min, excess ointment may be wiped off. Observe eyes for irritation. Explain treatment to parents.

■ Eye prophylaxis for ophthalmia neonatorum is required by law in all states of the United States.

Vitamin K: Phytonadione (AquaMEPHYTON, Konakion)

Action

- This intervention provides vitamin K, necessary because the newborn does not have the intestinal flora to produce this vitamin in the first week after birth. It also promotes formation of clotting factors (II, VII, IX, X) in the liver.

Indication

- Vitamin K is used for prevention and treatment of hemorrhagic disease in the newborn.

Neonatal Dosage

- Administer a 0.5- to 1-mg (0.25- to 0.5-ml) dose IM within 2 hr of birth; may be repeated if newborn shows bleeding tendencies.

Adverse Reactions

- Edema, erythema, and pain at injection site may occur rarely.
- Hemolysis, jaundice, and hyperbilirubinemia have been reported, particularly in preterm infants.

Nursing Considerations

- Wear gloves. Administer in the middle third of the vastus lateralis muscle using a 25-gauge, 5/8-inch needle. Inject into skin that has been cleaned, or allow alcohol to dry on puncture site for 1 min to remove organisms and prevent infection. Stabilize leg firmly, and grasp muscle between the thumb and fingers. Insert the needle at a 90-degree angle; aspirate, and inject medication slowly if there is no blood return.
- Massage the site with a dry gauze square after removing needle to increase absorption.
- Observe for signs of bleeding from the site.

Hepatitis B Vaccine (Recombivax HB, Engerix-B)

Action

- Hepatitis B vaccine induces protective antihepatitis B antibodies in 95% to 99% of healthy infants who receive the recommended three doses. The duration of protection of the vaccine is unknown.

Indication

- Hepatitis B vaccine is for immunization against infection caused by all known subtypes of hepatitis B virus (HBV).

Neonatal Dosage

- The usual dosage is Recombivax HB, 5 mcg/0.5 ml, or Engerix-B, 10 mcg/0.5 ml, at 0, 1, and 6 mo of age. An alternate dosing schedule is at 0, 1, 2, and 12 mo of age and is usually for newborns whose mothers were positive for hepatitis B surface antigen (HBsAg).

Adverse Reactions

- Common adverse reactions are rash, fever, erythema, swelling, and pain at injection site.

Nursing Considerations

- Parental consent must be obtained before administration. Wear gloves. Administer in the middle third of the vastus lateralis muscle by using a 25-gauge, 5⁄8-inch needle. Inject into skin that has been cleaned, or allow alcohol to dry on puncture site for 1 min to remove organisms and prevent infection. Stabilize leg firmly and grasp muscle between the thumb and fingers. Insert the needle at a 90-degree angle; aspirate, and inject medication slowly if there is no blood return.
- Massage the site with a dry gauze square after removing needle to increase absorption.
- If the infant was born to HBsAg-positive mother, hepatitis B immunoglobulin (HBIg) should be given within 12 hr of birth in addition to the HB vaccine. Separate sites must be used.
- Teach parents importance of completing the entire three injection vaccination series. Send documentation of first injection to clinic or office where baby will receive well-child care. Provide the correct address and telephone contact information for the parents to the office or clinic to enable follow-up to ensure that the baby receives the next two injections.

Hepatitis B Immunoglobulin

Action

- HBIG provides a high titer of antibody to HBsAg.

Indication

■ The HBIG vaccine provides prophylaxis against infection in infants born of HBsAg-positive mothers.

Neonatal Dosage

■ Administer one 0.5-ml dose intramuscularly within 12 hr of birth.

Adverse Reactions

■ Hypersensitivity may occur.

Nursing Considerations

■ Must be given within 12 hr of birth.
■ Wear gloves. Administer in the middle third of the vastus lateralis muscle using a 25-gauge, 5/8-inch needle. Inject into skin that has been cleaned, or allow alcohol to dry on puncture site for 1 min to remove organisms and prevent infection. Stabilize leg firmly, and grasp muscle between the thumb and fingers. Insert the needle at a 90-degree angle, aspirate, and inject medication slowly if there is no blood return.
■ Massage the site with a dry gauze square after removing needle to increase absorption.
■ May be given at same time as hepatitis B vaccine but at a different site.

Naloxone Hydrochloride (Narcan)

Action

■ Opioid antagonist that blocks both mu and kappa opioid receptors from the effects of opioid agonists.

Indications

■ Reverses opioid-induced respiratory depression in woman or newborn.
■ May be used to reverse pruritus from epidural opioids.

Dosage and Route

Adult

■ Opioid overdose: 0.4 to 2 mg IV, may repeat IV at 2- to 3-min intervals up to 10 mg; if IV route unavailable, IM or subcutaneous route may be used.

- Postoperative opioid depression: initial dose 0.1 to 0.2 mg IV at 2- to 3-min intervals up to three doses until desired degree of reversal obtained; may repeat dose in 1 to 2 hr if needed.

Newborn

- Opioid-induced depression: initial dose 0.1 mg/kg IV, IM, or subcutaneous; may be repeated at 2- to 3-min intervals up to three doses until desired degree of reversal obtained.

Adverse Effects

- Maternal hypotension and hypertension
- Tachycardia
- Hyperventilation
- Nausea and vomiting
- Sweating
- Tremulousness

Nursing Considerations

- Woman should delay breastfeeding until medication is out of her system.
- Do not give to mother or newborn if woman is opioid dependent—may cause abrupt withdrawal in woman and newborn.
- If given to woman for reversal of respiratory depression caused by opioid analgesic, pain will return suddenly.
- Monitor infant carefully for a return of respiratory depression approximately 45 min after giving naloxone. If the narcotic is still in the baby's system, respiratory depression will recur and the baby may need an additional dose of naloxone.

Selected Drugs Excreted in Breast Milk

DRUG	AAP RATING
Acetaminophen (Datril, Tylenol, Darvocet, Excedrin)	6
Alcohol (ethanol)	6
Aspirin (Bayer, Anacin, Bufferin, Excedrin, Fiorinal, Empirin)	5
Caffeine	6
Cocaine	2
Codeine	6
Heroin	2
Ibuprofen (Advil, Nuprin, Motrin)	6
Indomethacin (Indocin)	6
Ketorolac tromethamine (Toradol)	6
Marijuana	2
Medroxyprogesterone acetate (Depo-Provera)	6
Meperidine (Demerol, Mepergan)	6
Methadone	6
Morphine	6
Naproxen (Naproxyn, Anaprox, Naprosyn, Aleve)	6
Oxycodone	Not rated
Phenobarbital (Luminal, Donnatal, Tedral)	5
Phenytoin (Dilantin)	6
Propylthiouracil	6
Thyroid and thyroxine	6
Tolbutamide (Orinase)	6

American Academy of Pediatrics (AAP) Committee on Drugs rated drugs that transfer into human milk. The ratings are as follows:
1. Drugs that are contraindicated during breastfeeding
2. Drugs of abuse that are contraindicated during breastfeeding
3. Radioactive compounds that require temporary cessation of breastfeeding
4. Drugs with unknown effects on breastfeeding but may be of concern
5. Drugs that have been associated with significant effects on some breastfeeding infants and should be given to breastfeeding mothers with caution
6. Maternal medication usually compatible with breastfeeding
7. Food and environmental agents that have an effect on breastfeeding

APPENDIX C

English-Spanish Translations

ANTEPARTUM
BODY PARTS

Bone	hueso
Blood	sangre
Tongue	lengua
Head	cabeza
Arm	brazo
Finger	dedo
Leg	pierna
Neck	cuello
Elbow	codo
Foot	pie
Ear	oreja, oido
Nose	nariz
Mouth	boca
Bladder	vejiga
Back	espalda
Chest	pecho
Spleen	bazo
Gallbladder	vesícula biliar

DIET AND NUTRITION

You need to gain weight.	Usted necesita aumentar de peso.
You need to control your weight gain.	Usted necesita controlar su aumento de peso.
Eat nutritious foods.	Coma alimentos nutritivos.
Eat foods high in protein, calcium, vitamins, and iron.	Coma alimentos altos en proteínas, calcio, vitaminas, y hierro.
Eat a lot of fruits and vegetables.	Coma muchas frutas y vegetales.

Drink four glasses of milk each day.	Tome cuatro vasos de leche diariamente.
Drink low-fat instead of whole milk.	Tome la leche baja en grasa en lugar de la leche entera.
Avoid salty foods, such as sausage, hot dogs, and French fries.	Evite alimentos muy salados como calchichas, perros calientes, y papitas fritas.
Avoid fried foods.	Evite las frituras.
Avoid caffeine.	Evite la cafeína.
There is caffeine in Coca-Cola, tea, and chocolate.	Hay cafeína en la Coca-Cola, el té, y el chocolate.
Take prenatal vitamins.	Tome vitaminas prenatales.

HIGH RISK FACTORS

HIGH RISK ASSESSMENT		POTENTIAL PROBLEM
Have you had any problems with this pregnancy?	¿Ha tenido problemas con este embarazo?	General assessment
Have you had blurred vision?	¿Ha tenido visión borrosa?	Preeclampsia
Have you had severe headaches?	¿Ha tenido dolores fuertes de cabeza?	Preeclampsia
Have you had difficulty breathing?	¿Ha tenido dificultad para respirar?	Cardiac disease
Have you had heart palpitations?	¿Ha tenido palpitaciones del corazón?	Cardiac disease
Have you been vomiting?	¿Ha tenido vómitos?	Hyperemesis gravidarum
Have you had any infections?	¿Ha tenido alguna infección?	Sexually transmitted infections or vaginal infections
Have you had swelling?	¿Ha tenido hinchazón?	Preeclampsia
Were all your pregnancies term?	¿Llegaron a las cuarenta semanas todos sus embarazos?	Preterm labor
Have you ever had diabetes?	¿Ha tenido diabetes?	Diabetes

Have you ever had high blood pressure?	¿Ha tenido alta presión sanguínea?	Gestational hypertension/ chronic hypertension
Have you ever had anemia?	¿Ha estado anémica?	Anemia
Do you take drugs? Prescription medicine?	¿Usa drogas? ¿Medicina recetada?	Substance abuse
Do you drink alcohol? Smoke?	¿Toma bebidas alcohólicas? ¿Fuma?	Substance abuse

PELVIC EXAMINATION

Take off all your clothes, please.	Quítese toda la ropa, por favor.
Put on the gown, please.	Póngase la bata, por favor.
I am going to examine you.	Le voy a examinar.
You will feel less discomfort if you relax.	Se sentirá más cómoda si se relaja el cuerpo.
Lie down, please.	Acuéstese, por favor.
Put your feet in the stirrups.	Póngase los pies en los estribos.
Open your legs, please.	Sepárese las piernas, por favor.
I am going to take a sample from the lining of the cervix (Pap test).	Le voy a tomar una muestra del cuello uterino (el examen de Papanicolaou).
We will test this sample for cancer.	Haremos un análisis de esta muestra para determinar si hay cáncer.
It won't hurt.	No le va a doler.
Everything looks fine.	Todo está bien.
You may get dressed.	Puede vestirse.

PRENATAL INTERVIEW

Have you had a pregnancy test?	¿Ha tenido una prueba del embarazo?
When was your last menstrual cycle?	¿Cuándo fue su última menstruación (regla)?
Have you been pregnant before?	¿Ha quedado embarazada antes?
How many times?	¿Cuántas veces?
How many children do you have?	¿Cuántos hijos tiene usted?
Have you ever had a miscarriage (spontaneous abortion)?	¿Ha perdido un bebé alguna vez? (¿Ha tenido un aborto espontáneo?)

Have you ever had a therapeutic abortion?	¿Ha tenido un aborto provocado?
Have you ever had a stillborn?	¿Ha tenido un niño que nació sin vida?
Have you ever had a cesarean?	¿Ha tenido una operación cesárea?
Have you had any problems with past pregnancies?	¿Ha tenido problemas durante sus embarazos anteriores?
Do you take drugs? Prescription medicine?	¿Usa drogas? ¿Medicina recetada?
If so, which type of medicine do you use and for what?	¿Qué clases de medicina toma? ¿Para qué las toma?
Do you drink alcohol? Do you smoke?	¿Toma bebidas alcohólicas? ¿Fuma?

PRENATAL PHYSICAL EXAMINATION

Get on the scale, please.	Súbase a la balanza, por favor.
I need a urine sample.	Necesito una muestra de orina.
Go to the bathroom, please.	Vaya al baño, por favor.
I need to take your blood pressure.	Necesito verificar su presión sanguínea.
I am going to listen to the baby's heartbeat.	Voy a escuchar el latido del corazón del bebé.
The doctor is going to examine you.	El doctor le va a examinar.
Don't be afraid.	No tenga miedo.
Lie down, please.	Acuéstese, por favor.
Separate your legs, please.	Sepárese las piernas, por favor.
Relax.	Afloje los músculos.
Go to the laboratory for a blood test, please.	Vaya al laboratorio para un análisis de sangre, por favor.
Go to this office for your ultrasound, please.	Vaya a esta oficina para que se le haga el ultrasonido, por favor.

RECOGNIZING VIOLENCE IN A RELATIONSHIP

| ARE YOU IN A RELATIONSHIP IN WHICH YOU ARE … | ¿TIENE UNA RELACIÓN CON SU PAREJA EN LA QUE … |
| afraid of your partner's temper? | tiene miedo de que él pierda los estribos? |

afraid to break up because your partner has threatened to hurt someone?	tiene miedo de dejarlo porque él ha amenazado con pegar o lastimar a alguien?
constantly apologizing for or defending your partner's behavior?	constantemente tiene que disculparse por o defender el comportamiento de su pareja?
afraid to disagree with your partner?	tiene miedo de discutir con su pareja?
isolated from your family or friends?	está aislada de su familia o sus amigos?
embarrassed in front of others because of your partner's words or actions?	las palabras o acciones de su pareja delante de otra gente le dan vergüenza?
intimidated by your partner and forced into having sex?	su pareja le intimida a usted y le obliga a tener relaciones sexuales con él?
depressed and jumpy?	está deprimida y/o nerviosa?
A PERSON WHO IS VIOLENT IN A RELATIONSHIP OFTEN …	UNA PERSONA QUE TIENE UN CARÁCTER VIOLENTO EN UNA RELACIÓN A MENUDO…
has an explosive temper.	pierde los estribos.
is possessive or jealous of his partner's time, friends, or family.	es posesivo o tiene celos de que su pareja pase tiempo con la familia o los amigos.
constantly criticizes his partner's thoughts, feelings, or appearance.	critica constantemente los sentimientos, ideas, o apariencia física de su pareja.
pinches, slaps, grabs, shoves, or throws things at his partner.	pellizca, pega, agarra, empuja, o lanza objetos que pueden lastimar a su pareja.
forces his partner into having sex.	obliga a su pareja a tener relaciones sexuales.
causes his partner to be afraid.	causa que su pareja tenga miedo.

SPECIFIC CONDITIONS

Rubella	rubeola
Intensive care	cuidado intensivo
Menstrual period	menstruación
Birth control	anticonceptivo
Allergic reaction	reacción alérgica

WHAT TO DO IF SYMPTOMS OF PRETERM LABOR OCCUR

Empty your bladder.	Vacíese la vejiga.
Drink two to three glasses of water or juice.	Tome dos a tres vasos de agua o jugo.
Lie down on your left side for 1 hour.	Acuéstese del lado izquierdo por una hora.
Palpate for contractions like this.	Palpe por contracciones así.
If symptoms continue, call your health care provider or go to the hospital.	Si continúan los síntomas, llame a su proveedor de los servicios de salud/médico o vaya al hospital.
If symptoms abate, resume light activity, but not what you were doing when the symptoms began.	Si se alivian los síntomas, resuma sus actividades livianas, pero no haga lo que estaba haciendo cuando empezaron los síntomas.
If symptoms return, call your health care provider or go to the hospital.	Si se presentan de nuevo los síntomas, llame a su proveedor de los servicios de salud/médico o vaya al hospital.
If any of the following symptoms occur, call your health care provider immediately:	Si le sucede cualquier de los siguientes síntomas, llame inmediatamente a su proveedor de los servicios de salud/médico:

- Uterine contractions every 10 minutes or less for 1 hour or more
- Vaginal bleeding
- Odorous vaginal discharge
- Fluid leaking from the vagina

- Contracciones uterinas cada diez minutos o menos que duran por una hora o más
- Hemorragia vaginal
- Flujo vaginal con mal olor
- Flujo que le sale de la vagina

INTRAPARTUM

LABOR ASSESSMENT

What time did the contractions begin?	¿A qué hora le empezaron las contracciones?
How far apart are the contractions?	¿Con qué frecuencia tiene las?
Have the membranes ruptured? When?	¿Se le rompió la fuente? ¿Cuándo?
What color was the fluid? Red? Pink?	¿Qué color tenía el líquido? ¿Rojo? ¿Rosado?
Have you had bleeding?	¿Ha tenido hemorragia?

How much? A cupful? A table-spoon? A teaspoon?	¿Cuánto? ¿Una taza? ¿Una cucharada? ¿Una cucharadita?
When was the last time you ate or drank anything?	¿Cuándo fue la última vez que comió o tomó algo?
Have you had any problems with this pregnancy?	¿Ha tenido algún problema con este embarazo?
Are you taking any medications?	¿Toma algún medicamento?
Are you allergic to penicillin or other medicines?	¿Es alérgica a la penicilina u otras medicinas?
Please sign this consent form.	Por favor, firme este formulario de autorización.

CARE DURING LABOR

Lie down, please.	Acuéstese, por favor.
I am going to take your vital signs.	Voy a verificar sus signos vitales.
I am going to listen to the baby's heartbeat.	Voy a escuchar el latido del corazón del bebé.
This is a fetal monitor.	Este es un monitor fetal.
I need to examine you.	Necesito examinarle.
Do you need to use the bathroom?	¿Necesita usar el baño?
Would you like some pain medication?	¿Quisiera medicina para calmar el dolor?
Roll over on your side, please.	Póngase sobre un costado, por favor.
Relax.	Afloje los músculos.
Breathe deeply.	Respire profundamente.
Push.	Puje.
Do not push.	No puje.
Grab your knees, and push.	Agárrese las rodillas, y puje.
You are doing fine.	Bien. Muy bien.
Congratulations!	¡Felicidades!
You have a beautiful boy.	Usted tiene un niño precioso.
You have a beautiful girl.	Usted tiene una niña preciosa.

CESAREAN BIRTH

You need a cesarean.	Necesita una operación cesárea.
Has your doctor discussed with you the reason for needing a cesarean?	¿Ha hablado el doctor con usted sobre la necesidad de tener una operación cesárea?
Do you understand why you need a cesarean?	¿Entiende usted por qué necesita una operación cesárea?

| Your signature on this form will allow us to proceed with the surgery. | Su firma en este formulario nos permitirá seguir adelante con la operación. |
| Please sign this consent form. | Por favor, firme este formulario de autorización. |

INDUCTION OF LABOR/AUGMENTATION OF LABOR

Your labor is not progressing.	Su trabajo de parto no está progresando.
We need to stimulate the contractions.	Necesitamos provocar las contracciones.
I'm going to give you some medication to make your contractions stronger.	Le voy a dar una medicina para hacer más fuertes las contracciones.
I'm going to give you Pitocin through your IV.	Le voy a dar pitufina por medio del suero.

PAIN MANAGEMENT

Do you want to get up and walk?	¿Desea levantarse y caminar?
Do you want pain medication?	¿Quiere medicina para el dolor?
I am going to give you the pain medicine in an injection.	Le voy a dar la medicina para el dolor por inyección.
I am going to give you the pain medicine through an IV.	Le voy a dar la medicina para el dolor por el suero.
This is a pain reliever called Demerol/Stadol/Nubain.	Ésta es una medicina para aliviar el dolor que se llama Demerol/Stadol/Nubain.
The effects of this medicine are relatively short.	Los efectos de esta medicina son de corta duración.
The epidural is a stronger method of pain relief.	La anestesia epidural es un método más potente para aliviar el dolor.
You should not be able to feel the contraction pain.	No debe de sentir el dolor de las contracciones.

POSTPARTUM/INFANT CARE

POSTPARTUM PHYSICAL ASSESSMENT

| Are you planning to breastfeed or bottle feed? | ¿Piensa darle pecho o biberón al bebé? |
| Lie down, please. | Acuéstese, por favor. |

I am going to take your vital signs.	Le voy a tomar sus signos vitales.
Open your mouth.	Abra la boca.
Temperature	temperatura
Pulse	pulso
Heart rate	latido del corazón
Respiration	respiración
I need to take your blood pressure.	Necesito tomarle la presión sanguínea.
Do you need to use the bathroom?	¿Necesita usar el baño?
I need to examine you.	Necesito examinarle.
Please spread your knees and legs apart.	Por favor, abra las rodillas and las piernas.
Roll over on your side, please.	Póngase sobre un costado, por favor.
Where does it hurt?	¿Dónde le duele?
Would you like some pain medication?	¿Desea medicina para calmar el dolor?
Would you like to take a sitz bath?	¿Desea tomar un baño de asiento?
Are you sleeping well?	¿Está durmiendo bien?

BREASTFEEDING: LATCH

Do you want to breastfeed your baby?	¿Desea amamantar a su bebé?
I will help you.	Yo le ayudaré.
Hold your baby's head close to your breast.	Sostenga la cabeza del bebé cerca del pecho.
Lightly touch your nipple to lower lip until the baby opens his or her mouth.	Con el pezón, toque suavemente el labio inferior del bebé hasta que abra la boca.
Lift your breast to the baby's mouth.	Levante el seno hasta la boca del bebé.
Center your nipple and areola as far in the baby's mouth as possible.	Centre el pezón y la areola lo más que se pueda dentro de la boca del bebé.
Make sure the baby's tongue is under the nipple and the gums close around the areola.	Asegúrese de que la lengua del bebé esté debajo del pezón y que sus encías se cierren sobre la areola.
To change breasts, push one of your fingers into the corner of the baby's mouth.	Para cambiar al otro seno, métase un dedo en la comisura de los labios del bebé.

This will break the suction and prevent the baby from biting the nipple.

Esto interrumpe la aspiración e impide que el bebé muerda el pezón.

BURPING

Position #1
Hold your baby up, head on your shoulder.
Put one arm under the baby's bottom.
With the other hand, pat or rub the baby's back.

Posición #1
Ponga su bebé con la cabeza muy alta sobre su hombro.
Ponga un brazo debajo de las nalgas del bebé.
Con la otra mano, dé leves palmaditas o sobe la espalda del bebé.

Position #2
Sit your baby up in your lap.
Hold the head and back with one hand.
Hold the chin and front with the other.

Rock the baby's upper body back and forth.
Or pat the baby's back.

Posición #2
Siente al bebé sobre su regazo.
Con una mano, sostenga la cabeza y la espalda del bebé.
Con la otra mano, sostenga la barbilla y la parte delantera del bebé.

Mueva la parte superior del bebé hacia adelante y hacia atrás.
O dé suaves palmaditas a la espalda del bebé.

Position #3
Lay your baby face down on your lap.
Hold the baby's head with one hand.
Rub or pat the baby's back.

Posición #3
Coloque al bebé boca abajo sobre su regazo.
Con una mano, sostenga la cabeza del bebé.
Sobe o dé suaves palmaditas a la espalda del bebé.

ASSESS ADEQUACY OF INTAKE:
How many times did (he/she) urinate today?
How many wet diapers has (he/she) had?
How many dirty diapers?

¿Cuántas veces orinó hoy?
¿Cuántos pañales ha mojado?
¿Cuántos pañales sucios?

CONTRACEPTION

Do you plan to have more children?	¿Piensa tener más hijos?
Are you sexually active?	¿Tiene relaciones sexuales?
Do you have many partners?	¿Tiene muchas parejas sexuales?
Have you had many partners in the past?	¿Ha tenido muchas parejas sexuales en el pasado?
Do you presently use contraception/birth control?	¿Usa anticonceptivos/control de natalidad actualmente?
The pill? Condoms?	¿La píldora anticonceptiva? ¿Los condones (preservativos)?
The diaphragm? The IUD?	¿El diafragma? ¿El dispositivo intrauterino (DIU)?
Spermicides? The rhythm method?	¿Los espermaticidas? ¿El método del ritmo?
Injection (Depo-Provera)?	¿La inyección (Depo-Provera)?
How long have you used this method?	¿Por cuánto tiempo ha usado este método?
Do you like this method?	¿Le gusta este método?
Why did you stop using it?	¿Por qué dejó de usarlo?
Do you want to change to a different method?	¿Quiere cambiar a otro método?
Have you had a tubal ligation?	¿Ha tenido una ligadura de trompas?
Has he had a vasectomy?	¿Tuvo él una vasectomía?

DISCHARGE TEACHING FOR POSTPARTUM WOMAN

When you go to the bathroom, always wipe from front to back.	Cuando vaya al baño, séquese siempre de adelante hacia atrás.
Sit in a tub of warm water to relieve discomfort.	Siéntese en una bañera con agua tibia para aliviarse.
You will have moderate amounts of vaginal discharge.	Usted tendrá cantidades moderadas de sangrado vaginal.
It may last from 4 to 6 weeks.	Puede durar desde cuatro a seis semanas.
The color may vary from dark brown to red to pink.	El color puede variar entre café oscuro a rojo a rosado.
It may contain blood clots.	Es probable que contenga coágulos.

Use a sanitary pad instead of a tampon.	Use una toalla sanitaria en vez de un tampón.
Your menstrual period will not resume for 4 to 10 weeks.	Su regla no regrasará hasta cuatro a diez semanas más tarde.
If you are breastfeeding, it may take a little longer.	Si está amamantando, puede demorar un poco más.
It is possible to become pregnant while you are breastfeeding.	Es possible quedar embarazada mientras amamanta.
Avoid having sexual relations for 2 to 4 weeks after birth.	Evite las relaciones sexuales por dos a cuatro semanas después del parto.
Gradually increase activity to incorporate everyday routines.	Aumente las actividades gradualmente hasta llegar a su rutina normal.
Do your Kegel exercises.	Haga los ejercicios Kegel.
Do not lift heavy objects (more than 10 pounds).	No levante objetos pesados (de más de diez libras).
Rest as often as possible.	Descanse mucho.
Rest when your baby sleeps.	Descanse cuando duerma su bebé.
Eat four servings daily of bread/cereals, fruits/vegetables (green), milk or foods made from milk, and two servings of meat. You need to drink eight glasses of fluids each day to support breastfeeding.	Cómase diariamente cuatro porciones de pan/cereal, frutas/vegetales (verduras), leche o comidas del grupo de leche, y dos porciones de carne. Usted necesita tomar ocho vasos de líquidos diariamenta para soportar el dar de pecho.
Call your doctor (obstetrician) if you have:	Llame al médico de obstétricas si tenga cualquier de lo siguiente:

- Fever >38° C (>100.4° F)
- Increased vaginal bleeding (more than a regular period)
- Chills
- Painful, burning urination
- Foul-smelling vaginal discharge
- Increased pain or swelling
- Drainage or separation of incision (cesarean)

- Fiebre >38° C (>100.4° F)
- Aumento de desangre vaginal (más que una regla normal)
- Escalofríos
- Orin que le duele o le quema
- Desangre vaginal de muy mal olor
- Aumento de dolor o hinchazón
- Desangre o deshecho de la herida

PAIN MANAGEMENT

Please show me where it hurts.	Muéstrame dónde le duele, por favor.
When did it start?	¿Cuándo empezó?
Do you have pain?	¿Tiene dolor?
■ **Headache**	de cabeza
■ **Stomachache**	del estómago
■ **Backache**	de la espalda
■ **Chest pain**	en el pecho
■ **In the arm**	en el brazo
■ **In the legs**	en las piernas
■ **In the mouth**	en la boca
■ **In the eyes**	en los ojos
■ **In the bladder**	en la vejiga

EQUIPMENT

Diaper	pañal
Bulb syringe	bombilla
Antibiotic	antibiótico
Pacifier	chupón
Bottle (baby bottle or medicine bottle)	botella
Juice	jugo
Milk	leche

PROCEDURES

Injection	inyección
Lumbar puncture	punción lumbar
Start an IV	ponerle suero por vena
To breastfeed, nurse	amamantar
To burp	eructar
X-ray	radiografía

Bibliography

Abbott, J. (2007). Transcervical sterilization. *Current Opinion in Obstetrics and Gynecology, 19*(4), 325-330.

Academy of Breastfeeding Medicine Protocol Committee. (2008). Clinical Protocol No. 4: Mastitis. *Breastfeeding Medicine, 3*(3), 177-180.

Academy of Breastfeeding Medicine Protocol Committee. (2009). Clinical Protocol No. 3: Hospital guidelines for the use of supplementary feedings in the healthy term breastfed infant. *Breastfeeding Medicine, 4*(3), 175-182.

American Academy of Pediatrics. (AAP). (2006). *Textbook of neonatal resuscitation* (5th ed.). Elk Grove Village, IL: AAP.

American Academy of Pediatrics (AAP). (2008). *Pediatric nutrition handbook* (6th ed.). Elk Grove Village, IL: AAP.

American Academy of Pediatrics (AAP). (2009). *Caring for your baby and young child: Ages birth to age 5.* Available at www.healthychildren.org/ English/ages-stages/baby/feeding-nutrition/pages/Baby-Bottles-And-Bisphenol-A-BPA.aspx. Accessed February 27, 2010.

American Academy of Pediatrics Committee on Infectious Diseases. (2006). *Redbook: 2006 Report of the Committee on Infectious Diseases* (27th ed.). Elk Grove Village, IL: AAP.

American Academy of Pediatrics (AAP), Committee on Pediatric AIDS. (2008). HIV testing and prophylaxis to prevent mother-to-child transmission in the United States. *Pediatrics, 122*(5), 1127-1134.

American Academy of Pediatrics (AAP) & American College of Obstetricians and Gynecologists (ACOG). (2007). *Guidelines for perinatal care* (6th ed.). Washington, DC: ACOG.

American College of Obstetricians and Gynecologists (ACOG). (2010). *Management of intrapartum fetal heart rate tracings.* ACOG Practice Bulletin No. 116. Washington, DC: ACOG.

American College of Obstetricians and Gynecologists (ACOG). (2006). *Postpartum hemorrhage.* ACOG Practice Bulletin No. 76. Washington, DC: ACOG.

American College of Obstetricians and Gynecologists (ACOG). (2008). *Use of psychiatric medications during pregnancy and lactation.* ACOG Practice Bulletin No. 92. Washington, DC: ACOG.

Arnold, J., & Gemma, P. (2008). The continuing process of parental grief. *Death Studies, 32*(7), 658-673.

Association of Women's Health, Obstetric and Neonatal Nurses (AWHONN). (2009). Ethical decision making in the clinical setting: Nurses' rights and responsibilities. Available at www.awhonn.org/awhonn/content.do?name=05_HealthPolicyLegislation/5H_PositionStatements.htm. Accessed May 29, 2010.

Association of Women's Health, Obstetric and Neonatal Nurses (AWHONN). (2009). *Fetal heart monitoring: Principles and practice* (4th ed.). Dubuque, IA: Kendall/Hunt.

Baby-Friendly USA. (2010). *BFHI USA: Implementing the UNICEF/WHO baby friendly hospital initiative in the U.S.* Available at www.babyfriendlyusa.org. Accessed May 29, 2010.

Beck, C. (2008). State of the science on postpartum depression: What nurse researchers have contributed—part 1. *MCN The American Journal of Maternal/Child Nursing, 33*(2), 122-126.

Beck, C. (2008). State of the science on postpartum depression: What nurse researchers have contributed—part 2. *MCN The American Journal of Maternal/Child Nursing, 33*(3), 151-156.

Bennett, S., Litz, B., Lee, B., & Shira, M. (2005). The scope and impact of perinatal loss: Current status and future directions. *Professional Psychology, Research and Practice, 36*(2), 180-187.

Bina, R. (2008). The impact of cultural factors upon postpartum depression: A literature review. *Health Care for Women International, 29*(6), 568-592.

Blithe, D. (2008). Male contraception: What is on the horizon? *Contraception, 78*(4 Suppl 1), S23-S27.

Brier, N. (2008). Grief following miscarriage: A comprehensive review of the literature. *Journal of Women's Health, 17(3),* 451-464.

Centers for Disease Control and Prevention (CDC). (2006). Sexually transmitted diseases treatment guidelines, 2006. *MMWR Morbidity and Mortality Weekly Report, 55*(RR-11), 1-94.

Centers for Disease Control and Prevention (CDC). (2009). *Breastfeeding report card—United States, 2009.* Available at www.cdc.gov/breastfeeding/data/report_card.htm. Accessed February 27, 2010.

Chichester, M. (2007). Requesting perinatal autopsy: Multicultural considerations. *MCN: The American Journal of Maternal/Child Nursing, 32*(2), 81-86.

Cleveland, K. (2010). Feeding challenges in the late preterm infant. *Neonatal Network, 29*(1), 37-41.

Creasy, R., Resnik, R., Iams, J., Lockwood, C., & Moore, T. (Eds.). (2009). *Creasy and Resnik's maternal-fetal medicine: Principles and practice* (6th ed.). Philadelphia: Saunders.

Cunningham, F., Leveno, K., Bloom, S., Hauth, J., Rouse, D., & Spong, C. (Eds.). (2010). *Williams obstetrics* (23rd ed.). New York: McGraw-Hill.

D'Avanzo, C. (2008). *Mosby's pocket guide to cultural health assessment* (4th ed.). St. Louis: Mosby.

De La Rosa, I., Perry, J., & Johnson, V. (2009). Benefits of increased home-visitation services: Exploring a case management model. *Family and Community Health, 32*(10), 58-75.

Fehring, R., Schneider, M., & Barron, M. (2008). Efficacy of the Marquette method of natural family planning. *MCN The American Journal of Maternal/Child Nursing 33*(6), 348-354.

Fortinguerra, F., Clavenna, A., & Bonati, M. (2009). Psychotropic drug use during breastfeeding: A review of the evidence. *Pediatrics, 124*(4), e547-e556.

Frank, B., Lane, C., & Hokanson, H. (2009). Designing a postepidural fall risk assessment score for the obstetric patient. *Journal of Nursing Care Quality, 24*(1), 50-54.

Fretts, R. (2009). The study of stillbirth. *American Journal of Obstetrics and Gynecology, 201*(5), 429-430.

Gabbe, S., Niebyl, J., & Simpson, J. (Eds.). (2007). *Obstetrics: Normal and problem pregnancies* (5th ed.). Philadelphia: Churchill Livingstone.

Germano, E., & Jennings, V. (2006). New approaches to fertility awareness-based methods: Incorporating the Standard Days and TwoDay methods into practice. *Journal of Midwifery & Women's Health, 51*(6), 471-477.

Gilbert, E. (2011). *Manual of high risk pregnancy & delivery* (5th ed.). St. Louis: Mosby.

Hale, T. (2008). *Medications and mothers' milk* (13th ed.). Amarillo, TX: Hale Publishing.

Hatcher, R., Trussell, J., Nelson, A., Cates, W., Stewart, F., & Kowal, D. (Eds.). *Contraceptive technology* (19th rev. ed.). New York: Ardent Media, Inc.

Hofmeyr, G., Abdel-Alem, H., & Abdel-Aleem, M. (2008). Uterine massage for preventing postpartum haemorrhage. *The Cochrane Database of Systematic Reviews, 2008,* 3, CD006431.

Jenik, A., Vain, N., Gorestein, A., Jacobi, N., & Pacifier and Breastfeeding Trial Group. (2009). Does the recommendation to use a pacifier influence the prevalence of breastfeeding? *Journal of Pediatrics, 155*(3), 350-354.

Kaunitz, A., Arias, R., & McClung, M. (2008). Bone density recovery after depot medroxyprogesterone acetate injectable contraception use. *Contraception, 77*(2), 67-76.

King, J. (2007). Contraception and lactation. *Journal of Midwifery & Women's Health, 52*(6), 614-620.

Kliegman, R., Behrman, R., Jenson, H., & Stanton, B. (Eds.). (2007). *Nelson textbook of pediatrics* (18th ed.). Philadelphia: Saunders.

Kominiarek, M., & Kilpatrick, S. (2007). Postpartum hemorrhage: A recurring pregnancy complication. *Seminars in Perinatology, 31*(3), 159-166.

Lawrence, R., & Lawrence, R. (2005). *Breastfeeding: A guide for the medical profession* (6th ed.). Philadelphia: Mosby.

Levi, A., Simmonds, K., & Taylor, D. (2009). The role of nursing in the management of unintended pregnancy. *Nursing Clinics of North America, 44*(3), 1-14.

Limbo, R., & Kobler, K. (2009). Will our baby be alive again? Supporting parents of young children when a baby dies. *Nursing for Women's Health, 13*(4), 302-311.

Macones, G., Hankins, G., Spong, C., Hauth, J., & Moore, T. (2008). The 2008 National Institute of Child Health and Human Development Workshop Report on Electronic Fetal Monitoring: Update on Definitions, Interpretation, and Research Guidelines. *Journal of Obstetric, Gynecologic and Neonatal Nursing, 37*(5), 510-515.

Mahlmeister, L. (2008). Best practices in perinatal care: Evidence-based management of oxytocin induction and augmentation of labor. *Journal of Perinatal & Neonatal Nursing, 22*(4), 259-263.

McQueen, K., Montgomery, P., Lappan-Gracon, S., Evans, E., & Hunter, J. (2008). Evidence-based recommendations for depressive symptoms in postpartum women. *Journal of Obstetric, Gynecologic and Neonatal Nursing, 37*(2), 127-136.

Menon, S. (2008). Psychotropic medication during pregnancy and lactation. *Archives of Gynecology and Obstetrics, 277*(1), 1-13.

Milgrom, J., Gemmill, A., Bilszta, J., Hayes, B., Barnett, B., Brooks, J., et al. (2008). Antenatal risk factors for postnatal depression: A large prospective study. *Journal of Affective Disorders, 108*(1-2), 147-157.

National Women's Health Resource Center. (2008). Women and anxiety disorders. *National Women's Health Report, 30*(1), 1-7.

Navarro, P., Garcia-Esteve, L., Ascasco, C., Aguardo, J., Gelabert, E., & Martin-Santos, R. (2008). Non-psychotic psychiatric disorders after childbirth: Prevalence and comorbidity in a community sample. *Journal of Affective Disorders, 109*(1-2), 171-176.

O'Connor, N., Tanabe, K., Siadaty, M., & Hauck, F. (2009). Pacifiers and breastfeeding: A systematic review. *Archives of Pediatric and Adolescent Medicine, 163*(4), 378-382.

O'Leary, J., & Thorwick, C. (2006). Fathers' perspectives during pregnancy, postperinatal loss. *Journal of Obstetric, Gynecologic and Neonatal Nursing, 35(1)*, 78-86.

Pagana, K., & Pagana, T. (2009). *Mosby's diagnostic and laboratory test reference* (9th ed.). St. Louis: Mosby.

Pallone, S., & Bergus, G. (2009). Fertility awareness-based methods: Another option for family planning. *Journal of the American Board of Family Medicine, 22*(2), 147-157.

Practice Committee of the American Society for Reproductive Medicine. (2008). Hormonal contraception: Recent advances and controversies. *Fertility and Sterility, 90*(Suppl 3), S103-S113.

Remington, J., Klein, J., Baker, C., & Wilson, C. (Eds.). (2006). *Infectious diseases of the fetus and newborn infant* (6th ed.). Philadelphia: Saunders.

Riordan, J., & Wambach, K. (2010). *Breastfeeding and human lactation* (4th ed.). Boston: Jones and Bartlett.

Rios, E. (2009). Promoting breastfeeding in the Hispanic community. *Breastfeeding Medicine, 4*(Suppl 1), S69-S70.

Roy, P., & Payne, J. (2009). Treatment of bipolar disorder during and after pregnancy. In C. Zarate, & K. Husseini (Eds.), *Bipolar depression: Molecular neurobiology, clinical diagnosis and pharmacotherapy* (pp. 253-269). Cambridge, MA: Birkhauser.

Seidel, H., Ball, J., Dains, J., Flynn, J., Solomon, B., & Stewart, R. (2011). *Mosby's guide to physical examination* (7th ed.). St. Louis: Mosby.

Sharma, V., Burt, V., & Ritchie, H. (2009). Bipolar II postpartum depression: Detection, diagnosis, and treatment, *American Journal of Psychiatry, 166*(11), 1201-1204.

Simpson, K., Cesario, S., Morin, K., Trapani, K., Mayberry, L., & Snelgrove-Clark, E. (2008). *Nursing care and management of the second stage of labor: Evidence-based clinical practice guideline* (2nd ed.). Washington, DC: Association of Women's Health, Obstetric & Neonatal Nurses.

Simpson, K., & Creehan, P. (Eds.). (2008). *AWHONN's perinatal nursing* (3rd ed.). Philadelphia: Lippincott Williams & Wilkins.

Statistics Canada. (2008). Induced abortions. Available at www.statcan.gc.ca/daily-quotidien/080521/dq080521c-eng.htm. Accessed May 29, 2010.

Swanson, K., Chen, H., Graham, J., Wojnar, D., & Petras, A. (2009). Resolution of depression and grief during the first year after miscarriage: A randomized controlled clinical trial of couples-focused interventions. *Journal of Women's Health, 18*(8), 1245-1257.

Tucker, S., Miller, L., & Miller, D. (2009). *Mosby's pocket guide to fetal monitoring: A multidisciplinary approach* (6th ed.). St. Louis: Mosby.

U.S. Food and Drug Administration. (2009). *FDA approves Plan B One-Step emergency contraceptive; lowers age for obtaining two-dose plan B emergency contraceptive without a prescription*. Available at www.fda.gov/Drugs/DrugSafety/PostmarketDrugSafetyInformationforPatientsandProviders/ucm109775.htm. Accessed May 29, 2010.

Walker, M. (2008a). Breastfeeding the late preterm infant. *Journal of Obstetric, Gynecologic and Neonatal Nursing, 37*(6), 692-701.

Walker, M. (2008b). Conquering common breastfeeding problems. *Journal of Perinatal Nursing, 22*(4), 267-274.

World Health Organization Department of Reproductive Health & Research (WHO/RHR) and Johns Hopkins Bloomberg School of Public Health/Center for Communication Programs (CCP). (2007). *Family planning: A global handbook for providers*. Baltimore & Geneva: WHO & CCP.

Yranski, P., & Gamache, M. (2008). New options for barrier contraception. *Journal of Obstetric, Gynecologic and Neonatal Nursing, 37*(3), 384-389.

Zieman, M., Hatcher, R., Cwiak, C., Darney, P., Creinin, M., & Stosur, H. (2007). *A pocket guide to managing contraception.* Tiger, GA: Bridging the Gap Foundation.

Index

A

Abdomen, of newborn, 279t–311t
Abdominal muscles, round ligament pain/strain on, 18b
Abdominal ultrasonography, 33
Abnormal fetal heart rate, oxytocin and, 185b
ABO incompatibility, 368–369
Abruptio placentae, 68–72, 70t
Abstinence syndrome, 151b
Acceleration
  causes, clinical significance, interventions for, 132b
  definition of, 127–128
  example of, 132f
Acetabular dysplasia, 379
ACHES, 237
Acidemia, 144t
Acquired immunodeficiency syndrome (AIDS), 357
Acrodysesthesia, 19t–27t
Active phase
  of first-stage labor, 122b
  of second-stage labor, 159b
Acute pulmonary embolism, 252
Acyclovir, 356
Adolescent
  prenatal care for, 54–55
  response to pregnancy, 5
AIDS. See Acquired immunodeficiency syndrome (AIDS)
Airway obstruction, relieving, 312, 313b
Alcohol, 109
  breastfeeding and, 221
  methotrexate therapy, folic acid and, 63b

Alcohol (Continued)
  neonatal effects of, 363t–364t
  during pregnancy, effects of, 30–31
Allis sign, 379
Alpha-fetoprotein, 40
Ambiguous genitalia, 382
Ambulation, postpartum, 210–212, 212b
Amniocentesis, 36
Amnioinfusion, 144–145
Amniotic fluid volume index (AFI), 34–35
Amniotomy, 184, 184b
Amphetamines, 363t–364t
Analgesic, 196b
Anemia, 51, 104
Anencephaly, 373t–374t
Anesthesia, 196b
Ankle edema, 19t–27t
Antepartal assessment using electronic fetal monitoring, 42–43
Antepartum fetal assessment, 31–46
Anticoagulant therapy, 254, 254b
Antihypertensive medication, 95
Anus, of newborn, 279t–311t
Apgar score, 267–268, 268t
Apical pulse, of newborn, 279t–311t
Arms and hands, of newborn, 279t–311t
Arrhythmia, in newborn, 279t–311t
Arterial blood gas value, for neonate, 385t

Page reference followed by a *b* indicates box, *f* indicates figure or illustration, and *t* indicates table

449